PROGRESS IN CLINICAL AND BIOLOGICAL RESEARCH

See pages following the index for previous titles in this series.

VIRAL HEPATITIS
AND DELTA INFECTION

VIRAL HEPATITIS AND DELTA INFECTION

Proceedings of an International
Symposium on Viral Hepatitis
June 10–11, 1983
Torino, Italy

Editors

GIORGIO VERME
Division of Gastroenterology
Ospedale Molinette
Torino, Italy

FERRUCCIO BONINO
Division of Gastroenterology
Ospedale Molinette
Torino, Italy

MARIO RIZZETTO
Division of Gastroenterology
Ospedale Molinette
Torino, Italy

ALAN R. LISS, INC. • NEW YORK

Address all Inquiries to the Publisher
Alan R. Liss, Inc., 150 Fifth Avenue, New York, NY 10011

Copyright © 1983 Alan R. Liss, Inc.

Printed in the United States of America.

Library of Congress Cataloging in Publication Data

International Symposium on Viral Hepatitis (1983 :
    Turin, Italy)
    Viral hepatitis and delta infection.

    Bibliography: p.
    Includes index.
1. Hepatitis, Viral—Congresses. 2. Hepatitis, Non-A,
non-B—Congresses.I. Verme, Giorgio. II. Rizzetto,
Mario. III.Bonino, Ferruccio. IV. Title. V. Title:
Delta infection. [DNLM: 1. Hepatitis, Viral, Human—Congresses. W1 PR668E v.143 / WC 536 I613 1983v]
RC848.H43I58   1983   616.3′623   83-49050
ISBN 0-8451-0143-9

Contents

HEPATITIS A, B, NON-A, NON-B

THE DELTA AGENT: BIOLOGY AND EPIDEMIOLOGY

DELTA INFECTION: PATHOLOGICAL AND CLINICAL ASPECTS

x / Contents

PATHOGENESIS, PROPHYLAXIS, AND THERAPY

CONCLUDING REMARKS

Contributors

Giovanni C. Actis, Division of Gastroenterology, Ospedale Molinette, 10126 Torino, Italy [309]

Alfredo Alberti, Istituto di Medicina Clinica, Patologia Medica I, University of Padova, 35100 Padova, Italy [55,191,327]

Saleh Al-Kandari, Infectious Disease Hospital, Safat, Kuwait [161]

Basil Al-Nakib, Department of Medicine, Kuwait University, Faculty of Medicine, Safat, Kuwait [161]

Widad Al-Nakib, Department of Microbiology, Kuwait University, Faculty of Medicine, Safat, Kuwait [161]

Josef Altorfer, Department of Internal Medicine, City Hospital Waid, Zurich, Switzerland CH-8037 [181]

Elias Anzola, Ministry of Health, Caracas, Venezuela [177]

Marcello Aragona, Istituto di Clinica Medica II, Policlinico Gazzi, University of Messina, 98100 Messina, Italy [231]

Antonio Ascione, Division of Gastroenterology, Ospedale Cardarelli, Napoli, Italy [133]

Lucilla Badiali De Giorgi, Microscopia Elettronica Clinica, Università di Bologna, Via Massarenti 9, Bologna 40138, Italy [191]

Cristiana Barbera, II Pediatric Clinic, University of Torino, 10126 Torino, Italy [225]

Francesco B. Bianchi, Istituto di Patologia Medica Ia University of Bologna, 40138 Bologna, Italy [191]

Leonardo Bianchi, Department of Pathology, University of Basel, Basel, Switzerland CH-4056 [67,181]

Ferruccio Bonino, Division of Gastroenterology, Ospedale Molinette, 10126 Torino, Italy [79,91,337]

Flavia Bortolotti, Istituto di Medicina Clinica, Patologia Medica I, University of Padova, 35100 Padova, Italy [55,225]

Ana Bracho, South General Hospital, Marcaibo, Venezuela [177]

Christian Brechot, Unité de Recombinaison et Expression Génétique, Institut Pasteur, 75724 Paris, France [345]

Carlo Antonio Busachi, Istituto di Patologia Medica I°, University of Bologna, 40138 Bologna, Italy [55,191]

Maua Caltagirone, Cattedra di Patologia Medica R, Ospedale V. Cervello, University of Palermo, 90146 Palermo, Italy [231]

Renata Calzia, Institute for Infectious Diseases, University of Genova, Genova, Italy [225]

Maria Grazia Canese, Istituto di Anatomia Patologica, University of Torino, 10126 Torino, Italy [99]

Nicola Caporaso, Istituto di Semeiotica Medica Ia, Facoltà di Medicina, 80131 Napoli, Italy [133,139,225,237]

Francesco Caredda, Biomedical Sciences and Technologies, Infectious Diseases Clinic, University of Milano, 20157 Milano, Italy [237,245]

Antonietta Cargnel, Malattie Infettive, Ospedale L. Sacco, 20157 Milano, Italy [237]

Liliana Chemello, Istituto di Medicina Clinica, Patologia Medica I, University of Padova, 35100 Padova, Italy [327]

The number in brackets is the opening page number of that contributor's article.

Elisabetta Chiaberge, Division of Gastroenterology, Ospedale Molinette, 10126 Torino, Italy **[337]**

Kenneth P. Chin, USC Liver Unit, Rancho Los Amigos Hospital, Downey, CA 90242, USA **[235]**

Marilina Colombo, Istituto di Patologia Medica Ia, University of Bologna, 40138 Bologna, Italy **[191]**

Massimo Colombo, Clinica Medica III, University of Milano, 20122 Milano, Italy **[203]**

Mario Coltorti, Istituto di Semeiotica Medica Ia, Facoltà di Medicina, 80131 Napoli, Italy **[139]**

Antonio Craxi, Cattedra di Patologia Medica R, Ospedale V. Cervello, University of Palermo, Italy **[133,231]**

Osvaldo Crivelli, Division of Gastroenterology, Ospedale Molinette, 10126 Torino, Italy **[121,337]**

Antonella D'Arminio Monforte, Biomedical Sciences and Technologies, Infectious Diseases Clinic, University of Milano, 20157 Milano, Italy **[245]**

Ezio David, Istituto di Anatomia Patologica, University of Torino, 10126 Torino, Italy **[169]**

Gary L. Davis, Liver Diseases Section, NIADDK, National Institutes of Health, Bethesda, MD 20205, USA **[41]**

Friedrich Deinhardt, Max von Pettenkofer-Institute, University of Munich, 8000 München 2, Federal Republic of Germany **[3]**

Anne Dejean, Unité de Recombinaison et Expression Génétique, Institut Pasteur, 75724 Paris, France **[345]**

Camillo Del Vecchio-Blanco, Istituto di Semeiotica Medica Ia, Facoltà di Medicina, 80131 Napoli, Italy **[139]**

Maria De Monzon, South General Hospital, Marcaibo, Venezuela **[177]**

Katherin Denniston, Division of Molecular Virology and Immunology, Georgetown University, Rockville, MD 20852, USA **[91]**

Pietro Dentico, Clinic of Infectious Diseases, University of Bari, 70124 Bari, Italy **[133,145,237]**

Cristina Di Giacomo, Laboratorio di Immunologia, Ospedale S. Giacomo, 00186 Roma, Italy **[151]**

Nicola Dioguardi, Clinica Medica III, University of Milano, 20122 Milano, Italy **[203]**

Maria Francesca Donato, Clinica Medica III, University of Milano, 20122 Milano, Italy **[203]**

Adrian L.W.F. Eddleston, Liver Unit, King's College Hospital, London SE5, England **[299]**

Patrizia Farci, Division of Gastroenterology, Ospedale Molinette, 10126 Torino, Italy **[219,225,245]**

Stephen M. Feinstone, Laboratory of Infectious Disease, NIAID, National Institutes of Health, Bethesda, MD 20205, USA **[29]**

Stefano Ferrari, Istituto di Patologia Medica Ia, University of Bologna, 40138 Bologna, Italy **[191]**

Pierino Ferroni, Institute of Virology, University of Milano, 20133 Milano, Italy **[127]**

Verena Gauss-Müller, Max von Pettenkofer-Institute, University of Munich, 8000 München 2, Federal Republic of Germany **[3]**

Paolo Gerardo, Division of Gastroenterology, Ospedale Molinette, 10126 Torino, Italy **[133]**

Michael A. Gerber, Department of Pathology, Mount Sinai School of Medicine of the City University of New York, New York, NY 10029, USA **[177]**

Robert J. Gerety, Division of Blood and Blood Products, Bureau of Biologics, Bethesda, MD 20205, USA **[145]**

John L. Gerin, Division of Molecular Virology and Immunology, Georgetown University, Rockville, MD 20852, USA [23,79,91,107,113,369]

Gandolfo Giannuoli, Cattedra di Patologia Medica R, Ospedale V. Cervello, University of Palermo, 90146 Palermo, Italy [231]

Anthony Gimson, Liver Unit, Kings College Hospital Denmark Hill, London SE5 9RS, England [237]

Sugantha Govindarajan, Department of Pathology, Rancho Los Amigos Hospital, Downey, CA 90242, USA [235]

Fred Gudat, Department of Pathology, University of Basel, Basel, Switzerland CH-4056 [181]

Stephen C. Hadler, Division of Hepatitis and Viral Enteritis, CID, Centers for Disease Control, Phoenix, AZ, USA [177]

Stephanos J. Hadziyannis, Academic Department of Medicine, Hippokration General Hosptial, Athens 610, Greece [209]

Reginald G. Hanson, Liver Diseases Section, NIADDK, National Institutes of Health, Bethesda, MD 20205, USA [41]

Bengt-Göran Hansson, Department of Clinical Virology, University of Lund, Malmö General Hospital, Malmö, Sweden [155,161]

Paul V. Holland, Blood Bank Department, Clinical Center, National Institutes of Health, Bethesda, MD 20205, USA [357]

Jay H. Hoofnagle, Liver Diseases Section, NIADDK, National Institutes of Health, Bethesda, MD 20205, USA [41]

Bill Hoyer, Division of Molecular Virology and Immunology, Georgetown University, Rockville, MD 20852, USA [91]

Kamal G. Ishak, Armed Forces Institute of Pathology, Washington, D.C. 20012, USA [177]

Olafur Jensson, Blood Bank, Reykjavik, Iceland [155]

Gunthild Krey, Department of Pathology, University of Basel, Basel, Switzerland CH-4056 [181]

Krzysztof Krawczynski, Department of Immunopathology, National Institute of Hygiene, Warszawa, Poland [317]

Patrizia Landi, Istituto di Patologia Medica Ia, University of Bologna, 40138 Bologna, Italy [191]

Renzo Laschi, Microscopia Electronica Clinica, Università di Bologna, Via Massarenti 9, Bologna 40138, Italy [191]

Paul Leinikki, Department of Biomedical Sciences, University of Tampere, Tampere, Finland [155]

Anna S.F. Lok, Academic Department of Medicine, Royal Free Hospital, London N.W.3, England [219,379]

William T. London, Infection Diseases Branch, NINCDS, National Institutes of Health, Bethesda, MD 20205, USA [79]

Giuseppe Longo, Istituto di Clinica Medica II, Policlinico Gazzi, University of Messina, 98100 Messina, Italy [231]

Enrico Magliano, Institute of Virology, University of Milano, 20133 Milano, Italy [127]

Pier Mannuccio Mannucci, The Hemophilia and Thrombosis Centre Angelo Bianchi Bonomi, University of Milano, 20122 Milano, Italy [145]

Giuseppe Manzillo, IV Division "D. Cotugno" Hospital, 80100 Napoli, Italy [195]

Giovanni Marinucci, Laboratorio di Immunologia, Ospedale S. Giacomo, 00186 Roma, Italy [133,151]

Francesco Milazzo, Malattie Infettive, Ospedale L. Sacco, 20157 Milano, Italy **[237]**

Gian Ludovico Molaro, Immunoematologia, Ospedale Civile di Pordenone, 33170 Pordenone, Italy **[145]**

Franco Mollo, Istituto di Anatomia Patologica, University of Torino, 10126 Torino, Italy **[169]**

Alejandro Mondolfi, Ministry of Health, Caracas, Venezuela **[177]**

Daniela Morganti, Laboratorio di Immunologia, Ospedale S. Giacomo, 00186 Roma, Italy **[151]**

Mauro Moroni, Biomedical Sciences and Technologies, Infectious Diseases Clinic, University of Milano, 20157 Milano, Italy **[245]**

Francesco Negro, Division of Gastroenterology, Ospedale Molinette, 10126 Torino, Italy **[145,337]**

Judith Nelson, Division of Molecular Virology and Immunology, Georgetown University, Rockville, MD 20852, USA **[91]**

Jens O. Nielsen, Division of Epidemiology, Rigshospitalet, Copenhagen, Denmark **[155]**

Erik Nordenfelt, Microbiology, Kuwait University, Faculty of Medicine, Safat, Kuwait **[161]**

Gunnar Norkrans, Department of Infectious Diseases, University of Gothenburg, East Hospital, Gothenburg, Sweden **[155]**

Rosanna Novara, Istituto di Anatomia Patologica, University of Torino, 10126 Torino, Italy **[99]**

Franco Noventa, Istituto di Medicina Clinica, Patologia Medica I, University of Padova, 35100 Padova, Italy **[55]**

Luigi Pagliaro, Cattedra di Patologia Medica R, Ospedale V. Cervello, University of Palermo, 90146 Palermo, Italy **[231]**

George Papaevangelou, National Centre for Viral Hepatitis, Athens School of Hygiene P.O. Box 3085, Athens 618, Greece **[237]**

Robert L. Peters, Department of Pathology, Rancho Los Amigos Hospital, Downey, CA 90242, USA **[235]**

Francesco Peyretti, Banca del Sangue, Ospedale Molinette, 10126 Torino, Italy **[145]**

Felice Piccinino, Clinic of Infectious Diseases, 1st School of Medicine, University of Napoli, 80135 Napoli, Italy **[133]**

Emilio Pisi, Istituto di Patologia Medica Ia, University of Bologna, 40138 Bologna, Italy **[191]**

Giuseppe Poli, Division of Gastroenterology, Ospedale Molinette, 10126 Torino, Italy **[133]**

Patrizia Pontisso, Istituto di Medicina Clinica, Patologia Medica I, University of Padova, 35100 Padova, Italy **[327]**

Antonio Ponzetto, Division of Gastroenterology, Ospedale Molinette, 10126 Torino, Italy **[23,79,91,107,177]**

Hans Popper, The Stratton Laboratory for the Study of Liver Diseases, Mount Sinai School of Medicine of the City University of New York, New York, NY 10029, USA **[177,397]**

Robert H. Purcell, Laboratory of Infectious Diseases, National Institutes of Health, Bethesda, MD 20205, USA **[23,29,79,91,107,113,177,369]**

Giovanni Raimondo, Istituto di Clinca Medica II, Policlinico Gazzi, University of Messina, 98100 Messina, Italy **[133,231]**

Giuseppe Realdi, Istituto di Medicina Clinica, Patologia Medica I, University of Padova, 35100 Padova, Italy **[55,191,327]**

Allan G. Redeker, USC Liver Unit, Rancho Los Amigos Hospital, Downey, CA 90242, USA **[235]**

Angela Maria Rigoli, Istituto di Medicina Clinica, Patologia Medica I, University of Padova, 35100 Padova, Italy [55]

Dalia Rivera, South General Hospital, Marcaibo, Venezuela [177]

Mario Rizzetto, Division of Gastroenterology, Ospedale Molinette, 10126 Torino, Italy [79,121]

Roberto Rizzi, Division of Gastroenterology, Ospedale Molinette, 10126 Torino, Italy [169]

Giuseppe Rocca, Epidemiology Service, Ospedale Molinette, 10126 Torino, Italy [133,169]

Michael Roggendorf, Max von Pettenkofer-Institute, University of Munich, 8000 München 2, Federal Republic of Germany [3]

Adriana Rossi, Clinica Medica III, University of Milano, 20122 Milano, Italy [203]

Elio Rossi, Biomedical Sciences and Technologies, Infectious Diseases Clinic, University of Milano, 20157 Milano, Italy [245]

Massimo Rugge, Istituto di Anatomia Patologica, University of Padova, 35100 Padova, Italy [55]

Maria Grazia Rumi, Clinica Medica III, University of Milano, 20122 Milano, Italy [203]

Evangelista Sagnelli, Clinic of Infectious Diseases, 1st School of Medicine, University of Napoli, 80135 Napoli, Italy [195]

Giorgio Saracco, Division of Gastroenterology, Molinette, 10126 Torino, Italy [237,309]

Emma Schiavon, Istituto di Medicina Clinica, Patologia Medica I, University of Padova, 35100 Padova, Italy [327]

Wolf-Georg Schiller, Division of Infectious Diseases, Department of Internal Medicine, Bezirkskrankenhaus, Potsdam, German Democratic Republic [145]

Ozonio Schiraldi, Clinica Medica, University of Bazi, 70124, Bazi, Italy [133]

Martin Schmid, Department of Internal Medicine, City Hospital Waid, Zurich, Switzerland CH-8037 [181]

Fausto Sessa, Istituto di Anatomia Patologica, University of Pavia, 27100 Pavia, Italy [169]

James W.K. Shih, Division of Blood and Blood Products, Bureau of Biologics, Bethesda, MD 20205, USA [121]

Jens-Christian Siebke, Department of Virology, National Institute of Public Health, Oslo, Norway [155]

Antonina Smedile, Division of Gastroenterology, Ospedale Molinette, 10126 Torino, Italy [237,245]

Enrico Solcia, Istituto di Anatomia Patologica, University of Pavia, 27100 Pavia, Italy [169]

Hans-Peter Spichtin, Department of Pathology, University of Basel, Basel, Switzerland CH-4056 [181]

Giuseppe Squadrito, Istituto di Clinica Medica II, Policlinico Gazzi, University of Messina, 98100 Messina, Italy [231]

Alessandra Stacchiotti, Microscopia Elettronica Clinica, Università di Bologna, Via Massarenti 9, Bologna 40138, Italy [191]

Elisabeth Stöcklin, Department of Pathology, University of Basel, Basel, Switzerland CH-4056 [181]

Rosalba Suozzo, Istituto di Semeiotica Medica Ia, Facoltà di Medicina 80131 Napoli, Italy [139]

Elisabetta Tanzi, Institute of Virology, University of Milano, 20133 Milano, Italy [127]

Gianfranco Tappero, Division of Gastroenterology, Ospedale Molinette, 10126 Torino, Italy [245]

Bud C. Tennant, College of Veterinary Medicine, Cornell University, Ithaca, NY 14853, USA [23]

Howard C. Thomas, Academic Department of Medicine, Royal Free Hospital, London N.W.3, England [145,219,379]

Swan N. Thung, Department of Pathology, Mount Sinai School of Medicine of the City University of New York, New York, NY 10029, USA [177]

Pierre Tiollais, Unité de Recombinaison et Expression Génétique, Institut Pasteur, 75724 Paris, France [11,345]

Giovanni A. Touscoz, Division of Gastroenterology, Ospedale Molinette, 10126 Torino, Italy [309]

Federico Tremolada, Istituto di Medicina Clinica, Patologia Medica I, University of Padova, 35100 Padova, Italy [55]

Frank J. Tyeryar, NIAID, National Institutes of Health, Bethesda 20205 MD, USA [23]

Pentii Ukkonen, Department of Virology, University of Helsinki, Helsinki, Finland [155]

Pietro Vajro, II Pediatric Clinica, University of Napoli, 80131 Napoli, Italy [225]

Luciano Valeri, Preospedalizzazione, Ospedale S. Giacomo, 00186 Roma, Italy [133,151]

Angela Vegnente, Puericultura, University of Napoli, 80138 Napoli, Italy [225]

Giorgio Verme, Division of Gastroenterology, Ospedale Molinette, 10126 Torino, Italy [169]

Maria Vinci, Cattedra di Patologia Medica R, Ospedale V. Cervello, University of Palermo, 90146 Palermo, Italy [133]

Klaus von der Helm, Max von Pettenkofer-Institute, University of Munich, 8000 München 2, Federal Republic of Germany [3]

Simon Wain-Hobson, Unité de Recombinaison et Expression Génétique, Institut Pasteur, 75724 Paris, France [11]

Mats Weibull, Laboratory of Bacteriology, Falun Hospital, Falun, Sweden [155]

Ola Weiland, Department of Infectious Diseases, Roslagstull Hospital, Stockholm, Sweden [155]

Alessandro R. Zanetti, Institute of Virology, University of Milano, 20133 Milano, Italy [127]

Preface

Following the discovery of the Australia Antigen, research in viral hepatitis has rapidly escalated. Achievements have been rewarding, as the agents of hepatitis A and B, only suspected on epidemiological grounds two decades ago, are now fully characterized.

Once the etiological agents of infectious (HAV) and serum hepatitis (HBV) were identified, it became apparent that previously unsuspected non-A, non-B viruses had to exist to explain the multitude of hepatitis occurring in man. More unexpectedly, the pursuit of a chance immunofluorescence observation in liver of carriers of HBsAg led to the recognition of the delta agent, a new pathogen with seemingly unique biological properties.

Our knowledge of delta was born in Torino in the mid-seventies and soon adopted in the USA, where the current image of the delta agent was forged in the last few years. The relatively short time it took to change the low profile of an apparent HBV determinant to the semblance of a unique pathogen is the measure of the energy and enthusiasm that Italian and American scientists dedicated to the effort of establishing the identity and credibility of the new virus. Their success is demonstrated by the current interest in delta agent, which has fostered studies now in progress in many centers. These studies have transformed our concept of delta infection from an Italian phenomenon to one with world-wide importance.

The purpose of this Symposium is to present an update from leading world experts on recent developments in the biological and clinical aspects of viral hepatitis and to summarize the current knowledge and future perspectives of the delta agent. We gratefully acknowledge the contribution of the many sponsors which made this meeting possible and extend our special gratitude to A. Olivieri, President of USL 1-23, G. Poli, Vice-President of USL 1-23, W. Neri, Sanitarian Director of the Ospedale Molinette, and S. Bajardi, head of the Regional Health Administration, for encouragement to organize the Symposium and for providing the facilities to meet in the birth place of the discovery of delta agent.

The problems raised during the meeting far outnumber those that are solved. The hope is that the 1983 rendezvous in Torino may be the basis and stimulus for further and rapid research progress, so that a new meeting will soon be required to answer the many questions left unanswered these days.

The Editors

NOMENCLATURE: A PROPOSAL TO DESIGNATE THE DELTA AGENT AS
HEPATITIS D VIRUS

M. Rizzetto[1], F. Bonino[1], G. Verme[1],
R.H. Purcell[2], J.L. Gerin[3].
[1] Div. of Gastroenterology, Ospedale Molinette,
Torino, Italy; [2] National Institute of Allergy
& Infectious Diseases, NIH, Bethesda, MD;
[3] Dept. of Microbiology, Georgetown Univ. Med.
Ctr., Rockville, MD.

The term δ Ag was first introduced in 1977 to
designate a new antigen observed in the hepatocyte nuclei
of Italian HBsAg carriers with chronic liver disease; δ Ag
was considered to be an antigenic variant of HBcAg.
Subsequent epidemiologic data and transmission experiments
in chimpanzees, however, established that δ Ag was a marker
of an infectious agent, the delta agent (δ).

As documented in this volume, there is now a
considerable body of data to indicate that δ, although
dependent on HBV for its expression and replication,
represents a unique hepatitis agent, distinct from HBV.
This conclusion is based on the following evidence: 1) The
lack of cross-reactions between δ Ag/anti-δ and
HBV-specific Ag/Ab systems; 2) The lack of homology between
the δ-associated RNA and HBV DNA based on hybridization
analyses; 3) Terminal dilution experiments in chimpanzees
in which the dilution endpoint of δ in a serum far exceeds
that of the HBV and; 4) The successful transmission of δ of
human origin to WHV carrier woodchucks indicating that
other HBV-like viruses can provide the requisite helper
functions for δ infection.

Important observations based on clinical,
epidemiologic and histopathological features of patients
with acute and chronic δ infection, indicate that δ hepatitis
is a clinical entity separate from the underlying disease
related to HBV infection. Accordingly, we propose a new
nomenclature for δ consistent with the WHO recommendations
for hepatitis viruses (Table 1). Type D hepatitis is
recommended because 1) it is consistent with the δ

terminology and 2) Type C hepatitis was previously used in reference to non-A, non-B hepatitis.

Table 1. Nomenclature

Current	Recommended
Delta Hepatitis	Type D Hepatitis
Delta Agent (δ)	Hepatitis D Virus (HDV)
Delta Antigen (δ Ag)	Hepatitis D Antigen (HDAg)
Antibody to δ Ag (anti-δ)	Antibody to HDAg (anti-HD)

The proposed nomenclature for δ, of course, has no taxonomic implications in the classification scheme of vertebrate viruses. Its use by hepatitis researchers, however, should serve to clarify the presentation of this subject to the biomedical community.

List of Abbreviations

HAV = Hepatitis A Virus

HBV = Hepatitis B Virus

δ = delta agent

NANB = Non A, Non B (hepatitis viruses)

NANBH = Non A, Non B hepatitis

HBsAg = Hepatitis B surface antigen

HBcAg = Hepatitis B core antigen

HBeAg = Hepatitis B e antigen

δ-Ag, delta-ag = delta antigen

anti-HBs = antibody to HBsAg

anti-HBc = antibody to HBcAg

anti-HBe = antibody to HBeAg

anti-δ, anti-delta = antibody to δ-Ag

IgM anti-HAV, anti-HAV IgM = antibody to HAV of IgM type

IgM anti-HBc = antibody to HBcAg of IgM type

IgM anti-δ, IgM anti-delta = antibody to δ-Ag of IgM type

AH, AVH = acute viral hepatitis

ALH = acute lobular hepatitis

FH = fulminant hepatitis

CLD = chronic liver disease

CLH = chronic lobular hepatitis

CPH = chronic persistent hepatitis

CAH = chronic active hepatitis

AC = active cirrhosis

HCC = Hepatocellular carcinoma

RIA = Radioimmunoassay

ELISA = Enzyme linked immuno assay

IF, IFL = immunofluorescence

FITC = fluorescein-isothyocianate

HEPATITIS A, B, NON-A, NON-B

Viral Hepatitis and Delta Infection, pages 3–10
© 1983 Alan R. Liss, Inc., 150 Fifth Avenue, New York, NY 10011

HEPATITIS A VIRUS

Michael Roggendorf, M.D., Friedrich Deinhardt, M.D.,
Verena Gauss-Müller, Ph.D., Klaus von der Helm, Ph.D.
Max von Pettenkofer Institute for Hygiene and Medical
Microbiology, University of Munich
Munich, Western Germany

Hepatitis A virus (HAV) is a typical enterovirus, and has been classified in the family picornaviridae as type 72 of the enteroviruses (Melnick 1982). HAV has a icosahedral symmetry, 32 capsomeres, and the diameter is 28 nm. The buoyant density of the complete particles in CsCl is 1.33–1.34 g/ml, the sedimentation coefficient is 160 S, and the nucleic acid is a single-stranded RNA with a sedimentation coefficient of 33 S. The genome contains a 40-80 nucleotide sequence of poly A. The positive-stranded RNA has a molecular weight of about 2.25×10^6 dalton when measured under nondenaturating conditions and 2.8×10^6 dalton under fully denaturating conditions. So far, four distinct polypeptides typical of enteroviruses have been detected: VP1: 30,000-33,000, VP2: 24,000-26,500, VP3: 21,000-23,000, and VP4: 7,000-14,000. It is not known against which polypeptide antibodies to HAV (anti-HAV) in human convalescent sera are directed and which protein must be neutralized to prevent infection.

Several strains of HAV from all over the world have been isolated and propagated in cell culture, and as no antigenic differences between these isolated strains have been observed, it is assumed that only one antigenic type exists.

HAV has been propagated in tissue culture, and table 1 summarizes the cell lines which have been used.

Table 1

Cell lines in which HAV has been propagated

1. Liver explant cell culture of _Saguinus labiatus_
   Provost and Hilleman, 1979

2. Fetal rhesus kidney
   Frhk-6: Provost and Hilleman, 1979
   Frhk-4: Flehmig, 1980

3. Human hepatoma cell line (PLC/PRF/5)
   Frösner et al., 1979; Deinhardt et al., 1981

4. African green monkey cells
   AGMK: Feinstone et al., 1980; Daemer et al., 1981
   VERO: Lehmann et al., 1980; Locarnini et al., 1981;
   Kojima et al., 1981

5. Human amniotic tissue cells (FL)
   Kojima et al., 1981

6. Human embryo fibroblasts (HEF, WI-26)
   Gauss-Müller et al., 1981

   Human embryo lung fibroblasts (WI-38, MRC 5)
   Provost et al., 1981

   Human embryo kidney fibroblasts (HEKC)
   Flehmig, 1981

HAV infects man by the faecal-oral route. Figure 1 shows a typical course of virus excretion and development of antibodies in a hepatitis A infection in man. HAV is excreted in the feces for one to two weeks before the onset of disease and up to four weeks thereafter, and most virus is excreted before the onset of illness. Development of a chronic carrier state after infection with HAV has not been observed, nor have chronic infections, as have been observed in hepatitis B.

Figure 1

Typical course of hepatitis A infection

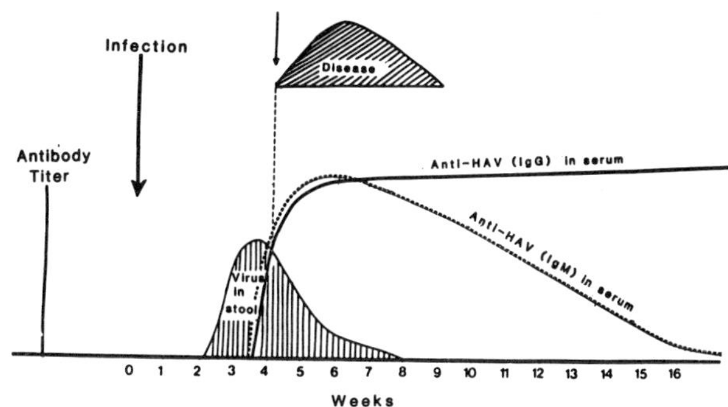

Hepatitis A infection is diagnosed serologically by demonstrating antibodies of the IgM class (anti-HAV IgM); anti-HAV IgM is always present at the onset of disease, and can be detected up to 6 months afterwards by sensitive RIA or ELISA tests, using the anti-µ capture system (Roggendorf et al 1980). This assay enables a diagnosis of acute hepatitis A to be made within 24 hours, and the sensitivity of the test system can be adjusted for diagnostic use so that antibodies of the IgM class are detectable only for three to four months.

TRANSLATION <u>IN VITRO</u> OF HAV-RNA

Growth of HAV in cell culture is atypical for a picornavirus. Viral antigens are expressed only after two or more weeks following infection, and no cytopathic effect has been observed. In contrast to other picornaviruses, HAV seems to have no major effect on host cell nucleic acid or protein synthesis. Study of the biosynthesis of HAV in cell culture by Locarnini and co-workers (1980) identified a few proteins of larger molecular weight than the structural proteins but detailed investigation of the biosynthesis and processing of viral proteins was hampered by the low production of HAV in cell culture, and a true precursor-endproduct relationship could not be established.

Translation _in_ _vitro_ of HAV-RNA offered the possibility of avoiding the difficulties, and the chance to study whether the low growth rate of HAV in cell culture was caused by a low translation rate of messenger RNA or poor processing of protein precursors (Gauss-Müller et al, in preparation). Virus particles propagated in a hepatoma cell line (PLC/PRF/5) were used as the source of HAV-RNA. Mock-infected cells (PLC/PRF/5) or poliovirus-infected cells were used as controls. The translation products of HAV-RNA or polio-RNA were analyzed by SDS-PAGE; poliovirus type 2 RNA translation products had molecular weights ranging from 95,000 to less than 15,000, corresponding to the weights described in the literature. The major translation products of HAV-RNA ranged from 150,000 to 27,000, and the most prominent proteins were those with molecular weights of 85,000, 65,000, 50,000 and 40,000. The products of mock-infected PLC/PRF/5 cells were similar to "endogenous" translation products without addition of RNA. Study of the kinetics of the translation rate established that 30 minutes at 30°C were sufficient to synthesize all products, a result similar to that obtained after translation of poliovirus type 2 RNA.

The processing _in_ _vitro_ of the synthesized proteins was studied by a pulse chase experiment. A 60 minute pulse was followed by a chase in the presence of excess unlabelled methionine for 5 hours. The pattern of HAV translation products showed only slight alterations after the chase. The protein of 85,000 disappeared while the intensity of the bands at molecular weights of 55,000, 28,000 and 27,000 increased. More dramatic changes occurred in the chase period during the processing of poliovirus type 2 proteins: precursor proteins lost in intensity and the proteins VP0, VP1 and VP3 increased.

Many of the products synthesized in vitro were HAV-specific, as was shown by immunoprecipitation with a serum containing antibodies to HAV. The precursors are not characterized yet, nor the processing into smaller proteins, but from the available data on the translation in vitro of HAV-RNA it can be concluded that:

1. HAV-RNA is plus-stranded
2. primary translation products are similar in size to those of other enteroviruses
3. the processing of HAV precursor molecules yields proteins corresponding to the structural proteins of native HAV.

VACCINATION AGAINST HEPATITIS A

In several countries, the prevalence of antibodies to HAV in the population is very low, so that individuals travelling into endemic areas of HAV, for example, run a high risk of acquiring hepatitis A. Three ways of producing a vaccine to hepatitis A are under investigation. HAV has been attenuated by passage in Frhk-6 and human diploid lung fibroblasts (Provost et al 1983). Chimpanzees inoculated with these attenuated HAV strains were challenged with virulent HAV; both animals produced anti-HAV and were resistant to HAV infection, indicating that these attenuated virus strains may be suitable vaccine candidates.

Another approach to the production of a vaccine would be the cloning and sequencing of the genome of HAV. One possibility would be to express HAV proteins in bacteria or eukaryotic cells containing cloned HAV genomes. Cloning of HAV-RNA is difficult, as the HAV genome is an RNA which can be cloned only after reverse transcription into double-stranded complementary DNA, and the limited amounts of HAV available from stools of infected persons or from cell cultures make it difficult to produce enough purified HAV genomic RNA for such experiments. Another difficulty is that the RNA (about 8,000 base pairs) is long, about 2.5 times longer than the HBV genome and that the reverse transcription of RNAs of a length greater than messenger RNAs (2,000 to 3,000 nucleotides) is difficult because the secondary structure of these RNAs apparently hinders the transcription of the full length of the RNA. Even so, DNA complementary to HAV-RNA has been prepared (von der Helm et al 1981) by reverse transcription of HAV-RNA, using oligo dT and limited digested calf thymus DNA as random primers (Ostermayer and von der Helm, unpublished data). These cDNAs were cloned into the plasmid pBR 322, cut by Pst 1. The clones obtained, although smaller than the full genome length, covered the entire RNA genome. The clones were mapped along the HAV-RNA by hybridizing them to each other and by restriction enzyme analysis. The overlapping fragments were hybridized by the southern blot technique. Nucleotides were sequenced by the method of Maxam-Gilbert, beginning with the clones proximal to the 3' end of the RNA genome, and at present about 1,500 nucleotides at the 3' end of the genome have been sequenced (Lezius et al, unpublished data).

HAV clones were also analyzed for antigen expression in bacteria, using the promotor of the ß-lactamase gene into which the HAV-cDNA had been cloned. The presence of HAV antigens in water shock lysates of bacteria carrying specific clones was sought by RIA, and two clones localized at the 5' end were weakly positive. At present, it is not known which of the viral proteins or part of them are expressed in the bacterial clones as the specific antigenicity of the various HAV proteins remain unknown.

Another possibility of producing a vaccine is to synthesize oligopeptides identical to HAV amino acid sequences but for the production of such oligopeptides, the nucleotide sequence of HAV-RNA must be known. With such oligopeptides, it might be possible to induce antibodies against HAV in a way similar to that shown for HBsAg (Dreesman et al 1982).

Daemer RJ, Feinstone SM, Gust ID, Purcell RH (1981). Propagation of human hepatitis A virus in African green monkey kidney cell culture: primary isolation and serial passage. Infection and Immunity 32:388.

Deinhardt F and Gust ID, on behalf of the participants in an informal WHO meeting (1982). Viral hepatitis. Bull WHO 60:661.

Dreesman GR, Sanchez Y, Ionescu-Matiu I, Sparrow JT, Six HR, Peterson DL, Hollinger FB, Melnick JL (1982). Antibody to hepatitis B surface antigen after a single inoculation of uncoupled synthetic HBsAg peptides. Nature 295:158.

Gauss-Müller V, von der Helm K, Deinhardt F (1983). Translation of hepatitis A virus *in* *vitro* (in preparation).

Flehmig B (1980). Hepatitis A virus in cell culture: I. Propagation of different hepatitis A virus isolates in a fetal rhesus monkey kidney cell line (Frhk-4). Med Microbiol Immunol 168:239.

Feinstone SM, Daemer R, Gust ID, Purcell RH (1980). Hepatitis A virus in cell culture. In: The 2nd Australasian symposium on viral hepatitis. J Clin Microbiol 11:710.

Flehmig B (1981). Hepatitis A virus in cell culture: II. Growth characteristics of hepatitis A virus in Frhk-4/R cells. Med Microbiol Immunol 170:73.

Kojima H, Shibayama T, Sato A, Suzuki S, Ichida F, Hamada C (1981) Propagation of human hepatitis A virus in conventional cell lines. J Med Virol 7:273.

Lehmann NI, Pringle RC, Gust ID (1980). Infection of cell culture of monkey kidney origin with hepatitis A virus. In: The 2nd Australasian symposium on viral hepatitis. J Clin Microbiol 11:710.

Lezius A, von der Helm D, von der Helm K, Winnacker EL, Deinhardt F (1983) unpublished data.

Locarnini SA, Coulepis AG, Westaway EG, Gust ID (1981). Restricted replication of human hepatitis A virus in cell culture: intracellular biochemical studies. J Virol 37:216.

Maxam AM, Gilbert W (1977). A new method for sequencing DNA. Proc Natl Acad Sci USA 74:560.

Melnick JL (1982). Classification of hepatitis A virus as enterovirus type 72 and of hepatitis B virus as hepadnavirus type 1. Intervirology 18:105.

Ostermayer R, von der Helm K (1983) unpublished data.

Provost PJ, Hilleman MR (1979). Propagation of human hepatitis A virus in cell culture *in* *vitro* (40422). Proc Soc Exp Biol Med 160:213.

Provost PJ, Giesa PA, McAleer WJ, Hilleman MR (1981). Isolation of hepatitis A virus *in* *vitro* in cell culture directly from human specimens. Proc Soc Exp Biol Med 167:201.

Provost PJ, Conti PA, Giesa PA, Banker FS, Buynak EB, McAleer WG, Hilleman MR (1983). Studies in chimpanzees of live attenuated hepatitis A vaccine candidates (41570). Proc Soc Exp Biol Med 172:357.

Roggendorf M, Frösner GG, Deinhardt F, Scheid R (1980). Comparison of solid-phase test systems for demonstrating antibodies against hepatitis A virus (anti-HAV of the IgM class). J Med Virol 5:47.

von der Helm K, Winnacker EL, Deinhardt F, Frösner GG, Gauss-Müller V, Bayerl B, Scheid R, Siegl G (1981). Cloning of hepatitis A virus genome. J Virol Methods 3:37.

Viral Hepatitis and Delta Infection, pages 11–22
© **1983 Alan R. Liss, Inc., 150 Fifth Avenue, New York, NY 10011**

STRUCTURE AND ORGANIZATION OF HEPATITIS B VIRUS DNA

Pierre Tiollais and Simon Wain-Hobson

Recombinaison et Expression Génétique
Inserm U 163
Institut Pasteur,28 rue du Docteur Roux, Paris

The human hepatitis B virus (HBV) belongs to the recently
designated group of animal DNA viruses and called the Hepadna
Viridae (Robinson et al, 1982). The importance and interest of
HBV come from the high prevalence of chronic HBV infection and
its relationship with liver cancer. HBV is one of the few viruses involved in the development of human cancer. The restricted host range of the virus and the lack of a cell culture system for its propagation has greatly impeded our understanding its molecular genetics. Turning to DNA recombinant
technology has opened up new possibilities, the structure of
the genome was deduced from cloning and sequencing of the viral DNA, and the basic genetic organization of the virus was
obtained by comparing the nucleotide sequences of different
HBV clones.

I - <u>STRUCTURE OF THE VIRION DNA</u>

The HBV genome is a small circular partly double-stranded DNA molecule. It has an unusual structure in that there
is a single-stranded region of variable length. The long of
L(-) strand is of fixed length of about 3,200 nucleotides and
has a nick or a gap of few nucleotides. The short or S(+)
strand, is of variable length ranging from 50 to 100% that of
the L strand. This structure, proposed by Summers et al.
(Summers, 1975), has been validated and refined by the determination of the physical map of both native and cloned HBV
DNA (Charnay et al, 1979; Sattler et al, 1979). The position
of the nick in the L(-) strand is fixed, and, if the single
EcoRI site is used as the origin of the restriction map, probably at nucleotide 1818 (Pasek et al, 1979)(Fig.1).

The position of the 5' end of the S(+) strand is fixed at approximately nucleotide 1560 while the position of the 3' end is variable. The maintenance of the circular structure is assured by base-pairing over a length of about 260 nucleotides. A DNA polymerase associated with the viral nucleocapsid is capable of repairing the single-stranded region by elongating the 3' end of the S(+) strand (Kaplan et al, 1973). A covalently linked protein has been found at the 5'end of the L strand but its biological role is undefined (Gerlich et al, 1980).

There are now six complete HBV sequences established : one is isolated in France, belongs to the ayw subtype (Galibert et al, 1979), another isolated in Great Britain, to the complex adyw subtype (Pasek et al, 1979), two others isolated in USA (Valenzuela et al, 1980) and Japan (Ono et al, 1983) to the adw subtype and a further two isolated in Japan (Ono et al, 1983; Miyanohara, personal communication) to the adr subtype. For the six genomes the lengths range from 3182 to 3221 base pairs (bp). The six genomes can be perfectly aligned, the variations in length are due to small deletions or insertions. A two by two analysis of these HBV sequences shows some degree of divergence. As expected the divergence is higher for viruses of different subtypes - about 8 to 10% - than for viruses of the same subtype - about 1.5% to 2%. A similar observation was reported previously for the restriction map of viruses of different subtypes (Siddiqui et al, 1979; Bichko et al, 1982). The existence of a correlation between the virus subtypes and specific sequences including restriction sites and/or insertions or deletions cannot yet be established. An analysis of a larger number of HBV clones is necessary to answer to this question. Concerning the homogeneity of the virus in a given carrier, the question is open. Although Sninsky et al. (1979) have not shown any difference in the restriction patterns of different clones derived from the same subtype, Ono et al. (1983) reported the existence of restriction site heterogeneity in the genome of HBV isolated from a single donor.

II - <u>GENETIC ORGANIZATION OF HBV</u>

A precise description of the transcription units and RNA processing cannot yet be given, not least in part due to the absence of a cell culture system for HBV replication. Nevertheless a general presentation of its genetic organization can be deduced from the comparative analysis

of the nucleotide sequences of cloned genomes (Tiollais et
al, 1981). Theoretical transcription of the two strands in
all three reading frames allows the definition of "open reading frames", which often represent potential genes or parts
of genes: An additional aid in defining the genetic organization is the conservation of such open reading frames amongst
several HBV genome sequences.

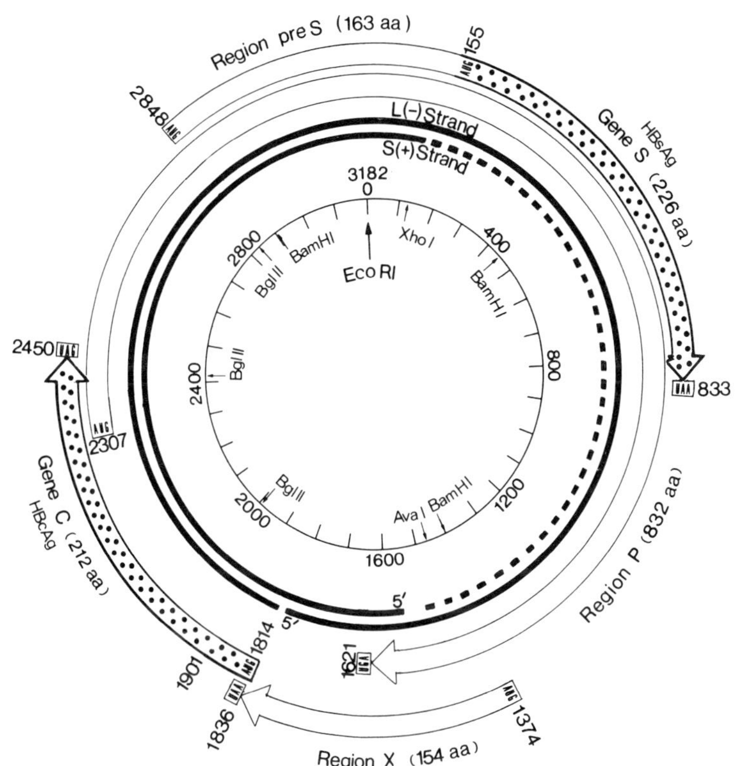

Fig.1. Genetic organization of the HBV genome : The cloned
HBV genome shown is that of the ayw subtype (Galibert et al,
1979). Some restriction sites present in this clone are indicated. The broad arrows surrounding the genome correspond to
the four large open regions of the L(-) strand transcript.
These four potential coding sequences are termed region S

(divided into pre S region and gene S), gene C, region P and
region X. The number of amino acids in brackets corresponds to
the length of the hypothetical polypeptides encoded by this
HBV clone. The two sequences coding for HBsAg and HBcAg are
stippled.

We define as a "region" an open reading frame delineated by
an AUG codon and a stop codon.

   For the L(-) strand transcript, four large regions are
conserved amongst all six genomes to date sequenced (Fig.1).
Moreover when these regions contain insertions or deletions,
they are always a multiple of three allowing conservation of
the reading frame. By contrast, there are no conserved open
reading frames in the S(+) strand transcript of any considerable length. The L(-) strand thus carries all or virtually
all of the protein coding capacity of the genome and can be
considered as the minus strand. The four large regions of the
L(-) strand transcript are termed S, C, P and X. All four regions possess a potential initiator AUG codon (FiG.1). All
overlap with at least another, region P overlapping with the
three other regions. The L(-) strand can be read one and a
half times. This is probably due to the fact that HBV, and
all the hepadna viruses, represent virtually the smallest
amongst mammalian DNA viruses, there being a recently described 1760 bp DNA virus in pigs (Tisher et al, 1982). By thus
employing extensively overlapping regions a small virus can
encode much more protein.

Region S : This region is subdivided into the pre-S region
and gene S. Gene S in fact corresponds to the coding sequence
of the major envelope protein related to the surface antigen
(HBsAg) (Pasek et al, 1979; Charnay et al, 1979; Valenzuela
et al, 1979). Gene S is of constant length in the six sequenced genomes, its translation product is 226 amino acids long
(Mr = 25,350) (Fig.2). Theoretical analysis of its primary
structure shows that the protein can be divided up into three
hydrophobic segments separated by two hydrophilic ones. Precise limits of these segments cannot be defined, but for the
three hydrophobic segments they could be amino acids 7 to 23
(segment I), amino acids 80 to 98 (segment II) and 170 amino
acids 170 to 226 (segment III). In addition, the hydrophobic
parameters of Segrest and Feldman (1974), suggest that they
penetrate a lipid bilayer. The presence of charge residues

at the boundaries of segments I and II as well as their lengths
suggest that these segments traverse the lipid bilayer of the
viral envelope. The hydrophobic segments I and II are strictly conserved and the amino acid variations in the hydrophobic segment III are generally conservative in nature. Interestingly most of the amino acid variations observed for the six
genomes occur in the two hydrophilic segments (Fig.2).By analogy with the distribution of antigenic determinants amongst
influenza heammaglutinnins (Wiley et al, 1981) and neuramidi-
nase (Colman et al, 1983) antigens, we argue that the two
hydrophilic segments carry most or all of the antigenic determinants of HBsAg. In addition some amino acid variations
are correlated with the HBsAg determinant, suggesting that
these amino acids are involved with the subtype antigenic
determinants. According to this hypothesis the subtype determinants would be distributed along the two hydrophilic
regions.

HBsAg is a dimer of the protein encoded by gene S and is
of some 49 K daltons in molecular weight (Misharo et al, 1980).
The dimer is stabilized by disulphide bonds which are essential for full antigenicity. The only chemical difference
between the two proteins of the dimer is that one is glycosylated - the site being asparagine 146 within the sequence
Asn-Cys-Thr (Machida et al, 1982).Combining all of the above
points we propose a model for the HBsAg dimer (Fig.3). The model considers HBsAg as being composed of two transmembrane
proteins symetrically arranged with respect to the membrane
and stabilized by intermolecular disulphide bonds. The two
hydrophilic segments carrying the HBsAg determinants point
out into solvent. The model shows that HBsAg determinants
are carried on both of the two hydrophilic segments, a result already demonstrated by the blocking of antisera to
HBsAg using synthetic peptides where sequences are contained
within these segments (Bhatnagar et al, 1982; Kennedy et al,
1983). The model can also explain why there is approximately
1 : 1 of glycosylated to non-glycosylated protein (Peterson
et al, 1981). Assuming that glycosylation occurs after assembly of the viral envelope only one of two asparagines 146 -
the site of glycosylation - points out. The other is poin-
ting inwards, protected by the particulate structure.

The conservation of the pre-S region, a long overlapping region, amongst six genomes is strong evidence in favor of its coding potential. Indeed there is evidence that
it, or at least part of it, is transcribed into mRNA.

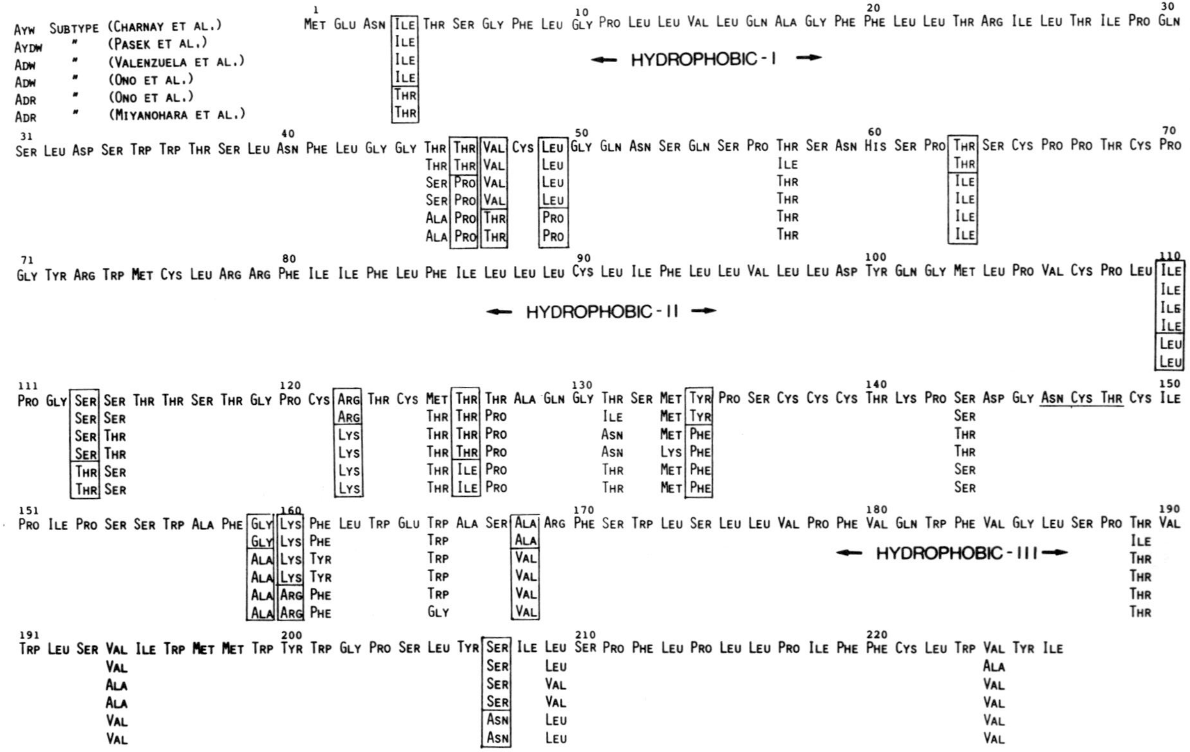
1 10 20 30
Ayw Subtype (Charnay et al.) Met Glu Asn Ile Thr Ser Gly Phe Leu Gly Pro Leu Leu Val Leu Gln Ala Gly Phe Phe Leu Leu Thr Arg Ile Leu Thr Ile Pro Gln
Aydw " (Pasek et al.) Ile
Adw " (Valenzuela et al.) Ile
Adw " (Ono et al.) Ile
Adr " (Ono et al.) Thr
Adr " (Miyanohara et al.) Thr
HYDROPHOBIC - I
31 40 50 60 70
Ser Leu Asp Ser Trp Trp Thr Ser Leu Asn Phe Leu Gly Gly Thr Thr Val Cys Leu Gly Gln Asn Ser Gln Ser Pro Thr Ser Asn His Ser Pro Thr Ser Cys Pro Pro Thr Cys Pro
Thr Thr Val Leu Ile Thr
Ser Pro Val Leu Thr Ile
Ser Pro Val Leu Thr Ile
Ala Pro Thr Pro Thr Ile
Ala Pro Thr Pro Thr Ile
71 80 90 100 110
Gly Tyr Arg Trp Met Cys Leu Arg Arg Phe Ile Ile Phe Leu Phe Ile Leu Leu Leu Cys Leu Ile Phe Leu Leu Val Leu Leu Asp Tyr Gln Gly Met Leu Pro Val Cys Pro Leu Ile
Ile
Ile
Ile
Leu
Leu
HYDROPHOBIC - II
111 120 130 140 150
Pro Gly Ser Ser Thr Thr Ser Thr Gly Pro Cys Arg Thr Cys Met Thr Thr Ala Gln Gly Thr Ser Met Tyr Pro Ser Cys Cys Cys Thr Lys Pro Ser Asp Gly Asn Cys Thr Cys Ile
Ser Ser Arg Thr Thr Pro Ile Met Tyr Ser
Ser Thr Lys Thr Thr Pro Asn Met Phe Thr
Ser Thr Lys Thr Thr Pro Asn Lys Phe Thr
Thr Ser Lys Thr Ile Pro Thr Met Phe Ser
Thr Ser Lys Thr Ile Pro Thr Met Phe Ser
151 160 170 180 190
Pro Ile Pro Ser Ser Trp Ala Phe Gly Lys Phe Leu Trp Glu Trp Ala Ser Ala Arg Phe Ser Trp Leu Ser Leu Leu Val Pro Phe Val Gln Trp Phe Val Gly Leu Ser Pro Thr Val
Gly Lys Phe Trp Ala Ile
Ala Lys Tyr Trp Val Thr
Ala Lys Tyr Trp Val Thr
Ala Arg Phe Trp Val Thr
Ala Arg Phe Gly Val Thr
HYDROPHOBIC - III
191 200 210 220
Trp Leu Ser Val Ile Trp Met Met Trp Tyr Trp Gly Pro Ser Leu Tyr Ser Ile Leu Ser Pro Phe Leu Pro Leu Leu Pro Ile Phe Phe Cys Leu Trp Val Tyr Ile
Val Ser Leu Ala
Ala Ser Val Val
Ala Ser Val Val
Val Asn Leu Val
Val Asn Leu Val

Fig.2. Correlation between the amino acid sequence of the
major envelope protein and the HBsAg subtypes : The amino
acid sequence of the protein is that derived from the nucleotide sequence of gene S of the ayw subtype (Galibert
et al, 1979). The tripeptide Asn (146)-Cys-Thr by which
the carbohydrate is attached is underlined. The three
hydrophobic sequences are indicated by arrows. The amino
acid changes observed in the aydw clone (Pasek et al, 1979)
the two adw clones (Valenzuela et al, 1980; Ono et al, 1983)
and the two adr clones (Ono et al, 1983; Miyanohara, personal communication) are respectively denoted below the sequence. Most of the variations observed are located in the
two hydrophilic regions. Amino acids are boxed when a direct
correlation between amino acid variation and the HBsAg
subtype is observed.

There are three interesting points regarding this region :
(i) The region is of variable length, the differences being
due to small deletions/insertions between the repeated sequences GCATGGG at the 5'end of the pre-S region and which
carry an in phase initiator methionine codon (underlined).
For both genomes of the ay subtype 33 nucleotides are dele-
ted while for only one of the four ad subtypes is there a
deletion and then of 21 nucleotides. Thus the pre-S region
encodes a putative protein of 163 or 174 aminoacids.(ii)
There is approximately twice the amino acid variability
within this region as there is in gene S. Furthermore while
some mutually exclusive pairs of amino acids following HBsAg
subtypes are found there is much more spontaneous or random
variation which would suggest that the amino acid sequence
of the putative product of this region, is not very critical.
(iii) Recently a minor-polypeptide derived from virions has
been purified and analyzed (Stibbe et al, 1983). This glyco-
protein shares all the antigenic determinants and structure
of the HBsAg dimer but has approximately 55 amino acids
residues extra at the NH$_2$ terminal. The structure of this
protein is consistant with an initiation of translation of
a methionine codon 55 amino acids upstream from that of gene
S. The translation initiation sequence GCCATGC does not
conform to that of strong initiation sites (Kozak et al, 1981)
though is similar to those of weak initiation sequences.

Region C : Region C encodes the HBV core antigen (HBcAg). For
the four genomes, not of the adw subtype, there is a small
deletion of six nucleotides in the 3'end of the region C

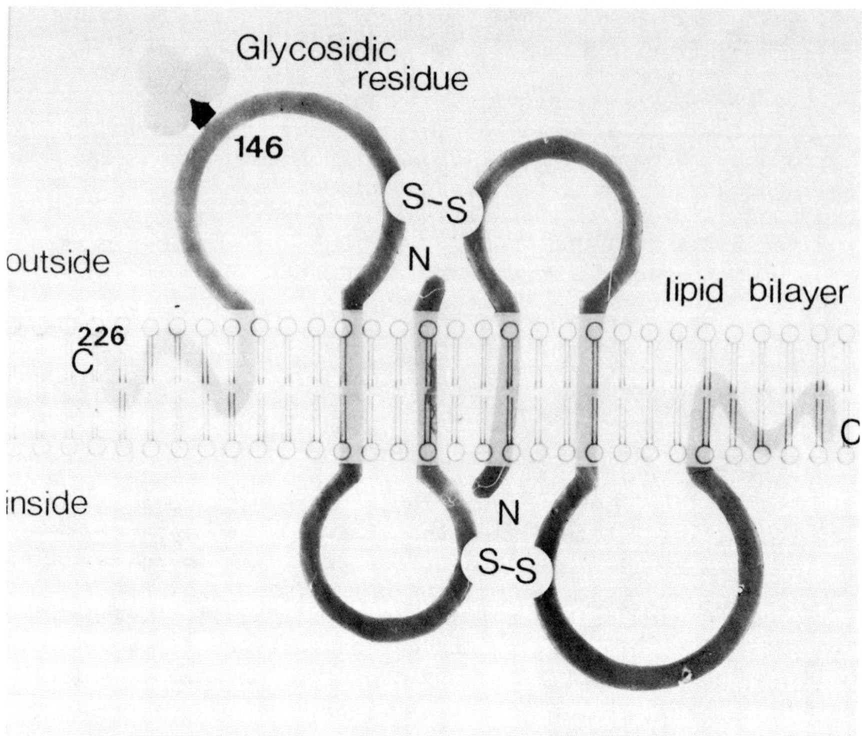

Fig.3. Model of the HBsAg structure : The dimer consists of
two transmembrane polypeptides symetrically arranged with
respect to the lipid bilayer and linked by disulphide bounds
(S-S). The two hydrophilic domains containing HBsAg determinants are alternatively inside and outside the lipid bilayer. The 50% glycosylation of the major envelope protein
could reflect a post assembly carbohydrate attachment of
only one of the two possible sites in the dimer.

(Fig.1). Four out of the six sequenced genomes, covering all subtypes show an AUG initiator just five bases before the site of the nick. This would give a polypeptide of 212-214 amino acids (MW = 22,300) depending on subtype. However for two other genomes, the aydw and one adr, the AUG initiator is 87 nucleotides downstream, so giving rise to a protein of 183 amino acids. For the aydw genome a point mutation eliminates translation from the first AUG, and for the adr genome a deletion of 33 nucleotides exactly before the nick eliminates the first AUG. Recently Feitelson et al (1982) have characterized a HBsAg 22kd polypeptide in infected liver. This polypeptide would be the precursor of the major 19kd HBcAg polypeptide present in the virion and which would derive from the 22kd polypeptide by cleavage of its COOH-terminus. The size of 22kd well agrees with the size of 212-214 amino acids of the gene C translation product. Three aspects of the HBcAg sequence deserve note. (i) Between residues 22 and 30 inclusive is an extremely hydrophobic nonapeptide Leu Cys Leu Gly Trp Leu Trop Gly Met flanked by charged residues. It could be that this sequence is in some way responsible for anchoring the lipid bilayer about the nucleocapsid.(ii) The COOH terminal sequence is remarkable in that is extremely rich in arginine, serine and proline. Presumably these arginine rich sequences. there is a tandem repeat of the octapeptide Ser Pro Arg Arg Arg Arg Ser Gln, are involved in interactions with the HBV DNA within the nucleocapsid. Such sequences resemble protamine and other DNA binding proteins. The DNA binding properties of HBcAg are as yet unknown. (iii) Compared to the amino acid variation amongst the pre-S and S regions (approximately 20% and 10% respectively amongst different subtypes) the HBcAg sequence is more highly conserved (up to 6% amongst different subtypes). Despite this, mutually exclusive pairs of amino acids can be discerned corresponding to the HBsAg subtype of the genome. It would be interesting to know if HBcAg subtype, or HBeAg subtypes (HBeAg is another post-transcriptional form of HBcAg) could be correlated with those of HBsAg.

Region P : Region P probably encodes the endogenous polymerase associated with virions and viral cores. It is extremely large and overlaps with all other regions. It can encode a basic protein unusually rich in histidine and of 832 to 845 amino acids depending on the subtype. A nucleotide sequence comparison between region P and the reverse transcriptase (pol gene product) of the oncogenic retrovirus, Rous sarcoma virus reveals tracts of homology. This,

together with the similar molecular weight of the RSV reverse
polymerase ($\simeq$ 92,000 daltons) and the fact that AMV reverse
transcriptase can repair <u>in vitro</u> the single-stranded region
of HBV (Summers et al, 1978) suggests that region P codes
for a RNA dependent reverse transcriptase. This agrees well
with the discovery of a reverse transcriptase activity associated with the endogenous viral polymerase.

<u>Region X</u> : Region X encodes a possible protein of 145-154
amino acids. There is a small insertion of six nucleotides
in the 3' end for the complex adyw subtype and a deletion
of 27 nucleotides eliminates 9 amino acids for the NH_2
region in one adr genome sequence. What HBV protein does
HBV correspond to ? The theoretical protein is not particularly hydrophobic and is therefore unlikely to be associated with the lipid bilayer. There exists a protein covalently bound to the 5' of the L(-) strand of the HBV genome
(Gerlich et al, 1980) and a protein kinase activity associated with HBcAg core peptides (Albin et al, 1980). As yet
there are no answers although the cloning of this region
into a gene expression vector will probably soon elucidate
this problem.

Albin C, Robinson WS (1980). Protein kinase activity in
     hepatitis B virus. J. Virol 34 : 297.
Bhatnagar PK, Papas E, Blum HE, Milich DR, Nitecki D,
     Karels MJ, Vyas GN (1982). Immune response to synthetic
     peptide analogues of hepatitis B surface antigen speci-
     fic for the determinant. Proc Natl Acad Sci USA 79 : 4440
Bichko VV, Kozlovskaya TM, Dishler A, Pumpen P, Janulatis A,
     Gren J (1982). Restriction map of the hepatitis B virus
     cloned in Escherichia coli. Gene 20 : 481.
Burrell CJ, Mackay P, Greenaway PJ, Hofschneider PH, Murray
     K (1979). Expression in Escherichia coli of hepatitis
     B virus DNA sequences cloned in plasmid pBR322. Nature
     279 : 43.
Charnay P, Pourcel C, Louise A, Fritsch A, Tiollais P (1979)
     Cloning in Escherichia coli and physical structure of
     hepatitis B virion DNA. Proc Natl Acad Sci USA 76 : 2222.
Charnay P, Mandart E, Hampe A, Fitoussi F, Tiollais P,
     Galibert F (1979). Localization of the viral genome and
     nucleotide sequence of the gene coding for the major
     polypeptide of the hepatitis B surface antigen (HBsAg)
     Nucl Acids Res 7 : 335.

Colman PM, Varghese JN, Laver WC (1983). Structure of the
    catalytic and antigenic sites in influenza virus neura-
    midinase Nature 303 : 41.
Feitelson MA, Marion PS, Robinson WS (1982). Core particles
    of hepatitis B virus and ground squirrel hepatitis
    virus. I. Relationship between hepatitis B core - and
    ground squirrel hepatitis core antigen - associated
    polypeptides by sodium dodecyl sulphate-polyacrylamide
    gel electrophoresis and tryptic peptide mapping. J Virol
    43 : 687.
Galibert F, Mandart E, Fitoussi F, Tiollais P, Charnay P.
    (1979). Nucleotide sequence of the hepatitis B virus
    genome (subtype ayw) cloned in E.coli. Nature 281 : 646.
Gerlich WH, Robinson WS (1980). Hepatitis B virus contains
    protein attached to the 5' terminus of its complete DNA
    strand. Cell 21 : 801.
Kaplan P; Greeman RL, Gerin JL, Purcell RH, Robinson WS
    (1973). DNA polymerase associated with human hepatitis
    B antigen. J Virol 12 : 995.
Kennedy RC, Dreesman GR, Sparrow JT, Cullwell AR, Sanchez Y
    Ionescu-Matio I, Hollinger FB, Melnick JL (1983).
    Inhibition of a common human anti-hepatitis B surface
    antigen by a cyclic synthetic peptide.J Virol 46 : 653.
Kozak M (1981). Possible role of flanking nucleotides in
    recognition of the AUG initiator codon by eukaryotic
    ribosomes. Nucl Acids Res 9 : 5233.
Machida A, Kishimoto S, Ohnuma H, Miyamoto H, Bata K, Oda K,
    Nakamura T, Funatsu G, Miyakawa Y, Mayumi M (1982).
    A glycopeptide containing 15 amino acids residues deri-
    ved from hepatitis B surface antigen particles : demons-
    tration of immunogenicity to raise anti-HBs in mice.
    Mol Immunol 19 : 1087.
Misharo S, Imai I, Takahashi K, Machida A, Gotanda T, Miya-
    kawa Y, Mayumi M (1980). A 49,000 dalton polypeptide
    bearing all the antigenic determinants and full immuno-
    genicity of 22 nm hepatitis B surface antigen particles.
    J Immunol 124 : 1589.
Miyanohara A. Personal communication.
Ono Y, Onda H, Sasada R, Igarashi K, Sugino Y, Nishioka K
    (1983). The complete nucleotide sequence of the cloned
    hepatitis B virus DNA; subtypes adr and adw. Nucl Acids
    Res 11 : 1747.
Pasek M, Goto T, Gilbert W, Zink B, Schaller H, Mackay P,
    Leadbetter G, Murray K (1979). Hepatitis B virus genes
    and their expression in E.coli. Nature 282 : 575.

Peterson DL (1981). Isolation and characterization of the major protein and glyco-protein of hepatitis B surface antigen. J Biol Chem 256 : 6975.

Robinson WS, Marion P, Feitelson M, Siddiqui A (1982). The hepadna virus group : hepatitis B and related viruses. In Viral Hepatitis (Eds Szmuness W, Alter HJ, Maynard JE) Franklin Institute Press, Philadelphia 57-68.

Sattler F, Robinson WS (1979). Hepatitis B viral DNA molecules have cohesive ends. J Virol 32 : 226.

Segrest JP, Feldmann RJ (1974). Membrane proteins : amino acid sequence and membrane penetration. J Mol Biol 87 : 853.

Siddiqui A, Sattler F, Robinson WS (1979). Restriction endonuclease cleavage map and location of unique feature of the DNA of hepatitis B virus, subtype adw_2. Proc Natl Acad Sci USA 76 : 4664.

Sninsky JJ, Siddiqui A, Robinson WS, Cohen SN (1979). Cloning and endonuclease mapping of the hepatitis B viral genome. Nature 279 : 346.

Stibbe W, Gerlich WH (1983). Structural relationship between minor and major proteins of hepatitis B surface antigen. J Virol 46 : 626.

Summers J, O'Connell A, Millman I (1975). Genome of hepatitis B virus : Restriction enzyme cleavage and structure of DNA extracted from Dane particles. Proc Natl Acad Sci USA 72 : 4597.

Summers J, Smolec J, Snyder R.(1978). A virus similar to human hepatitis B virus associated with hepatitis and hepatoma in woodchucks.Proc Natl Acad Sci USA 75 : 4533.

Tiollais P, Charnay P, Vyas G (1981). Biology of hepatitis B virus. Science 213 : 406.

Tisher I, Gelderblom H, Vettermann G, Koch MA (1982). A very small porcine virus with circular single-stranded DNA. Nature 295 : 64.

Valenzuela P, Gray P, Quiroga M, Zaldivar J, Goodman HM, Rutter WJ (1979). Nucleotide sequence of the gene coding for the major protein of hepatitis B virus surface antigen Nature 280 : 815.

Valenzuela P, Quiroga M, Zaldivar J, Gray P, Rutter WJ (1980). The nucleotide sequence of the hepatitis B viral genome and the identification of the major polypeptides. In Animal Viral Genetics (Eds Fields B, Jaenisch R, Fox CF) Academic Press, New York,57.

Wiley DC, Wilson IA, Skehel JJ (1981). Structural identification of the antibody binding sites of Hong-Kong influenza haemagglutinin and their involvement in antigenic variation. Nature 289 : 373.

Viral Hepatitis and Delta Infection, pages 23–28
© 1983 Alan R. Liss, Inc., 150 Fifth Avenue, New York, NY 10011

THE WOODCHUCK ANIMAL MODEL OF HEPATITIS B-LIKE VIRUS
INFECTION AND DISEASE

J.L. Gerin[1], B.C. Tennant[2], A. Ponzetto[3],
R.H. Purcell[4] and F.J. Tyeryar[4].
[1]Georgetown Univ., Rockville, MD, [2]Cornell
Univ., Ithaca, NY, [3]Osp. Molinette, Turin,
Italy and [4]NIAID, NIH, Bethesda, MD.

INTRODUCTION

In 1978, Summers, et al reported the discovery of a
hepatitis B-like virus in the eastern woodchuck (M.
monax). Soon thereafter, naturally-occurring infections
with HBV-like viruses were discovered in the Beechey
ground squirrel (Marion, 1980) and the Pekin duck
(Mason, 1980). Natural infection of these species with
viruses similar to HBV has major research implications
in that these species represent potential models of HBV
infection and disease in man.

HEPATITIS B-LIKE VIRUSES

Hepatitis B virus is the prototype of a unique
group of viruses. The other members of this group are
the woodchuck hepatitis virus (WHV), the ground squirrel
hepatitis virus (GSHV) and the duck hepatitis B virus
(DHBV). These viruses share many structural and
biological properties (Summers, 1981); one common
property of the HBV-like viruses is the capacity to
establish persistent infection in the natural host.
Despite similar virological features of chronic HBV-like
infection in the natural host, the association of
persistent infection with liver disease has not been
consistent (Table 1). Persistent infection in man is
associated with chronic hepatitis and hepatocellular
carcinoma and integration of the HBV genome into host
DNA appears to occur as part of the life cycle of virus
replication. HBV carrier chimpanzees have chronic

hepatitis but HBV DNA integration and hepatocellular carcinoma associated with HBV infection have not been observed. In woodchucks, however, chronic WHV infection is associated with chronic liver disease and hepatocellular carcinoma and WHV genome integration into woodchuck DNA has been detected in both tumor and non-tumor hepatic tissues. In contrast, neither significant liver pathology nor viral integration have been observed in chronic GSHV infection of ground squirrels. While the DHBV/Pekin duck model has yielded important information on vertical transmission and replication strategies of the DHBV, no studies to date have addressed the question of disease association and integrated forms of viral DNA in tissues have not been observed.

It appears, therefore, that WHV infection of woodchucks displays the major features of HBV-associated disease in man and represents the relevant model for the analysis of pathogenic mechanisms.

TABLE 1. MODELS OF HBV-INDUCED DISEASE

HOST	VIRUS	PERSISTENT INFECTION	DISEASE[1] CH	HCC	VIRAL DNA INTEGRATION
Human	HBV	+	+	+	+
Chimpan-zee	HBV	+	+	–	–
Woodchuck	WHV	+	+	+	+
Beechey Ground Squirrel	GSHV	+	–	–	–
Pekin Duck	DHBV	+	?	?	–

---

[1] CH, chronic hepatitis; HCC, hepatocellular carcinoma

THE WHV/WOODCHUCK MODEL

<u>Assays</u>. Successful application of the woodchuck model
requires the availability of sensitive and specific
markers of WHV infection and a great deal of research
has been dedicated to assay development in the early
phases of study. Current solid-phase radioimmunoassays
for WHsAg in our laboratory employ site-specific
monoclonal antibodies to WHsAg as substrates and probes
(Cote, 1983); anti-WHs is measured by double-antibody
precipitation using ^{125}I-WHsAg and rabbit anti-woodchuck
IgG. Serological assays for WHcAg and anti-WHc are
based on standard microtiter methods using anti-WHc
serum to coat wells and ^{125}I-woodchuck IgG as the probe.
Anti-WHc is performed by a blocking radioimmunoassay
using a standard quantity of WHcAg derived from liver
homogenates of WHV-infected animals and titers as high
as 10^6 are noted in some carrier animals. WHV DNA in
serum is determined by a "dot-blot" hybridization assay
using ^{32}P-labeled WHV DNA derived from a recombinant
plasmid as the probe. This probe is also used to detect
the presence and evaluate the state of WHV DNA in
tissues. Frozen liver biopsies are examined by direct
immunofluorescence for WHcAg or WHsAg using
FITC-conjugated IgG and standard methods.

<u>WHV Infection in Natural Populations</u>.

In 1978, the NIAID established an experimental
colony of woodchucks at Meloy laboratories using animals
trapped in central Maryland and southern Delaware. Over
a three year period, 72 woodchucks entering the colony
were analyzed for WHV-specific markers; 22% were chronic
WHV carriers, 40% were either anti-WHs positive or
undergoing self-limited infection and the remainder were
negative for WHV markers. A high prevalence of chronic
WHV infection in natural woodchuck populations from the
central eastern region of the country has also been
observed in other studies. In contrast, no markers of
WHV infection were detected in a large group of feral
woodchucks captured in Tomkins County, NY, although New
York animals were subsequently shown to be fully
susceptible to experimental WHV infection.
Obviously, additional studies are required to
define the patterns of WHV infection in natural
woodchuck populations from different geographic regions.

The data, however, do establish a high prevalence of WHV infection in certain regions of the United States and a high rate of persistent infection similar to that observed in certain human populations.

Three particulate forms of WHsAg circulate in the sera of chronic WHV carrier woodchucks; the major 20 nm form, filaments of varying lengths and virions. As in HBV, the virion core contains within its structure a circular partially double-stranded DNA genome and a DNA polymerase activity. Chronic WHV carriers exhibit all serum and hepatic markers of active viral replication and no equivalent of the asymptomatic human carrier has yet been observed in our studies.

Acute inflammation, chronic active hepatitis and hepatocellular carcinoma (HCC) were observed in chronic WHV carriers and not in recovered or seronegative animals (Popper, 1981). In a more recent summary (Mitamura, 1982), hepatocellular carcinoma was histologically confirmed in 13 of 62 animals from the NIAID colony; 11 of the 13 were long-time carriers and two animals with HCC were recovered from WHV infection. Thus, there appears to be an epidemiologic association between WHV infection and HCC.

In contrast to studies in man integrated forms of WHV DNA were detected in only 2 of 7 carriers with hepatomas. Multiple factors, therefore, may contribute to the process of carcinogenesis in this disease model and further analysis requires studies in a controlled environmental setting. To this end, a woodchuck breeding colony has been established at Cornell University in Ithaca, NY which will provide clean animals for research and further development of this model.

Transmission Studies.

Experimental transmission of WHV to susceptible wild-caught and colony-born woodchucks has established a number of important facts which are summarized below.

1. A standard WHV challenge pool, derived from the serum of a carrier animal, was titrated to end-point. It contains $10^{9.1}$ woodchuck ID_{50}/ml.

2. The pattern of WHV markers in acute and chronic infection is similar to those established for human HBV infection.

3. Woodchucks from the Maryland and New York regions
appear to be equally susceptible to WHV infection and
chronic sequelae.

4. Chronicity as an outcome of experimental infection
occurs in about 15% of woodchucks. No difference in the
incidence of chronic infection was observed between
adult and newborn animals suggesting that early exposure
may not represent a major factor in WHV persistence.

5. Markers of acute WHV infection were temporally
associated with histologic evidence of acute hepatitis,
thereby establishing a direct relationship between WHV
infection and liver disease.

SUMMARY

As a model of virus-induced disease, the
WHV/woodchuck system is at an early stage of
development; yet, much progress has been made and there
now exists considerable evidence that WHV causes serious
liver disease with major parallels to HBV infection of
man. The relatively short interval (4-5 yrs) from
infection to end-stage disease in this model provides
unique opportunities for definition of the natural
history of HBV disease and the evaluation of various
intervention strategies (e.g., vaccine prophylaxis and
anti-viral therapy). Such studies are currently in
progress in a number of laboratories.

REFERENCES

Cote P, Gerin J. (1983). Nonoverlapping antigenic sites
    of woodchuck hepatitis virus surface antigen and
    their cross-reactivity with ground squirrel hepatitis
    virus and hepatitis B virus surface antigen. J Virol
    47:15.
Marion P, Oshiro L, Regnery D, Scullard G, Robinson W.
    (1980). A virus of Beechey ground squirrels that is
    related to hepatitis B virus in humans. Proc Natl
    Acad Sci USA 77:2941.
Mason W, Seal G, Summers J. (1980). Virus of Pekin
    ducks with structural and biological relatedness to
    human hepatitis B virus. J. Virol 36:829.
Mitamura K, Hoyer B, Ponzetto A, Nelson J, Purcell R,
    Gerin J. (1982). Woodchuck hepatitis virus DNA in
    woodchuck liver tissues. Hepatology 2:47S.

Popper H, Shih J, Gerin J, Wong D, Hoyer B, London W, Sly D, Purcell R. (1981). Woodchuck hepatitis and hepatocellular carcinoma: correlation of histologic with virologic observations. Hepatology 1:91.
Summers J, Smolec J, Snyder R. (1978). A virus similar to hepatitis B virus associated with hepatitis and hepatoma in woodchucks. Proc Natl Acad Sci USA 75:4533.
Summers J. (1981). Three recently described animal virus models for human hepatitis B virus. Hepatology 41:179.

Viral Hepatitis and Delta Infection, pages 29–39
© **1983 Alan R. Liss, Inc., 150 Fifth Avenue, New York, NY 10011**

EVIDENCE FOR NON-A, NON-B VIRUSES

Stephen M. Feinstone and Robert H. Purcell

Laboratory of Infectious Diseases, NIAID
National Institutes Health, Bethesda, Md. 20205

Despite extensive world wide efforts, spanning at least 8 years the causative agent of non-A, non-B hepatitis (NANBH) remains unknown. Many approaches have been taken to detect the agent or a related antigen, but most techniques employed have been immunologic and have followed in a general way the methods used to identify hepatitis B and hepatitis A viruses. In addition, several non- immunologic methods for detection of viruses have been used in an attempt to find the NANBH agent. This paper will review and evaluate what has been learned from these studies as well as what has been learned about the nature of the agent itself from animal infectivity experiments.

Table 1 summarizes the catagories of serologic tests that have been applied to the NANBH problem, and the approximate sensitivity of these assays. Agar gel diffusion (AGD) and related immunoprecipition systems such as counterimmuno electrophoresis (CIEP) suffer from very low sensitivity. The chimpanzee infectivity titer of the most infectious inoculum reported in the literature is only 10^6 infectious doses/ml (Feinstone 1981). Even if there were a particle to infectivity ratio of 100:1, an immunodiffusion type assay would probably not be sensitive enough to detect these particles. All other infectious inocula that have been titered are reported to have infectivity titers of 10^3/ml or less. At these titers, the NANBH virus would not be detected by even the most sensitive radioimmunoassays unless there is a large excess of viral antigen present in the plasma as is the case in hepatitis B infections. In addition, both Suh and Hoofnagle have questioned the specificity of the AGD tests for NANBH (Suh 1981, Hoofnagle 1981). None of these tests have performed well on Alter's widely distributed coded panel that included known infectious NANBH plasmas as well as normal and disease controls (Alter 1982).

There have been several reports of nuclear fluorescence in liver biopsies from patients or chimpanzees with NANBH when these biopsies are reacted with certain convalescent sera in direct or indirect immunofluorescence systems (Kabiri 1979, Alberti 1981, Trepo 1981). Immunofluorescence has the advantage of detecting concentrated antigen within a few infected cells and even within certain subcellular areas or organelles such as nuclei. This may lead to high sensitivity, but the exact sensitivity is difficult to estimate in any individual case.

Immunoelectron microscopy (IEM) is a moderately sensitive technique with a lower limit of approximately 10^6 particles/ml. However, this sensitivity can only be achieved if the observer knows the morphology of the particle he is looking for and can distinguish that particle from the myriad of particulate forms that can be observed in biological fluids. IEM has the advantage of very high specificity once a morphologic entity is established because the antigen identity is determined both by reactivity with antibody and by the morphology of the antigen itself. IEM is generally not suitable for detecting soluble antigens. IEM experiments should always be controlled for both antigen and antibody and should always be performed "blind" to eliminate observer bias.

Radioimmunoassays (RIA) and the related enzyme immunoassays (EIA) have generally the highest sensitivity of the immunoassays. However, it is this high sensitivity that causes difficulty because non-specific reactions can often be detected with these assays that were not apparent with techniques of lower sensitivity. For instance, in 1978 we reported an antigen/antibody system based on RIA in which we detected an antigen in the plasma of patients with NANBH (Purcell 1978). This antigen had a close temporal relationship to the disease. However, we were unable to show any specific serologic responses to that antigen and therefore we felt it to be non-specific. Recently Roggendorf in Dr. Deinhardt's laboratory (Roggendorf 1983), and Shiraishi (in preparation) working with Drs. Alter and Purcell have shown that rheumatoid factor-like (RF) reactants frequently occur during NANBH. This may explain many of the false positive RIA results. These NANBH patients often do not have RF activity in their plasma as measured by conventional, less sensitive techniques. Furthermore, it is known that RF can bind to nuclear structures and be detected as nuclear fluorescence under some conditions

(Hannestad 1978). This may explain the common finding of
nuclear fluorescence in NANBH.

Neurath has reported the detection by RIA of a red blood
cell cytoplasmic alloantigen in the plasma of patients with
NANBH as well as other liver diseases (Neurath 1980, 1981).
Antibody to this antigen is found in many transfused patients.
Such an antigen could be confused with an antigen specifically
associated with NANBH.

The main point of this discussion is that immunoassays for
NANBH must be highly sensitive in order to detect the probably
very low level of antigen found in most clinical specimens. In
addition their specificity must be rigorously controlled
because, as some of these tests may very well be the most
sensitive assays available, even for non-specific reactants, it
becomes difficult to assess the presence of non-specificities
by any other less sensitive test. It is hard to imagine that
low sensitivity immunoassays have much value in NANBH, a
disease that is usually associated with a very low titer of
infectious virus in the plasma. It would also seem that both
the RF activity described by Roggendorf and the cytoplasmic
antigen of Neurath should always be excluded when high
sensitivity immunoassays yield seemingly positive results.

While low levels of viral antigen in the plasma may be the
most likely reason that the NANBH agent has not been detected
there are several other possibilities. One that has been
investigated is immune complexes composed of virus and specific
antibody (Dienstag 1979, Ohori 1982). Though immune complexes
may not be detected in an immunoassay designed to detect free
antigen, if these complexes are suspected it should not be a
difficult task to purify the complexes, separate them and
obtain free antigen and possibly specific antibody. Such
investigations have not, to my knowledge, yielded positive
results. It is also possible that while there may be virus or
viral antigen present in plasma, there may be no antibody
response or at least not antibody directed against a surface
component of the virus. NANBH is very commonly a chronic
infection and may possibly be chronic in all patients who are
infected. If, as in chronic hepatitis B virus infections,
there is no antibody produced to surface antigen, the virus
would not be detectable using an immunoassay. Very low levels
of antibody or antibody of low avidity may also be factors in
the failure to detect NANBH by immunoassays.

Table 1

Sensitivity of Immunoassays for Antigen and Antibody

Assay	Mass of Antigen	Number of Particles	Antibody
1) Agar Gel Diffusion	1000 pg	10^8	Low
2) Counter immuno-electrophoresis	50 pg	10^7	Low
3) Immunofluorescence	?	?	Moderate
4) Immunoelectron microscopy	particles only	10^6	Moderate
5) Radioimmunoassay and enzyme immunoassay	1 pg	10^5	High

Most viral infections do produce an immune response of some type and many chronic viral infections or latent, recurrent viral infections result in the production of very large quantities of antibody. Possibly analogous to the NANBH situation are the spongiform encephalopathies that include scrapie disease of sheep, transmissible encephalopathy of mink and kuru and Creutzfeld-Jacob disease of man (Gajdusek 1977). After extensive investigation there has been no antigen/antibody system defined for these chronic, progressive and fatal diseases that all seem to be caused by similar agents termed unconventional viruses. Because there is essentially no inflammation in these diseases, it is thought that there truly is no immune response. Although this analogy should not be overdrawn we should at least consider the possibility that NANBH is caused by an unconventional agent and may require unconventional methods to detect it. It is somewhat discouraging to note that the agents of these spongiform encephalopathies have not been identified after more than 20 years of searching.

Data exists that might indicate what sort of agent does cause NANBH. There are several infectivity experiments that weigh against NANBH being caused by an agent resembling kuru or scrapie. Published reports indicate that NANBH can be inactivated by heating to 60°C for 10 hrs or 100°C for 5 minutes (Yoshizawa 1982). Scrapie is very resistant to heat and it can only be reliably inactivated in the autoclave. Formalin at a dilution of 1:2000 has been shown to inactivate NANBH in 72 hrs at 37°C (Tabor 1980, Yoshizawa 1982) while scrapie resists inactivation in brain tissue fixed in 3.7% formaldehyde. We have shown that a plasma dilution that contained at least 10^4 chimpanzee infectious doses was completely inactivated by extraction with 10% chloroform (Feinstone 1983) Scrapie is generally not affected by lipid solvents. These inactivation experiments suggest that NANBH is caused by a conventional agent that probably contains lipid in an outer membrane. Prince reported that NANBH infectivity was filterable through a 220 nm filter (Prince 1978). However, the size of the agent remains unknown. Bradley has evidence that NANBH has a sedimentation coeficient greater than 200 S (Bradley, personal communication), but Shih believes it is smaller than 50S (Shih 1982). There have been numerous reports on the detection of particles by electron microscopy. These particles range in size and morphology from simple particles of 22mm, 25mm, 27mm and 35mm diameters to complex particles of a variety of sizes and shapes. None of these particles has been specifically associated with the causative agent of NANBH and many of these morphologic forms can be seen in normal plasma.

Table 2

Comparison of the NANBH Agent to Unconventional Viruses

	NANBH	Unconventional Viruses
Formalin	Sensitive	Resistant
Chloroform (10%)	Sensitive	Resistant
Heat (60°C, 10 hrs)	Sensitive	Resistant
Filtration 220 nm	Passed	Passed
Antigen/Antibody	No	No
Virus Particle	No	No
Chronic Infections	Yes	Yes
Inflammatory Response	Mild	No

One of the most interesting possibilities that has been suggested in the literature is that the agent of NANBH is a hepadnavirus, in reality a second type of human HBV resembling HBV as the woodchuck or ground squirrel hepatitis viruses resemble HBV. In fact there are enough clinical and epidemiological similarities between HBV and NANBH infections that make this possibility worthy of attention. Trepo and coworkers have reported a serologic cross reactivity between HBV and the NANBH agent at the levels of the core antigen and the e antigen. He also has found particles in the plasma of

NANBH patients that resemble all the morphologic forms associated with HBV infections. He has detected DNA polymerase activity in some of these plasmas (Trepo 1982) and, in collaboration with Charnay and colleagues of the Pasteur Institute, DNA hybridizable to cloned HBV DNA was detected in an integrated form in one liver and free in a second liver from patients with NANBH (Charnay 1982). These patients had no serologic or hepatic markers of HBV infection. Wands and colleagues also report there is a relationship between the NANBH agent and HBV (Wands 1982). Using an IgM monoclonal antibody produced against HBsAg they claim to detect NANBH cases and have found DNA in plasma from some chimpanzees that hybridized with cloned HBV DNA. In addition there is evidence from several studies of post transfusion hepatitis that donor blood positive for anti-HBc is approximately three times more likely to transmit NANBH than anti-HBc negative blood (Stevens 1981, Cossart 1982). Does this mean that these donors carry NANBH and the anti-HBc is really an anti-NANBH core that cross reacts in the anti- HBc test? Or does this mean that HBV and NANBH are simply epidemiologic fellow travelers?

I feel the shared epidemiology explanation is more likely the case. In the major post-transfusion hepatitis studies such as the Transfusion Transmitted Virus Study (TTVS) (Aach 1978), and those carried out by Dr. Alter at the NIH Clinical Center (Alter 1978), more than 90% of transfusion-associated hepatitis was NANBH and none of these patients developed anti-HBc. If they had, they would have been diagnosed as hepatitis B. The chimpanzees that have been infected with NANBH in our laboratory and in other laboratories have not developed anti-HBc. Prince also in collaboration with Tiollais' laboratory at the Pasteur Institute , could not find DNA homologous to HBV DNA in liver from chimpanzees with acute NANBH (Prince 1982). In addition, Fields and colleagues at the CDC have not found DNA hybridizable to HBV DNA nor have they detected DNA polymerase activity in the plasma from chimpanzees with NANBH (Fields 1983). Dr. Gerin has carefully studied concentrates of acute phase NANBH plasma including several of known infectious plasma. He could detect no DNA polymerase activity like that found in HBV plasma (Gerin, unpublished).

Several years ago in an attempt to detect a unique nucleic acid species in NANBH plasma we did find large quantities of host DNA (Feinstone, unpublished). This DNA is detectable in normal as well as hepatitis B plasma but it was present in very large quantities in plasma from several patients with NANBH.

It is possible that under conditions of low stringency or with
cloned HBV DNA probes contaminated with bacterial or plasmid
DNA, nucleic acid hybridization with this host DNA can occur.
Such studies must be rigidly controlled and probes carefully
prepared to prevent such false positive reactions.

Table 3
Reported Relationships Between NANBH and HBV

Serology	Test Methods	Investigator
HBsAg	RIA	Wands
HBcAg	IF, AGD	Trepo, Alberti
HBeAg	AGD	Trepo
Biochemistry		
DNA homology	Blot hybridization	Charnay, Wands
DNA polymerase	HBV DNA Polymerase	Trepo
Morphology		
HBsAg	Electron microscopy	Hantz, Trepo
Dane particles	Electron microscopy	Hantz, Trepo

The final consideration and perhaps the most interesting
possibility to be considered at this symposium is the
relationship between the NANBH agent and the delta agent.
Delta is in truth an NANBH agent, but the question remains if
it is in any way related to the agent that causes "classical"
NANBH. Rizzetto has found no serologic relationship between
Delta and NANBH (personal communication). Since the Delta
agent is felt to be defective with a very small genome and
requiring HBV as a helper (Rizetto 1981), it is somewhat
difficult to imagine how a non-defective, self-replicating form
of the same or a similar agent could exist without the presence
of a similar antigen/antibody system. It is quite possible
however, that this defective form (the Delta agent) has a
replication advantage over the non-defective NANBH virus. It
is known that the Delta infectivity may be present in very high
titers ($>10^{10}$) in the plasma and the Delta antigen may also
exist in extremely large quantities both in the plasma and
liver. If the problem in detecting NANBH is only one of
sensitivity due to very low titers of NANBH in the plasma then
there may be antigenic similarities to Delta that cannot now be
revealed.

As discussed above, it is thought that HBV and NANBH virus
are often epidemiologic fellow travelers. One can imagine then
how a defective NANBH virus may have arisen in a patient who
was coinfected with HBV, and this HBV replication provided the

necessary helper functions for the replication of the defective
NANBH virus.

While this scenario may seem far fetched there is some
direct evidence linking NANBH with Delta that will be covered
in detail in other papers in this symposium. Briefly, when
NANBH superinfects an HBV carrier patient or chimpanzee a
series of events occur which closely resemble those events when
Delta superinfects and HBV carrier. There is a general,
temporary supression of the HBV replication as determined by
the quantity of HBcAg in the liver and HBV DNA in the plasma.
At about the same time there is usually an exacerbation of the
clinical hepatitis. In chimpanzees the hepatitis that occurs
in HBV carrier chimpanzees that have normal ALT levels prior to
NANBH inoculation is usually more severe than the hepatitis
that occurs following the same NANBH inoculum in a chimpanzee
without a pre-existing chronic HBV infection.

Finally there are similar histopathologic lesions produced
by infection with the NANBH agent and the Delta agent which are
detectable at both the light and electron microscopic levels.
Canese and her colleagues in Italy and Kamimura and Dienes
working in Dr. Purcell's laboratory have both identified the
typical NANBH cytoplasmic tubular structures in chimpanzees
infected with the Delta agent.

The Delta/NANBH relationship should be a testable
hypothesis as soon as cDNA probes prepared from the Delta RNA
become available.

In summary the nature of the NANBH agent remains a
mystery. The failure of serologic tests to detect the agent
may be only a problem of sensitivity but other problems must
also be considered. Inactivation and physical characterization
experiments seem to indicate that NANBH is caused by some type
of relatively conventional virus. The relatedness of this
virus to hepatitis B virus seems unlikely. The possible
relationship to the Delta agent is intriguing but has not yet
been directly substantiated.

REFERENCES

Aach RD, Lander JJ, Sherman LA et al. (1978). Transfusion-
    transmitted viruses: interim analysis of hepatitis among
    transfused and nontransfused patients. In Vyas GN, Cohen SN,

Schmid R (eds): "Viral Hepatitis", Philadelphia: Franklin Institute Press, p. 383.

Alberti A, Realdi G, Bortolotti F, Cadrobbi P, Barbieri R, Tremolada F, Ongaro G (1981). Detection by immunofluorescence of an antigen-antibody system in patients with acute and chronic non-A, non-B hepatitis. Liver 1:183.

Alter HJ, Purcell RH, Feinstone SM, Holland PV, Morrow AG (1978). A review and interim report of an ongoing prospective study. In Vyas GN, Cohen SN, Schmid R (eds): "Viral Hepatitis", Philadelphia: Franklin Institute Press, p. 359.

Alter HJ, Purcell RH, Feinstone SM, Tegtmeier GE (1982). Non-A, non-B hepatitis: prologue, progress and prospects. In Szmuness W (ed): "Proceedings of the 1981 Internatinal Symposium on Viral Hepatitis", Philadelphia: Franklin Institute Press, p. 279.

Charnay P, Brechot C, Vitvitski L, Trepo C, Tiollais P (1982). Analysis by hybridization with HBV DNA of hepatocellular DNA from patients with chronic non-A, non-B hepatitis. In Szmuness W, Alter HJ, Maynard JE (eds): "Viral Hepatitis -- 1981 Symposium", Philadelphia: Franklin Institute Press p. 656 (abstract).

Cossart YE, Kirsch S., Ismay SL (1982). Postransfusion hepatitis in Australia. Lancet 1:208.

Dienstag JL, Bahn AK, Alter HJ et al. (1979). Circulating immune complexes in non-A, non-B hepatitis. Lancet 1:1265.

Feinstone SM, Alter HJ, Dienes HP, Shimizu Y, Popper H, Blackmore D, Sly D, London, WT, Purcell RH (1981). Non-A, non-B hepatitis in chimpanzees and marmosets. J Infect Dis 144:588.

Feinstone SM, Mihalik, KB, Kamimura T, Alter HJ, London WT, Purcell RH (1983). Infect Immun: in press.

Fields HA, Berninger M, Nath N, Davis CL, Hammer M, Margolis HS, McCaustland KA, Wheeler CM, Maynard JE, Bradley DW (1983). Unrelatedness of factor VIII-derived non-A/non-B hepatitis and hepatitis B virus. J Med Virol 11:59.

Gajdusek CK (1977). Unconventional viruses and the origin and disappearance of kuru. Science 197:943.

Hannestad K, Stollar BD (1978). Certain rheumatoid factors react with nucleosomes. Nature 275:671.

Hantz O, Vitvitski L, Trepo C (1980). Non-A, non-B hepatitis: idenLification of hepatitis-B-like virus particles in serum and liver. J Med Virol 5:73.

Hoofnagle JH (1981). Precipitin system detected in sera from patients with non-A, non-B hepatitis. J Med Virol 7:315.

Kabiri M, Tabor E, Gerety RJ (1979). Antigen-antibody system associated with non-A, non-B hepatitis detected by indirect immunofluorescence. Lancet ii:221.

Neurath AR, Stevens CE, Strick N, Szmuness W, Oleszko WR, Harley EJ (1980). An antigen detected frequently in human sera with elevated levels of alanine aminotransferase: a potential marker for non-A, non-B hepatitis. J Gen Virol 48:285.

Neurath AR, Strick N, Rowe AW, Rubinstein P, Fotino M (1981). Discovery of a cytoplasmic-dominant alloantigen prevalent in erythrocytes. Vox Sang 41:201.

Ohori H, Nagatsuka Y, Yamada E, Akiba T, Shirachi R, Shiraishi H, Ishida N (1982). Characterization of immune complexes in sera from patients with non-A, non-B hepatitis. In Szmuness W, Alter HJ, Maynard JE (eds): "Viral Hepatitis -- 1981 International Symposium," Philadelphia: Franklin Institute Press, p. 331.

Prince AM, Brechot C, Charney P, Brotman B, Richardson L, Tiollais P (1982). Absence of detectable HBV-like DNA sequences in chimpanzee liver infected with non-A, non-B hepatitis virus(es): a preliminary report. In Szmuness W, Alter HJ, Maynard JE (eds): "Viral Hepatitis -- 1981 International Symposium", Philadelphia: Franklin Instute Press, p. 657 (abstract).

Prince AM, Brotman B, Van Den Ende MC, Richardson L, Kellner A (1978). Non-A, non-B hepatitis: identification of a virus specific antigen and antibody. A preliminary report. In "Viral Hepatitis", Philadelphia: Franklin Institute Press, p. 419.

Purcell, RH, Feinstone, SM, Alter HJ, Wong DC (1978). Detection of a novel antigen in two cases of non-A, non-B hepatitis, a recently recognized persistent infection of probable viral origin. In Stevens JC, Todaro GJ, Fox CF (eds): "Persistent Viruses", Long-New York: Academic Press, p. 535.

Rizzetto M, Gerin JL, Purcell RH (1981). Delta antigen: evidence for a variant of hepatitis B virus or a non-A, non-B hepatitis agent? In Pollard M (ed): "Perspectives in Virology XI", New York: Alan R. Liss, p. 195.

Roggendorf M, Deinhardt F (1983). Demonstration of a rheumatoid factor like reaction in the acute phase of hepatitis non-A, non-B. In Deinhardt F (ed): "Second International Symposium on Viral Hepatitis", New York: Marcel Dekker, in press.

Shih, JW-K, Tabor E, Gerety RJ (1982). Sedimentation of a non-A, non-B hepatitis agent. Hepatitis Scientific Memorandum 8:35.

Stevens CE and Transfusion-Transmitted Viruses Study Group

(1981). Antibody to hepatitis B core antigen in donor blood and risks of non-A, non-B hepatitis in recipients. Transfusion 21:607.

Suh DH, White Y, Eddleston ALWF, Amini S, Tsiquaye K, Zuckerman AJ, Williams R (1981). Specificity of an immunoprecipitin test for non-A, non-B hepatitis. Lancet i:178.

Tabor E, Gerety RJ (1980). Inactivation of an agent of human non-A, non-B hepatitis by formalin. J Infect Dis 142:767.

Trepo C, Vitvitski L, Hantz O, Chevallier P, Lehman H, Schlaak M, Sepetjan M (1981). Detection by immunofluorescence of a new "core-like" Ag/Ab system in liver and serum of patients with NANB hepatitis. Liver 1:191.

Trepo C, Vitvitski L, Hantz O, Pichoud C, Blanchy B, Chevallier P, Trepo D, Babin S, Sepetjan M (1982). Characterization and detection of a virus related to HBV in NANB hepatitis. Philadelphia: Franklin Institute Press, p. 339.

Wands JR, Lieberman HM, Muchmore E, Isselbacher K, Shafritz DA (1982). Detection and transmission in chimpanzees of hepatitis B virus-related agents formerly designated "non-A, non-B hepatitis. Proc Natl Acad Sci USA 79:7552.

Yoshizawa H, Itoh Y, Iwakiri S, Kitajima K, Tanaka A, Tachibana T, Nakamura T, Miyakawa Y, Mayumi M (1982). Non-A, non-B (Type 1) hepatitis agent capable of inducing tubular ultrastructures in the hepatocyte cytoplasm of chimpanzees: inactivation by formalin and heat. Gastroenterology 82:502.

Viral Hepatitis and Delta Infection, pages 41–53
© **1983 Alan R. Liss, Inc., 150 Fifth Avenue, New York, NY 10011**

CHRONIC TYPE B HEPATITIS: CLINICAL COURSE

Jay H. Hoofnagle, M.D.
Gary L. Davis, M.D.
Reginald G. Hanson, M.B., F.R.A.C.P.
Liver Diseases Section, NIADDK, N.I.H.
Bethesda, Maryland   20205

INTRODUCTION

Chronic type B hepatitis is a major cause of chronic
liver disease and cirrhosis in the world and may be the
single most important cause of liver cell cancer. The
availability of serological assays for detecting the
hepatitis B virus and its antigens in serum has aided in
the understanding of the pathogenesis of this liver disease
and is beginning to clarify the natural history and
progression of chronic type B hepatitis (Hoofnagle et al.,
1981; Liaw et al., 1983; Norkrans et al., 1980; Realdi et
al., 1980; Viola et al., 1981).

PATIENTS AND METHODS

In the last five years, 140 patients with chronic type
B hepatitis have been seen and evaluated by the Liver
Diseases Section of the National Institutes of Health.
These patients were referred to this research institution
for possible antiviral or immunomodulating therapy for this
disease (Hoofnagle et al., 1983; Scullard et al., 1981).
This population has formed the basis of a long-term study
of the clinical, biochemical, histological and serological
course of this disease.

Patients were initially evaluated in the outpatient
clinic. They underwent a complete medical history and
physical examination. Serum laboratory tests were obtained
which included bilirubin, alanine aminotransferase (ALT,

SGPT), aspartate aminotransferase (AST, SGOT), alkaline phosphatase, lactic dehydrogenase (LDH), albumin, globulin, prothrombin time, complete blood count, immunoglobulins (IgG, IgA, IgM), rheumatoid factor and alpha-fetoprotein. Hepatitis B virus (HBV) serological testing included hepatitis B surface antigen (HBsAg) and antibody (anti-HBs) by radioimmunoassay, hepatitis B e antigen (HBeAg) and antibody (anti-HBe) by immunodiffusion and radio-immunoassay, HBV-DNA by molecular hybridization (Berninger et al., 1982) and DNA polymerase by measurement of tritiated thymidine incorporation after purification and disruption of Dane particles (Kaplan et al., 1973). Thereafter, patients were followed in the outpatient clinic at 1-3 month intervals. On each occasion, serum was obtained for routine biochemical liver tests (bilirubin, ALT, AST) as well as hepatitis B virus serology (HBsAg, anti-HBs, HBeAg, anti-HBe and DNA polymerase). Selected samples were tested for HBV-DNA, antibody to the HBV associated delta agent (anti-delta) by radioimmunoassay (courtesy of Dr. Antonio Ponzetto) (Rizzetto et al., 1980), IgM antibody to hepatitis A virus (anti-HAV) by radioimmunoassay (Decker et al., 1981) and antibody to hepatitis B core antigen (anti-HBc) by radioimmunoassay. Liver biopsy was not performed unless the patient entered a research protocol or was considered for corticosteroid therapy. Groups were compared using Chi square test; group means were compared using Student's t test.

Among the total of 140 patients evaluated during the past 5 years, 50 were excluded from this analysis. The reasons for exclusion were as follows: normal serum amino-transferase levels (6 patients), age below 21 years (5 patients), delta hepatitis (2 patients) and less than a complete year of follow-up evaluation (37 patients). The remaining 90 adult patients with chronic type B hepatitis who have been followed with frequent determinations of serum biochemical laboratory tests and hepatitis B virus serology and form the basis of this report.

RESULTS: INITIAL EVALUATION

DEMOGRAGPHIC FEATURES of the 90 patients in this analysis are shown in Table 1. Most patients were white men between the ages of 25-50 years. All patients were known to have chronic type B hepatitis of at least six

months and as long as thirteen years duration. Follow-up
at the National Institutes of Health ranged between one and
nine (2.4) years.

TABLE 1

DEMOGRAPHY OF PATIENTS WITH CHRONIC TYPE B HEPATITIS

FEATURE		NUMBER (PERCENT) OR MEAN AND RANGE
SEX	MALES	84 (93%)
	FEMALES	6 (7%)
AGE	MEAN	37 YRS
	RANGE	21-66 YRS
RACE	WHITE	79 (88%)
	ORIENTAL	6 (7%)
	BLACK	4 (5%)
	HISPANIC	1 (1%)
DURATION OF DISEASE	MEAN	5.1 YRS
	RANGE	0.5-13.5 YRS
DURATION OF FOLLOW-UP	MEAN	2.4 YRS
	RANGE	1-9 YRS

THE **SUSPECTED SOURCE OF INFECTION** in these 90 patients
is shown in Table 2. The majority of patients were
homosexual or bisexual men. Heterosexual contact was
presumed to be the source of infection in 13% of patients.
Occupational exposure in a medical or dental profession was
implicated in 6% of patients. Intrafamilial spread of
disease was known to account for 4% of cases and was
probably the origin of several cases classified as source
unknown. There was only one patient in this group of 90
who was an intravenous drug addict. This distribution of
patients reflects the type of person who is referred to a
research institution for evaluation. The patient
population was comprised largely of educated,
well-motivated and concerned individuals. The absence of a
large number of drug addicts and hemophiliac patients
probably accounts for the rarity of delta infection
(Rizzetto et al., 1979).

TABLE 2

SOURCE OF INFECTION IN 90 PATIENTS

SOURCE	NUMBER	(PERCENT)
HOMOSEXUAL CONTACT	51	(57%)
HETEROSEXUAL CONTACT	12	(13%)
MEDICAL OCCUPATION	5	(6%)
INTRAFAMILIAL SPREAD	4	(4%)
TRANSFUSION	3	(3%)
DRUG ABUSE	1	(1%)
UNKNOWN	14	(16%)

SYMPTOMS of chronic hepatitis were present in two-thirds of the patients in this study (Table 3). However, symptoms were usually mild and consisted largely of malaise or easy fatiguability. Twenty-three percent of patients complained of intermittent nausea and right upper quadrant pain in addition to chronic fatigue. Some described poor appetite and weight loss. In 9% of patients the major symptom was arthralgias. One patient had Raynaud's phenomenon. In follow-up, many of these symptoms improved or disappeared. Whether this reflected a natural tendency for symptoms in this disease to ameliorate with time or whether this merely reflected a more optimistic outlook on the part of the patient is difficult to assess. In paticular, the symptom of arthralgias was likely to disappear with time. All except one patient with arthralgias are currently asymptomatic of this complaint. The single case that remains symptomatic has clnical and serological evidence of Reiter's syndrome.

TABLE 3

SYMPTOMS IN 90 PATIENTS WITH CHRONIC TYPE B HEPATITIS

SYMPTOMS	NUMBER	(PERCENT)
MALAISE (FATIGUE) ONLY	30	(33%)
MALAISE, NAUSEA, PAIN	21	(23%)
ARTHRALGIAS	8	(9%)
NO SYMPTOMS	31	(35%)

PHYSICAL FINDINGS of chronic liver disease were
often minimal or absent in this group of patients. Only
18% had significant hepatomegaly and 23% splenomegaly. In
all cases the degree of hepatosplenomegaly was mild. Three
patients had clinically apparent muscle wasting and only
one had ascites. Spider nevi were present on 37% of
patients and palmar erythema was detected in 14%.
Gynecomastia, parotid enlargement and testicular atrophy
were rare. Ignoring the presence of occasional spider
nevi, 61 patients (68%) had an essentially normal physical
examination.

TABLE 4

PHYSICAL FINDINGS IN 90 PATIENTS

SIGN	NUMBER	(PERCENT)
HEPATOMEGALY	16	(18%)
SPLENOMEGALY	21	(23%)
ASCITES	1	(1%)
SPIDER NEVI	33	(37%)
PALMAR ERYTHEMA	13	(14%)
NO ABNORMALITIES	61	(68%)

Results of initial **SERUM BIOCHEMICAL TESTING** are
shown in Table 5. All patients had raised serum
aminotransferase levels. In every case the ALT was higher
than the AST. The average ratio of ALT/AST was 2:1. The
mean serum bilirubin was 0.9 mg/dl (range 0.4-3.9) and was
increased above 2.0 mg/dl in only five patients. The serum
albumin level averaged 4.1 gm/dl (range 2.5-4.9 and was
below 3.5 gm/dl in only 7 patients (8%). The patients with
abnormal serum bilirubin, alkaline phosphatase, LDH or
albumin usually had cirrhosis or had the onset of their
hepatitis within the preceding one year. Serum
immunoglobulins were raised in 25 patients (24 had raised
IgG and 5 raised IgM). In two cases (both of whom had
cirrhosis), immunoglobulins were greater than twice
elevated.

TABLE 5

LABORATORY VALUES IN 90 PATIENTS

LABORATORY TEST	PERCENT ABNORMAL	MEAN (RANGE)
ALT (u/l)	100%	246 (45-1370)
AST (u/l	95%	126 (20-1050)
Alkaline Phosphatase (u/l)	18%	93 (36-443)
LDH (u/l)	13%	207 (102-395)
Bilirubin (mg/dl)	6%	0.9 (0.4-3.9)
Albumin (gm/dl)	8%	4.1 (2.5-4.9)
IgG (mg/dl)	27%	1611 (590-3280)
IgM (mg/dl)	6%	160 (47-660)
Prothrombin time (sec)	10%	12.2 (10.1-16.2)

Results of **SEROLOGICAL TESTING** are shown in
Table 6. The HBsAg subtype was found to be adw in 89%,
ayw in 3% and adr in 8% of patients. All of the male
homosexual patients were adw and all Oriental patients
were adr subtype. The medical and transfusion related
cases were of the adw subtype. HBeAg was detected in 85
patients and anti-HBe in the remainder. HBV-DNA was
detectable in 84 and DNA polymerase activity in 83 of the
HBeAg positive specimens. In contrast, HBV-DNA was
detectable in only two and DNA polymerase in one of the
initial sera from the 5 anti-HBe positive patients.
These five patients have all become and remained

TABLE 6

HBV SEROLOGY IN 90 PATIENTS WITH CHRONIC TYPE B HEPATITIS

SEROLOGICAL TEST		NUMBER	(PERCENT)
HBsAg SUBTYPE:	adw	80	(89%)
	ayw	3	(3%)
	adr	7	(8%)
HBeAg		85	(94%)
Anti-HBe		5	(6%)
HBV-DNA		86	(96%)
DNA Polymerase		84	(93%)
Anti-HBs		33	(37%)

seronegative for both HBV-DNA and polymerase activity in
subsequent follow-up. Anti-HBs activity was present in
33 serum samples, but was invariably heterotypic - it was
directed against HBsAg of a different subtype (e.g.
anti-y in an HBsAg/adw serum) - and was usually present
in low titer.

Liver biopsy histopathology was available on 78
patients. Histological interpretations were made using
conventional criteria (International Group, 1977).
Twenty-seven (35%) biopsies revealed chronic persistent
hepatitis, 32 (41%) chronic active hepatitis and 19 (24%)
cirrhosis.

RESULTS: FOLLOW-UP EVALUATION

These 90 patients have now been followed for 1-9
years. Two of the 90 patients have died, both with
complications of cirrhosis and portal hypertension. Both
of these patients were older men (ages 55 and 60 years)
who were known to have cirrhosis and who had persistently
elevated serum aminotransferase levels and serological
markers of active viral replication (HBeAg and DNA
polymerase activity) up until the time of death.

On the other side of the spectrum, three patients
have become seronegative for HBsAg and concurrently had a
complete remission in disease. The disappearance of
HBsAg occurred 1, 3 and 4 years after the known onset of
illness. These three patients were males, aged 34, 35
and 62 years. Liver biopsy histopathology, obtained
before the loss of HBsAg revealed chronic persistent
hepatitis in two and chronic active hepatitis with
fibrosis in the third. All three are now asymptomatic,
have normal serum aminotransferase levels and are
seropositive for anti-HBs.

In the remaining 85 patients, the clinical course
and outcome of patients correlated with changes in
hepatitis B virus serological markers, particularly serum
levels of HBeAg, HBV-DNA and DNA polymerase activity.
For analysis, patients were categorized into three
groups: (1) those who remained persistently seropositive
for HBeAg; (2) those who became and subsequently remained
seronegative for HBeAg, HBV-DNA and DNA polymerase and

seroconverted to anti-HBe; (3) those who became
seronegative for HBeAg, HBV-DNA and DNA polymerase but
who subsequently redeveloped these serological markers of
hepatitis B virus replication (reactivation of chronic
type B hepatitis). A comparison of the subsequent course
of these three groups is shown in Table 7.

TABLE 7

COURSE OF CHRONIC TYPE B HEPATITIS IN 3 PATIENT GROUPS

FEATURE	PERSISTENT HBeAg	SEROCONVERSION TO ANTI-HBe	REACTIVATION
(No. Pts.)	(53)	(21)	(11)
SYMPTOMS (%)			
INITIALLY	78%	75%	88%
AT FOLLOW-UP	36%	5%*	88%
MEAN ALT (u/l)			
INITIALLY	195	412	222
AT FOLLOW-UP	179	46*	221
MEAN AST (u/l)			
INITIALLY	87	236	112
AT FOLLOW-UP	84	28*	144
MORTALITY (%)	2%	0%	9%

*$p < 0.01$

    Fifty-three (62%) of the 85 HBeAg positive patients
have remained persistently HBeAg positive during the
period of follow-up evaluation. Many of the patients in
this group have become asymptomatic; however, serum
aminotransferase levels have remained consistently
elevated. One patient in this group has died.

    Twenty-one patients (25%) have seroconverted from
HBeAg to anti-HBe. Serum HBV-DNA and DNA polymerase
activity invariably disappeared shortly before (1-8
months) or at the time of loss of HBeAg from serum.
Serum enzymes were often markedly elevated immediately
preceding this seroconversion (Liaw et al., 1983) (Table
7). Subsequent to this seroconversion these patients
uniformly demonstrated a remission in chronic hepatitis

disease activity concurrently with or shortly after the time of loss of HBeAg from serum. Most became asymptomatic and 71% of them now have normal serum enzymes. Thus, the seroconversion from HBeAg to anti-HBe with loss of serum markers of hepatitis B virus replication was associated with a good prognosis.

Eleven other patients (13%) seroconverted from HBeAg to anti-HBe and became seronegative for HBV-DNA and DNA polymerase but subsequently redeveloped one or more of these serum markers of hepatitis B virus replication. This serological pattern has been termed "reactivation" of chronic type B hepatitis (Davis et al., 1983). Patients in this group generally underwent a temporary clinical and biochemical remission in disease activity at the time of seroconversion from HBeAg to anti-HBe. In follow-up, however, there was an abrupt increase in serum aminotransferase levels which was accompanied by a return of serum HBV-DNA, DNA polymerase activity and, in ten cases, HBeAg. The clinical and serological course of one patient is shown in the figure. Episodes of reactivation were often severe; all but one patient became symptomatic, four patients developed either esophageal variceal bleeding or ascites and one patient died during an episode of reactivation. Reactivation invariably occurred within one year of the loss of HBeAg and lasted from 3-13 months. One patient has had three separate episodes of reactivation. Thus, a pattern of reactivation was associated with a poor prognosis and the development of progressive liver disease.

The cause of the reactivation in these 11 patients is not clear. Seven have received corticosteroids or antiviral agents in the past but none were being treated with these agents at the time of the reactivation. No other etiologic factor appeared to be associated with these episodes. None of these patients developed IgM anti-HAV or anti-delta antibody. All 11 patients were of the subtype adw and this subtype reactivity did not change with the return of active viral replication. Neither a superimposed hepatic injury nor reinfection appeared to be the cause of these episodes.

Comparison of patients who remained HBeAg positive with patients who seroconverted and those who suffered from an episode of reactivation is shown in Table 8.

FIGURE

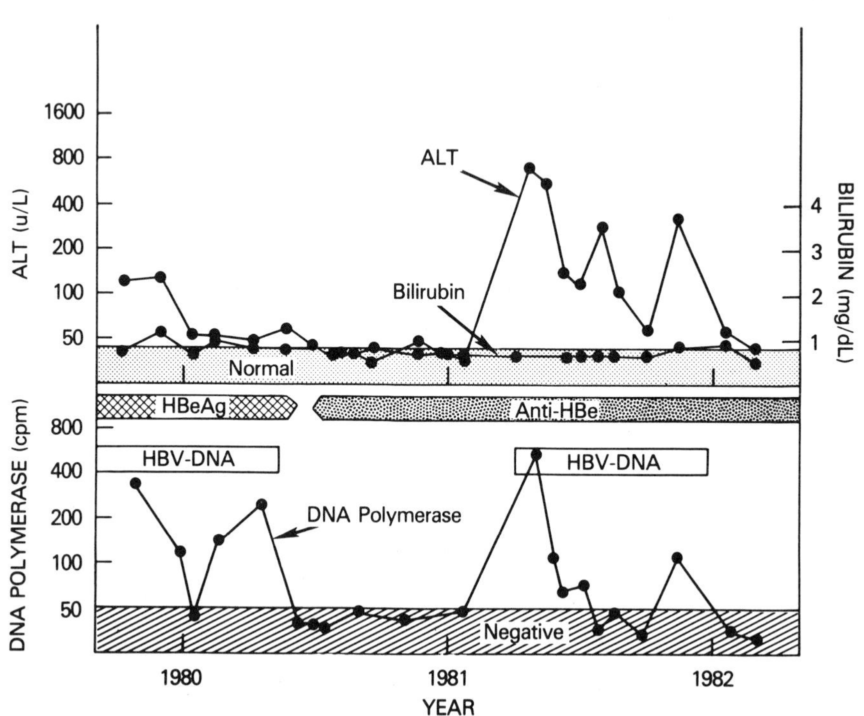

Clinical and serological course of a patient with chronic type B hepatitis and cirrhosis who underwent an episode of reactivation. In 1980 he became HBeAg, HBV-DNA and DNA polymerase negative and seroconverted from HBeAg to anti-HBe. Serum alanine aminotransferase (ALT) levels fell into the normal range. In early 1981 there was a sudden and marked increase in serum ALT levels associated with a return of serum HBV-DNA and DNA polymerase. This episode of reactivation lasted for 9 months.

Patients who underwent reactivation were older, had a
longer duration of chronic hepatitis and were more likely
to have cirrhosis. Similar numbers in all three groups
had previously received corticosteroid and/or antiviral
therapy.

TABLE 8

COMPARISON OF THREE GROUPS OF PATIENTS

FEATURE	PERSISTENT HBeAg	SEROCONVERSION TO ANTI-HBe	REACTIVATION
No Pts.	(53)	(21)	(11)
AGE			
MEAN (YRS)	37	34	44*
RANGE (YRS)	(22-66)	(21-61)	(30-65)
SEX (% MALE)	92%	91%	100%
DURATION OF			
DISEASE (YRS)	4.5	5.4	7.2*
MEAN (RANGE)	(1.5-13)	(2-13)	(3.6-11.5)
CIRRHOSIS			
(% WITH)	9%	28%	60%*
PREVIOUS THERAPY:			
CORTICOSTEROIDS	19%	38%	65%
ANTI-VIRAL AGENTS	40%	19%	27%
NEITHER**	41%	48%	36%

*Percentages add up to more than 100% because some
patients received both treatments.
*$p < 0.01$.

DISCUSSION

    These data demonstrate the spectrum of chronic type
B hepatitis. In the United States, chronic type B
hepatitis is largely a disease of young men. The disease
is often asymptomatic. If symptoms are present, they are
usually mild and tend to ameliorate with time. Testing
for hepatitis B virus serological markers demonstrates a
close association between active liver disease and the
presence of serum markers of active viral replication
such as HBV-DNA, DNA polymerase and HBeAg. The
persistence of these markers is associated with
persistence of the underlying chronic liver disease

activity. Disappearance of these markers and
seroconversion from HBeAg to anti-HBe is usually
accompanied by a remission of clinical symptoms and
biochemical evidence of disease activity. However, in
one-third of cases the remission may be transient and
followed by a return of chronic hepatitis disease
activity and hepatitis B virus replication.
Reactivation is particularly common among older patients
who have an underlying cirrhosis. Reactivation of
chronic type B hepatitis is associated with a poor
prognosis and frequent development of cirrhosis and its
complications. The underlying pathogenetic mechanisms
that lead to these various outcomes of this chronic viral
infection are unknown and are areas deserving of future
research.

REFERENCES

Berninger M, Hammer M, Hoyer B, Gerin JL (1982). An
    assay for the detection of the DNA genome of hepatitis
    B virus in serum. J Med Virol 9:57.
Davis GL, Hoofnagle JH, Waggoner JG (1983). Reactivation
    of chronic type B hepatitis. Gastroenterology 84:
    1370.
Decker RH, Kosakowski SM, Vanderbilt AS, Ling CM,
    Chairez R, Overby LR (1981). Diagnosis of acute
    hepatitis A by HAVAB-M, a direct radioimmunoassay
    for IgM anti-HAV. Am J Clin Path 76:140.
Hoofnagle JH, Dusheiko GM, Seeff LB, Jones EA, Waggoner
    JG, Bales ZB (1981). Seroconversion from hepatitis B
    e antigen to antibody in chronic type B hepatitis.
    Ann Intern Med 94:744.
Hoofnagle JH, Hanson RG, Minuk GY, Pappas SC, Schafer
    DF, Dusheiko GM, Straus SE, Popper H, Jones EA
    (1983). Randomized controlled trial of adenine
    arabinoside monophosphate for chronic type B
    hepatitis. Gastroenterology (in press).
International Group (1977). Acute and chronic hepatitis
    revisited. Lancet 2:914.
Kaplan PM, Greenman RL, Gerin JL, Purcell RH, Robinson
    WS (1973). DNA polymerase associated with human
    hepatitis B antigen. J Virol 12:995.
Liaw Y-F, Chu C-M, Su I-J, Huang M-J, Lin D-Y,
    Chang-Chien C-S (1983). Clnical and histological
    events preceding hepatitis B e antigen seroconversion
    in chronic type B hepatitis. Gastroenterology 84:216.

Norkrans G, Nordenfelt E, Hermodsson S, Iwarson S
(1980). Long-term follow-up of chronic hepatitis
patients with HBsAg, HBeAg and Dane particle
associated DNA polymerase in serum. Scand J
Infect Dis 12:159.
Realdi G, Alberti A, Rugge M, Bortolotti F, Rigoli AM,
Tremolada F, Ruol A (1980). Seroconversion from
hepatitis B e antigen to anti-HBe in chronic
hepatitis B virus infection. Gastroenterology
79:195.
Rizzetto M, Shih JW-K, Gerin JL (1980). The hepatitis
B virus-associated antigen: Isolation from liver,
development of solid-phase radioimmunoassays for
antigen and anti-δ and partial characterization of
δ antigen. J Immunol 125:318.
Rizzetto M, Shih JW-K, Gocke DJ, Purcell RH, Verme G,
Gerin JL (1979). Incidence and significance of
antibodies to delta antigen in hepatitis B virus
infection. Lancet 2:986.
Scullard GB, Pollard RB, Smith JL, Sacks SL, Gregory
PB, Robinson WS, Merigan TC (1981). Antiviral
treatment of chronic hepatitis B virus infection.
I. Changes in viral markers with interferon
combined with adenine arabinoside. J Infect Dis
143, 772.
Viola LA, Barrison IG, Coleman JC, Paradinas FJ, Fluker
JL, Evans BA, Murray-Lyon IM (1981). Natural history
of liver disease in chronic hepatitis B surface
antigen carriers. Lancet 2:1156.

Viral Hepatitis and Delta Infection, pages 55–66
© 1983 Alan R. Liss, Inc., 150 Fifth Avenue, New York, NY 10011

THE NATURAL HISTORY OF POST-TRANSFUSION AND SPORADIC NON-A,
NON-B HEPATITIS IN ITALY

G. Realdi, F. Tremolada, F. Bortolotti, A. Alberti
AM. Rigoli, F. Noventa, CA. Busachi, M. Rugge
Istituto di Medicina clinica, Patologia medica
Università di Padova
Padova (Italy)

Non-A, non-B hepatitis (NANBH) is currently defined as
an acute or chronic inflammatory liver lesion thought to be
caused by transmissible agents distinct from known hepatitis
viruses. The existence of this type of hepatitis infection
was initially suggested by two lines of observations. At first
came the finding of multiple attacks of hepatitis unrelated
to type A or B, particularly in drug addicts (Iwarson et al.
1973). Secondly, the incidence of post-transfusion hepatitis
has remained high despite the institution of sensitive screening procedures to eliminate HBV carriers from blood donation
(Prince et al., 1974). The exclusion of HAV, HBV and of other
hepatotropic viruses, such as cytomegalovirus (CMV) and Epste-
in Barr virus, as etiologic agents in some of these cases of
hepatitis, led to the identification of a new type of hepatitis, termed non-A, non-B hepatitis.

Inoculation experiments in chimpanzees established the
existence of transmissible agents in NANBH (Tabor et al. 1978).
Cross challange experiments have provided strong evidence for
implicating more than one etiologic agent in different forms
of NANBH (Bradley et al. 1980). Specific serologic markers for
NANBH have not been yet identified and the diagnosis is currently based on unspecific exclusion criteria. Despite these
limitations, several studies have already delineated some relevant epidemiologic and clinical features of the illness,
that appears as a world-wide entity.

The major route of NANB infection appears to be parenteral, polytransfused patients and drug-addicts being frequently affected. However NANBH also occurs as a sporadic illness

in patients having no evidence of parenteral exposure to blood
or to its derivates (Villarejos et al. 1975), and water-borne
epidemics have also been described (Khuroo et al. 1980). It
remains to be established whether these distinct epidemiologic forms of the illness recognize a single or different NANB
etiologic agents.

DIAGNOSTIC CRITERIA

Exclusion of known viral agents and of other non-viral
causes of liver damage is the only way to identify NANBH in a
patient with acute or chronic liver disease. The level of diagnostic accuracy varies therefore in relation to the anamnestic and serologic data that are available. The diagnosis may
be easily made during prospective studies of transfused patients. The diagnostic accuracy is still good if there is a
history of recent exposure to blood or to its derivates, even
in the absence of pretransfusion evaluation. On the contrary,
the spectrum of possible etiologic factors becomes wider when
evidence of parenteral exposure is lacking and it may be difficult, in the individual case, to rule out all non-viral causes of liver damage; in fact, the diagnosis of NANBH in this
setting remains truly presuntive.

On the basis of these considerations, it seems conceivable that, in the current absence of specific markers, the best
way to define the natural history of NANBH is to rely on prospective studies of well defined groups of patients presenting
with acute illness. We have recently conducted two distinct
prospective studies of parenterally acquired and of sporadic
NANBH and will review here the results obtained, mainly in
relation to the clinical features and to the long-term outcome of our patients.

PROSPECTIVE STUDIES OF NANBH

Post-transfusion NANBH

Since 1980 we have conducted a prospective study of post-
transfusion (PT) NANBH in open-heart surgery patients (Tremolada et al.,1983). Of the 297 patients enrolled, 21.2% (63 cases) developed PT hepatitis, with a NANBH prevalence of 84.1%.
The remaining PT hepatitis cases were identified as hepatitis

B (2 cases;3.2%) and as CMV related (8 cases;12.7%), as they became positive in serum for HBsAg or anti-HBc and for IgM-anti-CMV respectively. The incidence of PT hepatitis was significantly higher among 51 patients who received blood units and clotting factor concentrates compared to that of 246 patients treated only with blood units from single donors (Table 1). The rate of hepatitis attack in our patients was significantly influenced by the number of blood units (p<0.05). Patients treated with clotting factors received an average number of blood units significantly higher than the patients not treated with these products. However, the incidence of PT hepatitis, calculated as the number of PT hepatitis cases per 1000 blood units, remained significantly higher in the former compared to the latter cases (Table 1).

Table 1 - Incidence of PT hepatitis in cardiac-surgery patients receiving only blood or also clotting factor concentrates.

Product transfused	N° Cases	Blood units (mean±SD)	Recipients with PT hepatitis		
			N°	%	N/1000 units
Only blood	246	6.1±3.1	34	13.8	22.5
Blood units and clotting factors	51	10.5±8.8[*]	29	56.8[*]	54.0[*]

[*]p<0.001

When patients with NANBH and those with CMV infection were compared, the incubation period was significantly shorter in the latter (mean weeks ± SD: 7.5±4.4 vs. 5.4±1.8; p<0.05), who also showed a higher incidence of fever and pleural effusion. The incidence of icteric cases and mean peak of alanine-aminotransferase (ALT) levels did not differ between the two groups; however, transaminases normalized within 12 months of follow-up in 75% of CMV cases, but only in 25% of NANBH cases (p<0.01).

Sporadic NANBH

In order to evaluate prevalence and clinical features of NANBH in patients without evidence of parenteral exposure (spo

radic NANBH) we studied 565 consecutive patients presenting
with symptomatic acute viral hepatitis. The diagnostic criteria used in this study have been reported elsewhere (Bortolotti et al.,1982). Ninety-four patients were classified as NANBH.
After exclusion of cases with recent blood transfusions (25
cases), or admitting drug addiction (25 cases) or having frequent contacts with blood samples (2 laboratory employees),42
cases were left in whom parenteral exposure could not be identified. Thus these sporadic NANBH cases reached in our series
a 7.4% prevalence among symptomatic acute viral hepatitis cases. A high number of elderly women concurred to this group,
a finding similar to that reported by Dienstag et al. (1977)
in the United States. Acute clinical features in the 42 sporadic NANBH cases did not differ significantly compared to those
observed in patients with type A or type B hepatitis. Acute
liver failure did not occur in our series and extrahepatic manifestations were rare (Bortolotti et al., 1982).

LONG TERM EVOLUTION OF NANBH IN TWO EPIDEMIOLOGIC SETTINGS

The 53 patients who developed PT NANBH during our prospective study of open-heart surgery patients, and the 42 cases of
sporadic NANBH identified among symptomatic acute viral hepatitis cases, were followed prospectively for 12-39 months (mean $\pm$
SD: 23+8) and for 24-43 months (mean+SD: 34+7), respectively.
During this longitudinal study, all patients underwent periodical clinical and biochemical evaluation. Patients who continued to show abnormal transaminase levels for more than 12
months after presentation, were considered to have progressed
to a chronic phase of the illness. Figure 1 shows the cumulative probability of ALT normalization in the two groups, calculated according to the follow-up data. The expected rate of
biochemical resolution was 92% in sporadic cases at 12 months
of follow-up and did not change afterwards, while a different
trend was observed in PT hepatitis cases. In these patients a
plateau value of 43% was obtained only after 24 months of follow-up, indicating the existence of a subgroup of cases showing delayed biochemical resolution of the illness.

Acute phase features were analyzed in PT hepatitis cases
in relation to the outcome. As shown in Table 2, the only differences noted between patients who recovered and those with
chronic evolution related to the ALT profile.

Of the 42 sporadic cases enrolled, 38 have completed 36

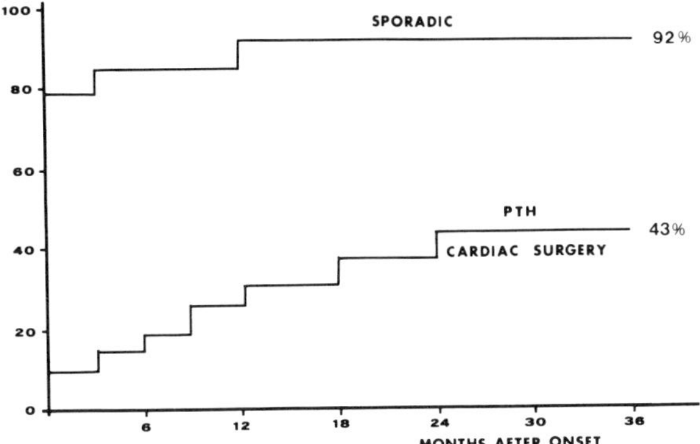

Figure 1 – Cumulative probability, expressed as a function of time, of spontaneous normalization of ALT in the two groups of patients prospectively followed after acute hepatitis.

months of follow-up. Three patients in this group (8%) have progressed to chronic hepatitis. The histologic diagnosis in liver biopsies taken during chronic phase, was of chronic lobular hepatitis in 2 cases and of chronic persistent hepatitis in the remaining one. In contrast to the mild histologic lesions observed in this group, most PT hepatitis patients who have progressed to chronic hepatitis and have undergone liver biopsy, showed features of active disease (see below).

SPECTRUM OF LIVER DISEASE IN CHRONIC PT NANBH

In order to define the long term outcome of PT NANBH, follow-up data were analyzed in 61 patients. These included the 40 patients showing persistence of abnormal ALT levels for more than 12 months during our prospective study and 21 further non-consecutive open-heart surgery patients observed between 1975 and 1979. Also these patients had progressed to chronic hepatitis after acute PT NANBH and were followed for a mean period of 68 months, with a range of 42 and 90 months.

Symptoms of chronic liver disease were relatively rare in these patients (19.6). In 10 patients (16.3%) a moderate sple-

Table 2 - Acute phase clinical and biochemical features in patients with PT hepatitis in relation to the outcome.

	Patients who recover (13 cases)		Patients with chronic evolution (40 cases)
Months of follow-up ($\overline{M}$)	19+6		23+7
Treated with clotting factors	54%		50%
Jaundice	23%		35%
ALT peak ($\overline{M}$ IU/1)	648	p<0.01	1180
Gammaglobulin ($\overline{M}$ g%)	1.59		1.62
ALT pattern during acute phase (number of patients)			
- monophasic	12		0
- polyphasic	5	p<0.02	32
- plateau	0		8

nomegaly was felt. Oesophageal varices developed in 3 patients, one of whom died of gastrointestinal bleeding.

Up to now, 41 patients have been evaluated histological-ly, with liver biopsy taken 1 to 6 years after acute onset. Several patients had serial liver biopsies during follow-up to assess further evolution of histologic lesions. As shown in figure 2 a wide spectrum of morphologic features was observed.

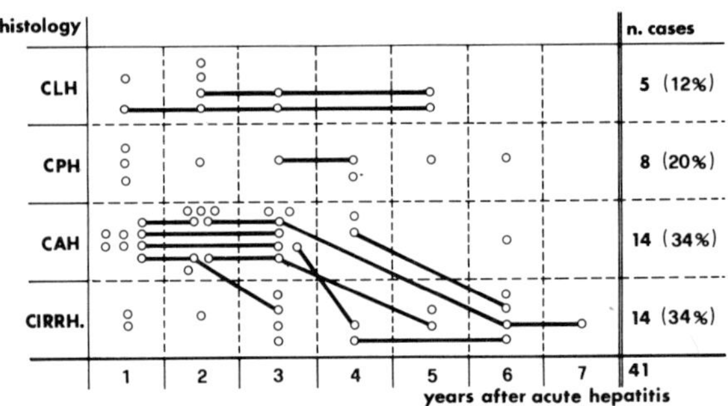

Figure 2 - Histologic features in 41 patients with chronic PT NANBH in relation to time of liver biopsy. Continuous lines indicate serial liver biopsies during follow-up in the same patient.

A minority of the patients showed non-progressive liver disease, including 5 cases (12%) with chronic lobular hepatitis (CLH) and 8 (20%) with chronic persistent hepatitis (CPH). It was of interest to note that all patients in this group who underwent serial histologic assessment showed no progression to severe lesions. Two patients who underwent liver biopsy 12 months after onset on the basis of persistence of abnormal transaminase values, eventually normalized enzyme levels during the subsequent follow-up. Liver histology in these patients was consistent with CLH in one and CPH in the other.

The remaining 28 patients had features of chronic active hepatitis (CAH)(14 cases; 34%) or of liver cirrhosis (14 cases; 34%). Thus, about two thirds of the patients studied showed progressive liver disease. Five patients with CAH on first biopsy developed histologic evidence of cirrhosis during follow-up. In the whole group, liver cirrhosis was observed mainly in biopsies obtained between the third and the sixth year of follow-up. Two patients however already had cirrhotic features when biopsied only one year after acute onset.

Our data indicate the existence of two distinct patterns of chronic evolution of PT NANBH. About 30% of the patients showed mild, non-progressive liver lesions, while the remaining 70% had severe, progressive disease. In these two groups of patients we noted a different behaviour of the transaminase profile. Figure 3 shows an example of the transaminase pattern observed during follow-up in most patients with CLH or CPH on biopsy. Marked fluctuations of enzyme levels occurred in these cases, often with short periods of normalization. No worsening of liver lesions occurred, even after 7 years of florid biochemical activity.

On the contrary patients with an active histology tended to show more stable transaminase levels after the acute phase, as shown in the example of figure 4. In this patient, as well as in several others, transaminases progressively decreased during follow-up, thus mimicking a slow resolution of the disease. This contrasted, however, with liver histology that progressively worsened during follow-up, with development of cirrhosis.

In order to better define these two distinct clinical entities observed in chronic PT NANBH, we have tried to identify risk factors that could predict the severity of chronic liver lesions. As shown in Table 3, among the various parame-

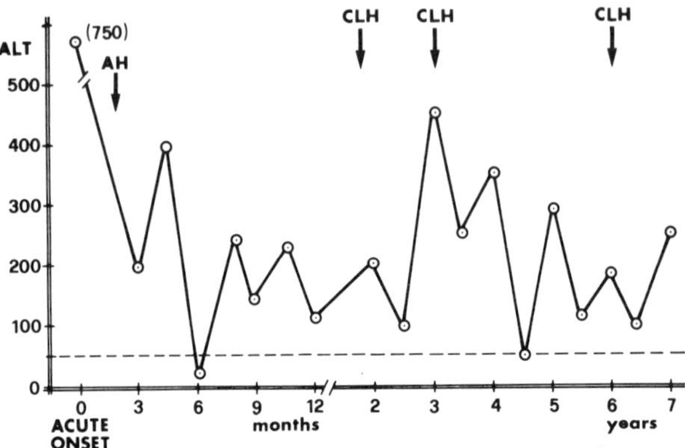

Figure 3 - Transaminase behaviour in a patient with chronic lobular hepatitis (CLH) followed for 7 years after acute PT NANBH. Arrows indicate liver biopsies. AH denotes acute hepatitis.

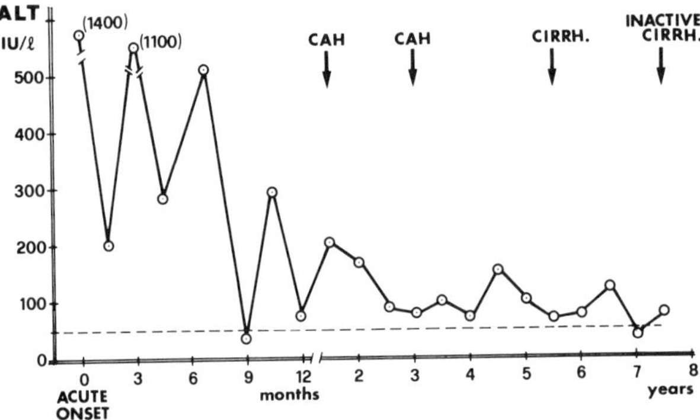

Figure 4 - Transaminase behaviour in a patient with chronic active hepatitis (CAH) followed for more than 7 years after acute PT NANBH. Arrows indicate liver biopsies.

ters here considered, only the use of clotting factors during surgery was statistically associated with the development of severe and progressive disease.

Table 3 - Risk factors and chronic evolution in PT NANBH

Histologic lesions:	Non-progressive (CPH-CLH)		Progressive (CAH-Cirrh)
Number of cases	13		28
Months of follow-up ($\overline{M}$ and range)	28 (12-58)		29 (12-91)
Events before surgery(number of patients)			
- Congestive heart failure	2		5
- Hepatitis B virus markers	4		3
- Alcohol abuse (>80 g/die)	3		8
- Previous blood transfusions	0	p=0.06	7
Patients receiving clotting factors during surgery	2	p<0.01	17

This observation suggests that the virus load or a coinfection with more than one virus strain could influence the outcome of chronic PT NANBH. This assumption appears to be further supported by the comparison of the biochemical outcome observed in our open-heart surgery patients and in 25 further PT NANBH cases, selected on the basis that they had received a small number of blood units and no blood derivates. The cumulative probability of ALT normalization at 12 months was, in this latter group, of 62% and of the 4 patients who underwent liver biopsy during chronic phase, 2 had features of CPH and 2 of CAH without bridging necrosis.

TWO CANDIDATE MARKERS OF PT NANBH

The clinical data obtained in our prospective studies clearly outlined the existence of several differences between parenterally acquired and sporadic forms of the illness. These differences could relate to the existence of distinct etiologic agents and this assumption appears also supported by the results we obtained when studying two candidate NANB markers in liver biopsies of patients with chronic NANBH.

Biopsy specimens obtained from 9 patients with chronic PT NANBH and from 9 additional cases of HBsAg negative chronic hepatitis (including the 3 patients who presented with sporadic NANBH and 6 further patients with no recognizable causes of liver damage) were studied by immunofluorescence for a NANB nuclear antigen (Alberti et al.,1981) and by electron microscopy

for the presence of intranuclear particles of the type originally described by Shimizu et al. (1979). Only PT NANBH cases
were found positive for NANB antigen (7 out of 9) and for intranuclear particles (7 out of 9). None of the patients with sporadic NANBH, nor a control group of 20 patients with HBsAg positive, delta negative, chronic hepatitis showed nuclear antigen or particles in the liver.

CONCLUSIONS

Our prospective studies on the natural history of NANBH
indicate that the illness, as currently diagnosed by exclusion
criteria, is an heterogeneous clinical entity with a wide spectrum of histologic features and of biochemical profiles.
Chronic evolution is a rare event in sporadic NANBH with no
evidence of parenteral exposure, while it is quite frequent
in NANBH acquired after blood transfusion. In these cases,
both mild, slowly resolving, as well as severe and progressive chronic liver lesions are observed (Realdi et al.,1982).
The entity of virus load, or coinfection with more than one
agent, may be one of the relevant factors in determining the
severity of chronic PT NANBH.

In the patients with chronic NANBH the biochemical profile often reflects the type of liver lesions, marked fluctuations of transaminase levels over time being characteristic of chronic, non-progressive liver disease, with histologic features of chronic lobular hepatitis or of chronic persistent hepatitis. In contrast, patients with more progressive liver lesions usually show more stable ALT levels during
the course of their illness.

The clinical differences observed in sporadic and post-
transfusion NANBH may suggest the existence of distinct etiologic agents in these two forms of liver disease. Although
this assumption is only presumptive, due to the current absence of reliable specific markers to identify NANBH agents,
it appears supported by the results we have obtained when two
candidate NANB tissue markers were studied by immunofluorescence and by electron microscopy in the liver of NANBH cases
having a different epidemiologic background. However, further
characterization of the nature and specificity of these markers is required before a definitive answer to this important
issue could be obtained.

REFERENCES

Alberti A, Realdi G, Bortolotti F, Cadrobbi P, Barbieri R, Tremolada F, Ongaro G (1981). Detection by immunofluorescence of an antigen-antibody system in patients with acute and chronic non-A, non-B hepatitis. Liver 1:183

Bortolotti F, Cadrobbi P, Carretta M, Meneghetti F, Pornaro E, Realdi G (1982). Epidemiological aspects on acute viral hepatitis in Northern Italy. Scand J Infect Dis 14:161

Bortolotti F, Realdi G, Cadrobbi P, Crivellaro C, Pornaro E (1982). Clinical features and evolution of non-A, non-B hepatitis in relation to the epidemiological background. Ital J Gastroenterol 14:86

Bradley DW, Maynard JE, Cook EH, Ebert JW, Gravelle CR, Tsiquaye KN, Zuckerman AJ, Miller MF, Ling CM, Overby LR (1980). Non-A, non-B hepatitis in experimentally infected chimpanzees: crosschallenge and electron microscopic studies. J Med Virol 6:185

Dienstag JL, Alaama A, Mosley JW, Redeker AG, Purcell RH (1977). Etiology of sporadic hepatitis B surface antigen-negative hepatitis. Ann Intern Med 87:1

Iwarson S, Lundin P, Holmgren J, Hermodsson S (1973). Multiple attacks of hepatitis in drug addicts: biochemical, immunochemical and morphologic characteristics. J Infect Dis 127:544

Khuroo MS (1980). Study of an epidemic of non-A, non-B hepatitis. Possibility of another human hepatitis virus distinct from post-transfusion non-A, non-B type. Am J Med 68:818

Prince AM, Brotman B, Grady GF, Kuhns WJ, Hazzi C, Levine RW, Milliam SJ (1974). Long-incubation post-transfusion hepatitis without serological evidence of exposure to hepatitis-B virus. Lancet 2:241

Realdi G, Alberti A, Rugge M, Rigoli AM, Tremolada F, Schivazappa L, Ruol A (1982). Long-term follow-up of acute and chronic non-A, non-B post-transfusion hepatitis: evidence of progression to liver cirrhosis. Gut 23:270

Shimizu JK, Feinstone SM, Purcell RH, Alter HJ, London WT (1979). Non-A, non-B hepatitis: ultrastructural evidence of two agents in experimentally infected chimpanzees. Science 205:197

Tabor E, Drucker AJ, Hoofnagle MJ, April M, Gerety RJ, Seeff LB, Jackson DR, Barker LF, Tamondong G (1978). Transmission of non-A, non-B hepatitis from man to chimpanzees. Lancet 1:463

Villarejos VM, Visona KA, Eduarte CA, Provost PJ, Hilleman MR (1975). Evidence for viral hepatitis other than type A or type B among persons in Costa Rica. New Engl J Med 293:1350

Tremolada F, Chiappetta F, Noventa F, Valfrè C, Ongaro G, Realdi G (1983). Prospective study of post-trasfusion hepa-

titis in cardiac-surgery patients receiving only blood or
also blood products. Vox Sang 44:25

titis in cardiac-surgery patients receiving only blood or
also blood products. Vox Sang 44:25

Viral Hepatitis and Delta Infection, pages 67–76
© 1983 Alan R. Liss, Inc., 150 Fifth Avenue, New York, NY 10011

HISTOPATHOLOGY OF VIRAL HEPATITIS

Leonardo Bianchi, M.D.

Department of Pathology
University of Basel
CH-4056 Basel (Switzerland)

Infection of the liver with hepatitis viruses causes a wide spectrum of histologic alterations occurring singly or in various combinations. Based mainly on observations in hepatitis B, a morphologic classification has emerged (*Table 1*) and has met with a fair measure of agreement (De Groote et al 1968; Fogarty International Center Criteria Committee 1976; Bianchi et al 1971, 1977).

Table 1. Morphologic classification of viral hepatitis.

1. *ACUTE VIRAL HEPATITIS (AVH)*

   1.1. *AVH with spotty necrosis*
   1.2. *AVH with piecemeal necrosis*
   1.3. *AVH with confluent bridging hepatic necrosis*
   1.4. *AVH with confluent panlobular (massive) necrosis*

2. *CHRONIC VIRAL HEPATITIS*

   2.1. *"True" hepatitis B virus carrier (no inflammation or nonspecific reactive hepatitis)*
   2.2. *Chronic non-aggressive hepatitis (chronic persistent, chronic lobular, chronic septal hepatitis)*
   2.3. *Chronic aggressive (active) hepatitis*
        - with minimal/moderate activity (a)
        - with severe activity   (b)

As a general rule, in acute forms of hepatitis diffuse lobular changes predominate over portal lesions while chronic hepatitis is characterized by conspicuous alterations of portal (and periportal) areas. Exact staging of viral hepatitis by histologic criteria is an important tool in the evaluation of prognosis, indication and control of therapy, as well as for comparison with immunologic findings.

1. ACUTE VIRAL HEPATITIS

1.1. Acute Spotty Necrotic Hepatitis.

Main histologic features include a combination of spotty liver cell necrosis of the acidophilic and lytic type with a lympho-histiocytic intralobular and portal inflammation giving rise to the characteristic variegated picture with marked lobular disarray, described in textbooks (Bianchi et al 1979). Except for very early preclinical stages of disease hepatitis B viral (HBV) antigens (e.g. HBsAg-containing groundglass cells) are not demonstrable in liver tissue (*Elimination type*: Gudat et al 1975; Bianchi, Gudat 1979). The outcome of this form in almost all cases is healing without sequelae through immunologic elimination of infected liver cells by means of spotty necrosis.

Clinical features may not reliably differentiate this benign spotty necrotic acute hepatitis from forms with more severe prognostic implications such as acute hepatitis with piecemeal necrosis or confluent bridging/massive necrosis (*Table 1*). Liver biopsy thus is justified not only in chronic but also in acute forms of viral hepatitis.

1.2. Acute Viral Hepatitis with Piecemeal Necrosis

most often occurs in drug addicts or in the elderly. The histologic lesion combines features of spotty necrotic hepatitis with a periportal reaction similar to chronic active hepatitis including piecemeal necrosis. This has given rise to the term "*acute hepatitis with possible transition to chronicity*" (Bianchi et al 1971, 1977). Histological features in acute hepatitis suggesting chronicity are listed in *Table 2*.

Table 2. Histologic features in acute hepatitis suggesting chronicity.

- Disproportionately severe degree of
  portal inflammation
- *Piecemeal necrosis*
- Predominance of *lymphocytes and plasma cells*
  in portal and intralobular infiltrates
- *Lymph follicle formation*
- *Bile duct lesions* of the hepatitic type
- Presence of *viral antigens in tissue*
- *Centro-portal bridging necrosis,* particularly
  if accompanied by piecemeal necrosis
- *Trapped viable liver cells* in periportal loca-
  tion or within zones of confluent necrosis.

Although AVH with piecemeal necrosis may regress spontaneously (Fauerholdt et al 1977), evolution to chronic hepatitis or at least a markedly prolonged course is the rule.
In a 3 years follow-up of drug addicts with biopsy-proven
AVH with piecemeal necrosis 40% of cases revealed chronic
active hepatitis (CAH) of minimal or moderate activity, 60%
had chronic persistent hepatitis (CPH). None of the patients
showed complete histologic resolution (Aenishänslin et al
1975).

Interpretation and pathogenesis of this variant are
controversial. Co- or superinfection with the delta agent
appears to be more frequent in drug addicts (Stöcklin et al
1981). It has been suggested that a finely graded immune insufficiency in these patients may allow persistent viral replication and result in chronic hepatitis (Gudat et al 1975).

*1.3. Acute Hepatitis with Confluent Bridging Hepatic
     Necrosis (BHN)*

Necrosis affecting substantial groups of adjacent liver
cells is referred to as confluent necrosis (Bianchi et al
1971). Such necrosis may bridge neighboring hepatic venules
(*centro-central bridging*) or central veins and portal tracts
(*centro-portal bridging*) (Bianchi, Gudat 1983). Bridging he-

patic necrosis may vary in extent from lobule to lobule and also the alterations in the remaining parenchyma may be extremely variable. This has a bearing on the evolution of the lesion. While centro-central bridging usually heals without sequelae or with insignificant scars, centro-portal bridging - particularly if accompanied by piecemeal necrosis and/or trapped liver cells (*Table 2*) - often leads to CAH and cirrhosis.

In their classical follow-up study, Boyer and Klatskin (1970) first drew attention on the significance of bridging necrosis reporting death in hepatic coma in 19% and evolution to cirrhosis in 37% of their cases.

Pathogenesis of bridging necrosis is yet poorly understood.

1.4. *Acute Hepatitis with Massive Necrosis*

is characterized by confluent necrosis involving whole liver lobules (*panlobular necrosis*) in a substantial part of the liver (Bianchi 1983). The clinical correlate is fulminant hepatitis. Survival largely depends on the remaining intact liver mass capable of regeneration. Interestingly, fulminant hepatitis, if survived, usually heals without functional sequelae and without evolution to cirrhosis (Desmet et al 1972).

2. *CHRONIC VIRAL HEPATITIS*

Chronic viral hepatitis results from persistence in the liver of viral antigens which cannot be efficiently eliminated by host defense systems. Etiologically, this applies to hepatitis B and to non-A, non-B (NANB) agents, but not to hepatitis A. In chronic HBV infection, a fairly good correlation of three different expression patterns of viral antigens (notably HBcAg) in liver tissue and type and degree of inflammation has been established (Bianchi, Gudat 1979).

2.1. "True" HBV Carrier

Histologically, the HBV carrier is characterized by lack of inflammation or minor inflammatory changes (nonspecific reactive hepatitis; *Table 1*). HBs-containing groundglass cells as a rule are present in large numbers.

For their different biological implications it is recommended to distinguish two types of "healthy" carriers (Bianchi, Gudat 1979):

The *HBcAg-free HBsAg Type of Carrier*, exhibiting groundglass cells usually in widespread areas in the absence of HBcAg expression. This is the carrier type commonly seen in the Western world. The course is stable over years. Because of integration of HBV-DNA into the host genome, however, there is the risk of developing hepatocellular carcinoma in the long run.

The *Generalized HBcAg Type of Carrier*, occurring mostly in immunosuppressed patients or after vertical transmission from mother to child, usually shows less HBsAg-containing groundglass cells but HBcAg expression in almost all liver cell nuclei as a result of ongoing viral replication. Excessive nuclear core accumulation may even be recognized in conventional H+E preparations by the appearance of "*sanded nuclei*" (Bianchi, Gudat 1976). Inflammation may be slightly more pronounced than in the HBcAg-free type and the course is less stable; deteriorations to chronic aggressive hepatitis are documented.

This type reflects a full, unrestricted active viral replication with episomal viral DNA, without interference of the immune response of the host. Indeed, a sequential nuclear/cytoplasmic/submembraneous flow of core has been observed (Gudat, Bianchi 1977). This observation may be of interest in the speculation on candidate target antigens for the immune attack on the cell membrane and for the concept of Dane particle formation.

*2.2. Chronic Non-Aggressive Hepatitis
      (Chronic Persistent Hepatitis, and variants thereof)*

Histologic hallmark of CPH is a dense, predominantly lymphocytic inflammation restricted to enlarged portal tracts, leaving the parenchymal limiting plate preserved.

In general, CPH is considered to have a good prognosis, with histological features persisting for years without deterioration to more aggressive forms (De Groote et al 1968). However, complicating acute exacerbations, even with confluent necrosis may occur at any time and then progression to CAH may be the result. In some cases, lobular alterations with features of acute spotty necrotic hepatitis may be pronounced. For this, the term *"chronic lobular hepatitis"* seems appropriate (Popper, Schaffner 1976). This applies mainly to infections with NANB agents, including HBV infection with delta. Another variant, said to have a much poorer prognosis, is *"chronic septal hepatitis"* (Gerber, Vernace 1974), characterized by the formation of extensive porto-portal septa with conspicuous inflammatory activity. CPH, particularly the chronic septal form may also represent a regressive stage of CAH after immunosuppressive therapy (Czaja et al 1981).

The histologic and prognostic variability of CPH is reliably reflected in the occurrence of different types of viral antigen expression. Cases with demonstrable core in tissue (*Generalized* or *Focal HBcAg Type*: Bianchi, Gudat 1979) as a rule carry a higher risk of deterioration to CAH. Presence of the *HBcAg-free HBsAg Type* of viral antigen expression with abundance of groundglass cells in light microscopy on the other hand is associated with the more stable course in which inflammation may even regress.

2.3. Chronic Active (Aggressive) Hepatitis (CAH)

is characterized histologically by portal and periportal inflammation with erosion of the limiting plate by piecemeal necrosis and fibrosis. Peripolesis and rosetting of liver cells are key features distinguishing true piecemeal necrosis from mere spillover of inflammatory cells from portal tracts which may be seen also in severe acute hepa-

titis. For prognostic and therapeutic reasons a graduation
of activity of the destructive inflammatory process has been
proposed (Bianchi et al 1977; Bianchi, Gudat 1983; *Table 1.*)

Viral antigen expression in CAH interestingly is always
of the *Focal HBcAg Type* (Bianchi, Gudat 1979): A focal nuclear core expression in immunofluorescence studies is often
together with a diffuse *membraneous* staining for HBsAg. The
same pattern is observed in most cases of acute hepatitis
with piecemeal necrosis.

By definition, CAH is a progressive destructive inflammatory lesion which ultimately ends-up in cirrhosis with a
high frequency. However, remissions, spontaneous or more
often as an effect of therapy may occur in some instances,
histologically presenting with a regression to CPH (Czaja
et al 1981). The spead of evolution is extremely variable,
probably according to the degree of the patient's immune
deficiency state. A deviation from the regular immunopathology may be induced also by co- or superinfection with other
viruses, e.g. the delta agent (Rizzetto et al 1977, Stöcklin
et al 1981), by (viral-induced?) autoimmune phenomena (Thomas et al 1982) and by therapeutical immunomanipulation
(Bianchi, Gudat 1983).

THE THREE TYPES OF HEPATITIS VIRUSES

Serological tests may recognize acute infection with
the HA virus as well as acute and chronic forms of HB but
there is still no commercial test system available to identify NANB infections. Liver biopsy interpretation offers some
hints as to the possible underlying viral infection.

<u>Hepatitis B</u>. Histologic features in acute and chronic HB are
those usually described in textbooks. In chronic forms, the
presence of HBs-containing groundglass cells and, in rare
instances, of sanded nuclei may prove the etiology.

<u>Hepatitis A</u>. At least in early stages of acute hepatitis A
a marked periportal predilection of the lobular lesions with
severe periportal necrosis of the lytic type and a periportal inflammatory infiltrate rich in plasma cells contrasts
to acute HB or NANB infection (Teixeira et al 1982; Bianchi

1983). Despite the severity of the histological changes complete restoration without sequelae is the rule. There is no evidence for chronic liver disease after HA infection.

Hepatitis NANB. In analogy to findings in experimentally infected chimpanzees (Popper et al 1980) and based on the limited experience with human cases (Dienes et al 1982), particularly in hemophiliacs, some histological features in favor of NANB hepatitis have emerged (*Table 3*; under study).

Table 3. Histologic features in favor of NANB hepatitis.

- *Acute/chronic hepatitis difficult to distinguish*
- *Histology often borderline CPH/CAH*
- *Bile duct lesions more frequent than in HB*
- *Acidophilic bodies with little if any surrounding mesenchymal reaction ("naked" acidophilic bodies), and often showing crumbling of cytoplasm (Mallory body-like)*
- *Acidophilic rhomboid-shaped hepatocytes in large amounts*
- *Presence of fat in fully developed hepatitic stage, not otherwise explained*
- *Accentuated liver cell borders (clear cells)*
- *Accumulation of lymphocytes in sinusoids in a beadfile manner (mononucleosis-like), with little liver cell damage*
- *Squeezed, boomerang-shaped sinusoidal-lining cells*
- *Giant cell hepatitis in adults.*

REFERENCES

Aenishänslin HW, Stalder GA, Bianchi L, Gudat F, Carmann H (1975). Hepatitis bei Drogensüchtigen. Verlaufskontrollen anhand bioptisch-histologischer Kriterien. Dtsch med Wschr 100: 857
Bianchi L (1983). Liver biopsy interpretation in hepatitis. Path Res Pract (In press)
Bianchi L, Gudat F (1976). Sanded nuclei in hepatitis B. Lab Invest 35: 1

Bianchi L, Gudat F (1979). Immunopathology of hepatitis B. In Popper H, Schaffner F (eds): "Progress in Liver Diseases", Vol 6, New York: Grune and Stratton, p 371

Bianchi L, Gudat F (1983). Histo- and immunopathology of viral hepatitis. In Deinhardt F, Deinhardt J (eds): "Viral hepatitis", New York: Marcel Dekker, p·343

Bianchi L, De Groote J, Desmet VJ, Gedigk P, Korb G, Popper H, Poulsen H, Scheuer PJ, Schmid M, Thaler H, Wepler W (1971). Morphological criteria in viral hepatitis. Lancet i: 333

Bianchi L, De Groote J, Desmet VJ, Gedigk P, Korb G, Popper H, Poulsen H, Scheuer PJ, Schmid M, Thaler H, Wepler W (1977). Acute and chronic hepatitis revisited. Lancet ii: 914

Bianchi L, Zimmerli-Ning M, Gudat F (1979). Viral hepatitis. In Mac Sween RNM, Anthony PP, Scheuer PJ (eds): "Pathology of the liver", Edinburgh: Churchill-Livingstone, p 164

Boyer JL, Klatskin G (1970). Pattern of necrosis in acute viral hepatitis. Prognostic value of bridging (subacute hepatic necrosis). New Engl J Med 283: 1063

Czaja AJ, Ludwig J, Baggenstoss AH, Wolf A (1981). Corticosteroid-treated chronic active hepatitis in remission: uncertain prognosis of chronic persistent hepatitis. New Engl J Med 304: 5

De Groote J, Desmet VJ, Gedigk P, Korb G, Popper H, Poulsen H, Scheuer PJ, Schmid M, Thaler H, Uehlinger E, Wepler W (1968). A classification of chronic hepatitis. Lancet ii: 626

Desmet VJ, De Groote J, van Damme B (1972). Acute hepatocellular failure. A study of 17 patients treated with exchange transfusion. Human Path 3: 167

Dienes HP, Popper H, Arnold W, Lobeck H (1982). Histologic observations in human hepatitis non-A, non-B. Hepatology 2: 562

Fauerholdt L, Asnaes S, Ranek L, Schiødt T, Tygstrup N (1977). Significance of suspected "chronic aggressive hepatitis" in acute hepatitis. Gastroenterology 73: 543

Fogarty International Center Criteria Committee (1976). Standardization of nomenclature, diagnostic criteria and diagnostic methodology for diseases of the liver and biliary tract, Basel: Karger

Gerber MA, Vernace S (1974). Chronic septal hepatitis. Virchows Arch Path Anat A 363: 303

Gudat F, Bianchi L (1977). Evidence for phasic sequences in nuclear HBcAg formation and cell membrane-directed flow of core particles in chronic hepatitis B. Gastroenterology 73: 1194

Gudat F, Bianchi L, Sonnabend W, Thiel G, Aenishänslin W, Stalder GA (1975). Pattern of core and surface expression in liver tissue reflects state of specific immune response in hepatitis B. Lab Invest 32: 1

Popper H, Schaffner F (1976). Chronic hepatitis: Taxonomic, etiologic, and therapeutic problems. In Popper H, Schaffner F (eds): "Progress in Liver Diseases", Vol 5, New York: Grune and Stratton, p 531

Popper H, Dienstag JL, Feinstone SM, Alter HJ, Purcell RH (1980). Lessons from the pathology of viral hepatitis in c̄himpanzees. In Bianchi L, Gerok W, Sickinger K, Stalder GA (eds): "Virus and liver", Lancaster: MTP Press, p 137

Rizzetto M, Canese MG, Arico S, Crivelli O, Trepo C, Bonino F, Verme G (1977). Immunofluorescence detection of new antigen-antibody system (δ/anti-δ) associated to hepatitis B virus in liver and in serum of HBsAg carriers. Gut 18: 997

Stöcklin E, Gudat F, Krey G, Dürmüller U, Gasser M, Schmid M, Stalder G, Bianchi L (1981). δ antigen in hepatitis B: immunohistology of frozen and paraffin-embedded liver biopsies and relation to HBV infection. Hepatology 1: 238

Teixeira MR jr, Weller IVD, Murray A, Bamber M, Thomas HC, Sherlock S, Scheuer PJ (1982). The pathology of hepatitis A in man. Liver 2: 53

Thomas HC, Montano L, Goodall A, De Koning R, Oladapo J, Wiedman KH (1982). Immunological mechanisms in chronic hepatitis B virus infection. Hepatology 2, Suppl. 2: 116S

THE DELTA AGENT:
BIOLOGY AND EPIDEMIOLOGY

Viral Hepatitis and Delta Infection, pages 79–89
© 1983 Alan R. Liss, Inc., 150 Fifth Avenue, New York, NY 10011

EXPERIMENTAL TRANSMISSION OF THE DELTA AGENT TO CHIMPANZEES

Robert H. Purcell, M.D.[1], John L. Gerin, Ph.D.[2], Mario
Rizzetto, M.D.[3], Antonio Ponzetto, M.D.[3], Ferruccio
Bonino, M.D.[3], and William T. London, D.V.M.[4]

[1]Laboratory of Infectious Diseases, NIAID
National Institutes of Health, Bethesda, Md. 20205

[2]Division of Molecular Virology and Immunology
Georgetown U. Medical School, Rockville, Md. 20852

[3]Division of Gastroenterology, Ospedale Molinette
10126 Torino, Italy

[4]Infectious Diseases Branch, NINCDS
National Institutes of Health, Bethesda, Md. 20205

INTRODUCTION

The discovery of a new pathogen of major medical importance is a significant event in medical research. It is
surprising that, in this age of scientific sophistication, such
basic discoveries continue to be made. One such "new" agent is
the delta agent (Rizzetto, 1981), the cause of a severe form of
viral hepatitis that has sometimes been attributed erroneously
to infection with the hepatitis B virus (HBV).

In order to establish the pathogenicity of a newly
recognized agent it has been necessary since the time of Koch
to demonstrate the recovery and transmissibility of the agent
and its association with the disease it is suspected of
causing. The transmissibility and pathogenicity of the delta
agent were confirmed by transmission studies in chimpanzees
(Rizzetto, 1980). This species of primate has also played an
important part in the characterization of the delta agent. A
summary of these and other studies follows.

HOST RANGE

Extensive studies of the host range of the delta agent have not been performed. The defective nature of the agent and its requirement for coinfection with hepatitis B virus have discouraged a systematic evaluation of animal species. It is probable that the delta agent can replicate in all primate species believed to be capable of supporting the replication of hepatitis B virus, including, in addition to chimpanzees, orangutans, gorillas and gibbons. Of this group, only chimpanzees are available in sufficient numbers to be considered useful for transmission studies and virtually all of the animals employed at present come from breeding colonies.

Marmosets are the only other primate species extensively used for hepatitis studies, principally with hepatitis A virus (Holmes, 1969; Mascoli, 1973). Marmosets are not susceptible to infection with hepatitis B virus but may have a limited susceptibility to non-A, non-B hepatitis agents (Feinstone, 1981). We took advantage of this differential susceptibility of marmosets to determine if the delta agent could undergo at least limited replication in the absence of HBV replication. Marmosets (Saguinus mystax) were inoculated with chimpanzee plasma that contained 10^3 infectious doses of HBV and at least 10^8 infectious doses of delta agent. The animals did not develop biochemical evidence of hepatitis or serologic evidence of infection with the delta agent or HBV. Thus, S. mystax marmosets do not appear to be useful for the study of the delta agent.

Evidence that, in the presence of appropriate helper viruses, the host range of the delta agent may be quite broad comes from transmission studies carried out by Ponzetto (these Proceedings) in woodchucks chronically infected with a virus taxonomically and serologically related to HBV, the woodchuck hepatitis virus (WHV). In these studies the delta agent was transmitted from a chimpanzee chronically infected with HBV to woodchucks chronically infected with WHV. Attempts to transmit the delta agent to other non-primate species that harbor HBV-like "hepadnaviruses" are being planned.

TRANSMISSION STUDIES IN CHIMPANZEES

To date, 23 chimpanzees have been successfully infected with the delta agent. These include 13 chimpanzees acutely infected with HBV and 10 animals that were chronic carriers of

HBsAg (Table). The studies were carried out from 1978 to the present (Rizzetto, 1980, 1980b, 1981a, 1982; Bonino, 1983; Ponzetto, unpublished; Purcell and Gerin, unpublished).

Table

Attempts to Transmit the Delta Agent to Chimpanzees

HBV status of chimps	No. Tested	No. of Studies	No. infected with δ agent
Acute	15	15	13
Chronic	10	15	10
Immune	5	5	0
Other*	3	3	0
TOTAL	33	38	23

*Includes susceptible animals and an animal post-HBsAg but pre-anti-HBs that were inoculated with plasma containing delta agent but not HBV.

Delta Agent and Acute Type B Hepatitis

Acute HBV infection in the chimpanzee can support replication of the delta agent if the latter is introduced at the same time as HBV or after an interval of several weeks, when HBsAg has appeared in the serum. When simultaneous infection with the two agents occurs, the delta antigen is not detected until after HBsAg is detected in the serum.

Since, in some of these experiments, the number of hepatocytes available for infection far exceeded the number of infectious particles present, the chance of dual infection of the same hepatocyte with both viruses at the time of inoculation was very small. The delta agent must therefore be able to survive, either extracellularly or intracellularly, until sufficient numbers of hepatocytes have been infected with HBV to assure coinfection of the same hepatocyte with both viruses. We do not yet know how long the delta agent can survive prior to coinfection with HBV but such a strategy would obviously be beneficial to the perpetuation of the delta agent in nature.

Simultaneous infection with delta agent and HBV can result in simultaneous expression of the two viruses as measured by detection of delta antigen and hepatitis B core antigen (HBcAg) respectively. Alternatively, expression of HBcAg and the delta antigen can occur sequentially. In the latter case, HBcAg may precede or follow delta antigen and each is sometimes individually associated with hepatitis, resulting in a bimodal disease.

Superinfection of HBsAg-carrier Chimpanzees with the Delta Agent

The availability of chimpanzees chronically infected with HBV provided an opportunity to study the delta agent in a setting that is probably more analogous to the typical infection in man than is simultaneous coinfection. In these studies, chimpanzees whose chronic HBV infection had been well characterized (Thung, 1981) were sequentially infected with the delta agent. Such serial passage resulted in a progressive shortening of the incubation period to appearance of delta antigen and a progressive increase in the severity of associated hepatitis. Delta antigen was detected by immunofluorescence in an increasing proportion of hepatocytes after an incubation period of as little as one week. This was accompanied by a decrease in the number of hepatocytes that contained HBcAg detectable by immunofluorescence. In parallel with peak expression of delta antigen in the liver, delta antigen was detected in the plasma in association with 35-37 nm particles. Delta antigen in the plasma could not be detected directly but required disruption of the particles with detergent. Thus, delta antigen was an internal component of the particles. Shedding of delta antigen-containing particles in the plasma was generally detectable for only two or three weeks and peak shedding lasted only a few days. Hepatitis, as measured by elevation of liver enzymes and histologic changes, appeared coincident with or slightly following the peak of delta antigen in the liver and plasma. The hepatitis resulting from inoculation of chimpanzee-adapted delta agent was the most severe disease observed in extensive collaborative studies of experimental viral hepatitis in chimpanzees (Popper, 1980). None of the experimentally infected chimpanzees developed chronic infection with the delta agent. However, one chimpanzee did have a prolonged infection, associated with expression of delta antigen in the liver for approximately six months.

The disappearance of delta antigen from the liver and plasma was paralleled by the appearance of anti-delta in the serum in a pattern similar to the appearance of antibody to

HBcAg in HBV infections. In chimpanzees, as in man, anti-delta
following acute, self limiting delta-associated hepatitis was
often transient and of relatively low titer. Smedile et al.
(1982) recently demonstrated that transient anti-delta was of
the IgM class. Thus, seroepidemiologic studies of the delta
agent probably underestimate the true prevalence of infection.

We have been unable to detect serologic evidence for an
antigen on the surface of delta antigen-containing particles
that is unique to these particles and not characteristic of the
HBsAg coat that incapsidates the delta agent. This failure to
detect a unique surface antigen, coupled with the transient
nature of anti-delta in acute infections, suggests that
reinfection with the delta agent might occur. However,
attempts to reinfect HBsAg carrier chimpanzees with the same
inoculum of delta agent used for the first infection have been
unsuccessful to date (Rizzetto, 1981). One explanation for the
resistance of these chimpanzees may be the development of
antibody to one or more antigenic specificities of HBsAg that
were not shared by the HBsAg of the chronically infected host
and the HBsAg coat of the experimentally introduced delta
agent. Indeed, the HBsAg coat of newly synthesized delta
antigen-containing particles has the complement of antigens of
the host-associated HBsAg and not that of the introduced HBsAg
(Rizzetto, 1980b; Bonino, 1983). This strategy of constantly
changing coat antigens might also provide the delta agent with
survival advantages.

SIMILARITIES BETWEEN DELTA ASSOCIATED HEPATITIS AND NON-A,
NON-B HEPATITIS

The ability to transmit both the delta agent and non-A,
non-B hepatitis agents to chimpanzees has permitted a
comparison of the host response to these two partially
characterized agents. Some interesting similarities have been
observed.

Histopathology

In collaborative studies with Drs. H. Dienes and H. Popper
a detailed analysis of light microscopic changes occurring in
delta-associated hepatitis was completed (Dienes, 1981).
Briefly, changes consisted of diffuse hydropic swelling of
hepatocytes, sometimes associated with varying degrees of
steatosis and cholestasis, infiltration by inflammatory cells

of portal tracts, and eosinophilic granulation of hepatocytes.
The eosinophilic changes were indistinguishable from those seen
in chimpanzees experimentally infected with non-A, non-B
hepatitis viruses but did not resemble hepatitis in chimpanzees
infected with hepatitis A virus or hepatitis B virus. The
histologic changes seen in chimpanzees infected with the delta
agent closely resembled those seen in patients with
delta-associated hepatitis (Rizzetto, 1983).

Studies of electron micrographic changes occurring during
delta-associated hepatitis, (Rizzetto, 1980; Dienes, 1981;
Canese, 1983; Kamimura, 1983) demonstrated that the
similarities between delta agent-associated hepatitis and
non-A, non-B hepatitis detected by light microscopy were
paralleled by similarities of ultrastructure. Thus, the
peculiar cytoplasmic membranous alterations and aggregates of
nuclear particles first detected in chimpanzees infected with
non-A, non-B hepatitis (Shimizu, 1979) were also found in
chimpanzees infected with delta agent. In contrast, these
changes were never found in chimpanzees infected with HAV or
HBV. In general, the appearance of these electron micrographic
changes, especially the cytoplasmic changes, appeared to
parallel the appearance of liver damage and not the appearance
of delta antigen in the liver or plasma, suggesting that they
represent a unique pathologic response of the host to infection
and not necessarily actual viral components (Kamimura, 1983).
Thus, hepatitis caused by the delta agent was indistinguishable
by light or electron microscopy from hepatitis caused by non-A,
non-B agents but was quite different from hepatitis caused by
HAV or HBV, suggesting that the former two agents are
taxonomically similar or share similar pathways to cell damage.

Lack of Cross Protection Between Delta Agent-associated
Hepatitis and Non-A, Non-B Hepatitis.

Despite the similarities described above, infection with
the delta agent does not protect against subsequent infection
with non-A, non-B hepatitis virus and vice versa although
rechallenge with each homologous virus has generally
demonstrated solid immunity (Rizzetto, 1981; Feinstone, 1981).
However, limited experiments in which chimpanzees were
simultaneously infected with the delta agent and non-A, non-B
hepatitis virus suggested that one virus might interfere with
synthesis of the other (Purcell, unpublished). Such
interference might suggest taxonomic similarity between the two
viruses or simply competition for shared metabolic pathways.

Franklin Institute Press, p 355.

Rizzetto M, Verme G, Recchia S, Bonino F, Farci P, Arico S, Calzia R, Picciotto A, Colombo M, Popper H (1983). Chronic HBsAg hepatitis with intrahepatic expression of the delta antigen. An active and progressive disease unresponsive to immunosupressive treatment. Ann Intern Med 98:437.

Shimizu YH, Feinstone SM, Purcell RH, Alter HJ, London WT (1979). Non-A, non-B hepatitis: ultrastructural evidence for two agents in experimentally infected chimpanzees. Science 205:197.

Smedile A, Lavarini C, Crivelli O, Raimondo G, Fassone M, Rizzetto M (1982). Radioimmunoassay detection of IgM antibodies to the HBV-associated delta (δ) antigen: clinical significance in δ infection. J Med Virol 9:131.

Thung SN, Gerber MS, Purcell RH, London WT, Mihalik KB, Popper H (1981). Animal model: chimpanzee carriers of hepatitis B virus. Am J Path 105:328.

Viral Hepatitis and Delta Infection, pages 91–97
© 1983 Alan R. Liss, Inc., 150 Fifth Avenue, New York, NY 10011

PROPERTIES OF DELTA-ASSOCIATED RIBONUCLEIC ACID

B. Hoyer[1], F. Bonino[2], A. Ponzetto[2], K. Denniston[1],
J. Nelson[1], R. Purcell[3], and J.L. Gerin[1]
[1]Georgetown Univ., Rockville, MD 20852, [2]Ospedale
Maggiore S. Giovanni 10126 Torino, and [3]NIH,
Bethesda, MD 20205

Ribonucleic acid extracted from the particles
associated with infection with the delta agent (Rizzetto
1980; Bonino 1981) appears to have properties as unique
as those of the delta syndrome itself. The RNA and its
associated delta antigen (δ-Ag) are dependent upon a
concomitant hepatitis B virus (HBV) infection. The
particle found in serum prior to the appearance of delta
antibody (anti-δ) "borrows" hepatitis B surface antigen
(HBsAg) as a coat component; the RNA, uncoated, is
highly susceptible to RNAase and its existence in serum
is probably dependent upon the integrity of its HBsAg
coat.

The RNA associated with the delta particle (DAR)
is larger (1.75kb) than that of viroids and smaller than
that of the picornaviruses. The delta agent is, indeed,
so unusual that the term virus is not appropriate and
the appellation "pseudovirus" may be justifiable
or required; use of HBsAg from a DNA virus to supply the
coat of the δ-particle which contains RNA is also
unusual. Capsid exchange between Coxsackie viruses and
polioviruses is well known as are envelope protein
exchanges from leukemia viruses to defective sarcoma
viruses; the latter are all RNA viruses. A helper
function exists between adenoviruses (and some other DNA
viruses) and adeno-associated viruses, all DNA viruses.
Hence, the δ-particle occupies a unique niche in
virology and we will briefly summarize what is currently
known about its associated RNA.

The delta particle

DAR and δ-Ag are sequestered in a particle (Fig. 1)
with an HBsAg coat which isolates and/or protects the
RNA and δ-Ag from the surrounding environment (Rizzetto,
1980). The HBsAg is specified by HBV-DNA and it is
likely that DAR specifies δ-Ag; therefore the δ-particle
has a hybrid composition which apparently contributes to
some instability. Serum or plasma preparations exposed
to repeated freeze thaw cycles or prolonged exposure to
room temperature yield degraded or no DAR upon
extraction. The usual treatment for exposing δ-Ag from
serum, 0.3% NP40, not only unmasks the antigen but
results in the loss of DAR by nuclease degradation.

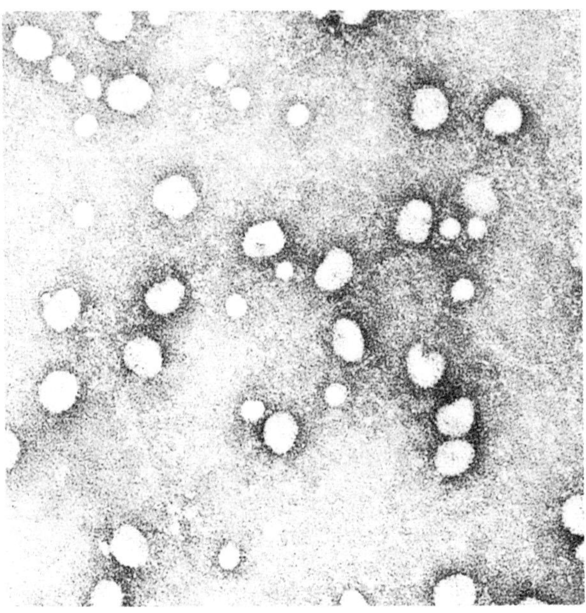

Figure 1. An electron micrograph of the 35-37 nm
delta-associated particle isolated from the serum of a
delta-infected chimpanzee. The preparation was
negatively-stained with 1% phosphotungstic acid; 150,000
X magnification.

DAR Size and Implied Structure

Native DAR, compared to bacteriophage lambda DNA fragments prepared by digestion with HindIII, has a size of 1.2 kb by agarose gel electrophoresis and ethidium bromide staining. Subsequent agarose gel electrophoresis of DAR and lambda HindIII DNA marker fragments denatured with glyoxal (McMaster 1977) yielded a size of 1.75 kb which is now our best estimate. Formaldehyde treatment of DAR and 28S and 18S ribosomal RNA coupled with comparative electrophoresis (Rave 1979), indicated that DAR is not 18S ribosomal RNA as its migration rate was greater than that of the 18S RNA. This is of some importance since ribosomal RNA might conceivably be released from degenerated hepatocytes along with δ-Ag and be coated with HBsAg because of the probable affinity between these two antigens. The lack of comigration of DAR and 18S RNA rules out this possibility and strengthens the conclusion that DAR is a unique type of RNA which is associated with an infectious agent.

The more rapid migration of DAR in its undenatured form, compared with that of denatured DAR, as well as preferred sites for RNAase digestion (see Rizzetto 1980, Fig 7), indicate that DAR, is strongly base paired; the specific cleavage site, indicated by two distinct fluorescent bands in the lane treated with DNAase, was due to a contamination of the DNAase with sufficient RNAase to cause the cleavage. An enzyme which adds a poly(A) tail to the 3' end of RNA readily adds poly(A) tracts to DAR. This indicates that a free 3' end exists and that DAR is probably linear rather than a closed circular RNA such as that found in viroids.

Detection of DAR

Delta RNA was first observed by ethidium bromide staining of an agarose gel. DAR from at least 0.5 ml of serum or plasma from a sample containing peak δ-Ag is necessary for detection by this relatively insensitive procedure. However, avian myeloblastosis virus reverse transcriptase may be used to make ^{32}P-labeled cDNA from DAR. The ^{32}P-cDNA may then be used to probe high salt transfers (Thomas 1980) of DAR

from formaldehyde-agarose gels (Rave 1979) to
nitrocellulose; microliter quantities of serum yield
sufficient DAR for rapid detection by autoradiography.
We have also developed plasmids containing DAR sequences
which may be ^{32}P-labeled by nick translation; this
^{32}P-labeled DNA is also useful as a probe for DAR
transferred from agarose gels and/or spotted on
appropriate matrices such as nitrocellulose.

In the chimpanzee model system, the appearance of
anti-δ coincides with the disappearance of δ-Ag and DAR
from serum. Chronic δ-infection has not been observed
in chimpanzees but it is relatively common in humans.
Anti-δ titers are often high in δ-carriers and the
presence of this antibody makes serological detection of
δ-Ag difficult. Certain diagnosis of chronic
δ-infection now requires liver biopsies coupled with
immunofluoresence assays; however, detection of DAR from
serum may provide an alternative and noninvasive
diagnostic method. It is known that sera from humans
may transmit δ-infection to other humans or chimpanzees;
this indicates the presence of δ-particles if these
particles are, indeed, the infectious units. Therefore
use of sufficient volumes of serum for preparation of
DAR, combined with sensitive probes and autoradiography,
may allow recognition of chronic δ-infection through its
associated nucleic acid rather than protein.

DAR as a biological molecule

DAR does not have a 3' poly(A) tail as determined
by lack of binding to oligo-dT cellulose. This
indicates that the delta agent either has the properties
of a negative strand virus (where the DAR is not
messenger RNA but its complementary strand serves this
purpose) or that it resembles histone or plant RNAs
which serve as messengers but lack a poly(A) tail. If
the negative strand hypothesis is true, an RNA
complementary to DAR may eventually be found.

The δ-particle could contain an enzyme similar to
the reverse transcriptase of the retroviruses.
Therefore, we looked for reverse transcriptase using
techniques developed by RNA tumor virologists; no
evidence for the presence of transcriptase was found.

This negative result is not unexpected since DAR is only
of sufficient size to specify δ-Ag and not the usually
larger transcriptases.

DAR is not homologous to HBV-DNA

One of the easily foreseen possibilities is that
DAR may be homologous to part of HBV (about half of one
HBV strand) and need the lacking DNA to supply "helper"
functions. We have examined numerous transfers from
agarose gels which contain DAR and HBV. When these
transfers are probed with ^{32}P HBV DNA, radioactive
regions appear which are unique to HBV and not DAR; when
the same transfer is probed with ^{32}P-cDNA from DAR or a
cloned portion of DAR, radioactive regions unique to DAR
appear. Therefore, no sequence homology between DAR and
HBV is indicated.

Effect of the δ-agent on HBV DNA

Animals co-infected with the delta agent all have
chronic or developing HBV infections. When the delta
particle is present in the blood of infected animals,
the amount of HBV-DNA in serum (presumably from Dane
particles) decreases; this decrease continues as the
amount of δ-Ag in serum increases. When peak
concentrations of DAR and δ-Ag are reached little or no
HBV-DNA is detected by ^{32}P HBV DNA probes and
autoradiography. After anti-δ appears, the amount of
HBV DNA gradually returns to its original level. This
decrease of HBV DNA may possibly be the result of the
use of HBsAg as the delta particle coat. About 300
HBsAg molecules (average M.W. 25,000) would be required
for each delta particle. If one RNA molecule is present
in each delta particle, as many as 3×10^{14} HBsAg
molecules would be required to form the HBsAg coats for
one microgram of DAR; about 1 ug of DAR is present per
ml of serum at the δ-Ag peak as inferred from
comparative ethidium bromide staining of DAR and
ribosomal RNA. The quantity of HBsAg usurped by the
delta particle may cause an HBsAg deficit which
could interfere with the coating and/or transport of the
hepatitis B virions; other factors, of course, may be
involved in the decrease, during δ-infection, of HBV DNA
in serum.

Presence of DAR in liver

     Quick frozen needle biopsies of chimpanzee liver
were used to prepare RNA. This RNA was subjected to
agarose gel electrophoresis in the presence
of formaldehyde and transferred to nitrocellulose.
Probing with ^{32}P nick translated, cloned cDNA derived
from DAR indicated radioactive regions in the agarose
gels of RNA from some biopsies which corresponded to the
size of DAR derived from serum. Some of the biopsies
expected to yield a DAR signal failed to do so; this
suggests that the ability to detect DAR in liver is
closely related to the quality of the preparative
procedures (rapidity of sampling, quick freezing and no
freeze-thaw of the sample) as well as the actual
presence of DAR. The presence of DAR in delta-infected
liver, along with δ-Ag, supports the concept that DAR
specifies (directly or indirectly) δ-Ag.

Reactivity of DAR probes

     Nearly all of our work has been done with DAR
initially derived from the serum of one patient. Our
^{32}P-labeled probes have also been derived from this same
source. The sequence similarity of DAR is indicated by
the fact that the probe also reacts with RNA from the
serum of another delta infected patient (Bonino 1981).
The antigenic similarity of δ-Ag from various patients
from many different geographic regions has been amply
demonstrated by their reaction with anti-δ. Sequence
analysis of DAR or its cloned cDNA may be used to
determine possible variations in the amino acid
sequences of polypeptides of δ-Ag from various patients.
The availability of δ-probes will also be useful for the
clinical diagnosis of delta infection and the study of
associated molecular biological reactions.

REFERENCES

Bonino F, Hoyer B, Ford E, Shih J, Purcell R, Gerin J.
   (1981). The δ-agent: HBsAg particles with δ-antigen
   and RNA in the serum of an HBV carrier. Hepatology
   1:127.

McMaster G, Carmichael G. (1977). Analysis of single-and double-stranded nucleic acids in polyacrylamide and agarose gels by using glyoxal and acridine orange. Proc Natl Acad Sci USA 74:4835.

Rave N, Crkvenjakov R, Boedtker, H. (1979). Identification of procollagen mRNAs transferred to diazobenzyl-oxymethyl paper from formaldehyde agarose gels. Nucleic Acid Res 6:3559.

Rizzetto M, Hoyer B, Canese M, Shih J, Purcell R, Gerin J. (1980). The δ-agent: Association of δ-antigen with hepatitis B surface antigen and RNA in serum of δ-infected chimpanzees. Proc Natl Acad Sci USA 77:6124.

Thomas P. (1980). Hybridization of denatured RNA and small DNA fragments transferred to nitrocellulose. Proc Natl Acad Sci USA 77:5201.

ULTRASTRUCTURAL ASPECTS OF DELTA (δ) INFECTED LIVER
BIOPSIES

Maria Grazia Canese and Rosanna Novara
Instituto Anatomia Patologica, Torino
Italy

The ultrastructural aspects of δ infection were
analyzed by electron and immunoelectron microscopy in
liver biopsies of experimentally infected chimpanzees
and naturally infected patients.

Electron Microscopy

a) Chimpanzee liver biopsies.
Electron microscopy studies in serial weekly
biopsies of 9 chimpanzees inoculated with serum from
human hepatitis B surface antigen (HBsAg) carriers with
intrahepatic δ-antigen (δ-Ag) did not demonstrate
ultrastructural aspects that were specific to δ
infection (Canese et al., 1983). Virus-like particles
other than the hepatitis B virus (HBV) subunits were not
observed. Post-inoculation liver samples often showed
cytoplasmic and nuclear alterations that were not seen
in pre-inoculation samples. The cytoplasmic alterations
consisted of structures composed of double-unit
membranes with electron dense material, that were formed
by the opposition of smooth endoplasmic reticulum
membranes on the cytoplasmic face and displayed an
undulating, loop, ring or double-ring shape. They
projected into or were enclosed by into the cisternae of
smooth endoplasmic reticulum (Fig. 1). Besides these
cytoplasmic alterations, bundles of microtubules with a
diameter of 23 nm and an internal channel of 10 nm were
frequently observed (Canese et al., 1983). These
changes occurred concomitantly with an increase of fatty
changes in the liver.

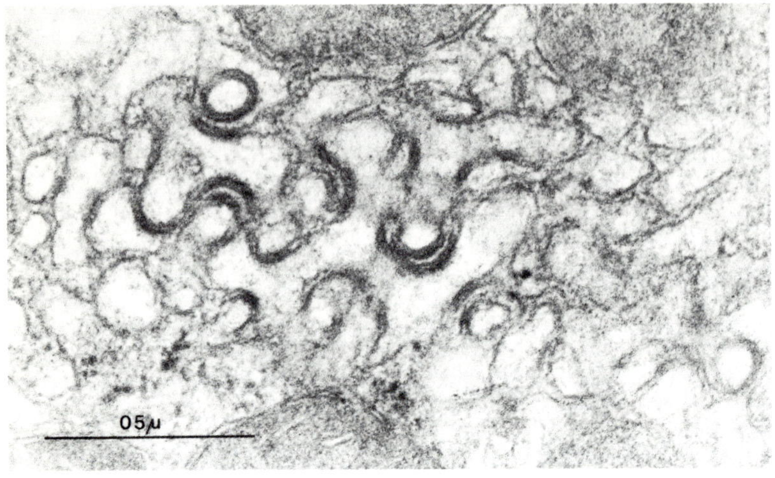

Fig. 1. Liver biopsy of δ-infected chimpanzee:
cytoplasmic alteration.

The nuclear alteration consisted of aggregates of
irregular dense particles of 20-30 nm in diameter (Fig.
2). One or two aggregates of particles were usually
observed in a single nucleus; occasionally up to 6 or7
were counted. The nuclei with this change had an
irregular outline and clumped chromatin. In the
majority of chimpanzees both types of alterations could
be detected in the same biopsy or in different serial
specimens. The ultrastructural changes were maximal in
coincidence with the intrahepatic synthesis of δ-Ag and
aminotransferase elevation, but were also observed
independently of these two events (Fig. 3).

b)   Human liver biopsies.
    A previous ultrastructural study of human liver
biopsies containing δ-Ag had also failed to demonstrate
aspects specific to δ infection. Electron dense 20-30
nm particles of irregular shape were frequently observed
in the human material. The particles were free or
aggregated in chains and clusters. They did not exhibit
any feature allowing distinction from the granular
material ascribed to normal nuclear components

or degenerative phenomena (Canese et al., 1979). To
establish the significance of the nuclear alterations in
δ infection, 23 liver biopsies from HBsAg chronic
carriers with δ-infection were reviewed and compared
with a group of 7 liver biopsies from patients with
chronic HBV hepatitis and a group of 11 patients with
non A-non B hepatitis. Of the 23 patients with
δ infection, 17 had δ-Ag in the liver; 6 had antibody to
δ in serum but were negative for intrahepatic δ-Ag. In
the non A-non B group were included the liver biopsies
from 3 drug addicts and 8 polytransfused patients, all
with hepatitis by histology but without evidence in the
serum and liver of infection with known hepatitis
viruses. Aggregates of intranuclear particles similar
to those observed in chimpanzees with experimental
δ infection (Fig. 4) were found in all groups with a
prevalence varying from 29% in hepatitis B, to 61% in
HBsAg-positive hepatitis with δ infection, to 91% in non
A-non B hepatitis (Table 1).

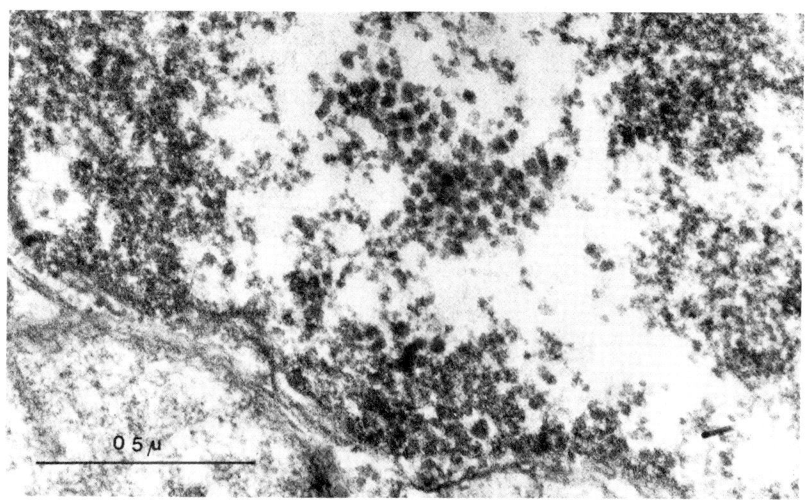

Fig. 2. Liver biopsy of δ-infected chimpanzee: group
of round particles in a nucleus.

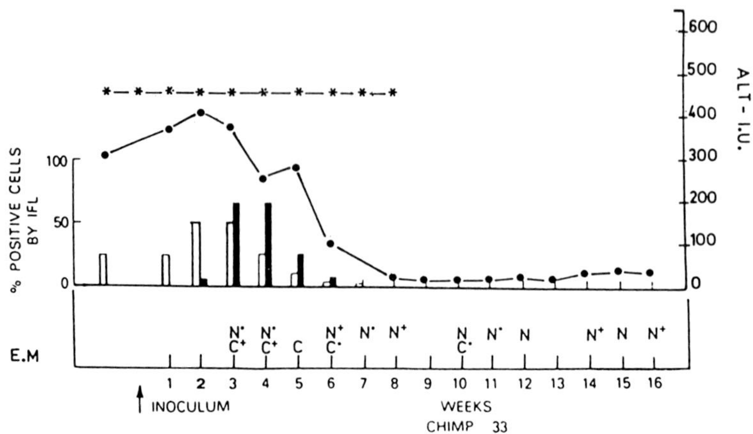

Fig. 3. Correlation between infectious events, hepatitis and the ultrastructural liver aspects in a chimpanzee inoculated with δ agent. From top to bottom: (*---*): HBsAg in blood; (---): alanine aminotransferase level in blood. Solid vertical and open vertical bars are respectively δ-Ag and HBcAg in the liver by immunofluorescence. The corresponding ultrastructural changes are reported over the time-line divided in weeks: C = cytoplasmic alterations; N = nuclear alterations; + = large quantity; . = small quantity.

Table 1.

Prevalence of nuclear changes (NC) in human biopsies.

Type of Hepatitis	N° of Biopsies	Biopsies Positive for NC
δ-Hepatitis	23	14 (61%)
Hepatitis B	7	2 (29%)
Non A-non B	11	10 (91%)

Both in δ and non A-non B hepatitis the nuclear
alterations were occasionally observed also in
sinusoidal cells and in epithelial cells of biliary
ducts in the portal tracts. The particles were
contained in dysplastic nuclei and in cells that
displayed ultrastructural features of cytological
damage. Their presence was not correlated with
expression of δ-Ag in liver; many biopsies with a large
number of nuclei positive for δ-Ag in immunofluorescence
showed only a few altered nuclei by EM, while 2 of the 6
biopsies negative for δ-Ag displayed a large number of
nuclei with the aggegated particles. No cytoplasmic
alterations similar to those observed in δ and in non
A-non B infected chimpanzees (Shimizu et al., 1979,
Pfeifer et al., 1980) were observed in human samples.

<u>Immunoelectronmicroscopy</u>

    Liver biopsies containing δ-Ag were stained with
IgG or Fab$_1$ anti-δ labelled with horse-radish peroxidase
(HRPO). Results were similar in man (Canese et al.,
1979) and in chimpanzee (Rizzetto et al., 1980). In the
different biopsies examined a variable proportion of
nuclei were stained by the HRPO conjugate. The product
of the peroxidase reaction was deposited with an
irregular granular morphology all over (Fig. 5a) or in
part of the nucleus, usually with a perichromatin and
interchromatin distribution. The granular material was
amorphous, with a soft, often indistinct outline. The
HRPO-positive granules were isolated or grouped in
clusters of chains, connected by thin filaments (Fig.
5b). They probably represent aggregates of intranuclear
δ-Ag. No reaction was observed in the cytoplasm of
hepatocytes.

CONCLUSIONS

    Electron and immunoelectronmicroscopy of liver
biopsies from patients and chimpanzees with δ-infection
have not shown ultrastructural aspects unique to this
infection.
    The intranuclear aggregates of particles observed
in humans and animals were repeatedly noted also in
natural and experimental non A-non B hepatitis (Shimizu
et al., 1979, Cabral et al., 1981). We have observed
identical nuclear particles in human HBV disease without

δ and Spichtin et al. (Dr. F. Gudat, personal
communication) have recently reported an analogous
finding in liver biopsies from healthy volunteers.
Probably this nuclear change represents a non-specific
degenerative feature of the liver cell, occurring in
different liver diseases. Cytoplasmic alterations
similar to those observed in δ infected chimpanzees were
often described in chimpanzees infected with non A-non B
strains (Shimizu et al., 1979, Jackson et al., 1979,
Pfeifer et al., 1980). These changes were not
detectable in human liver biopsies from patients with
δ and non A-non B hepatitis. Ultrastructural data
provided additional evidence to the hypothesis that
δ agent is distinct from HBV and may possibly share
characteristics of non A-non B viruses of hepatitis.

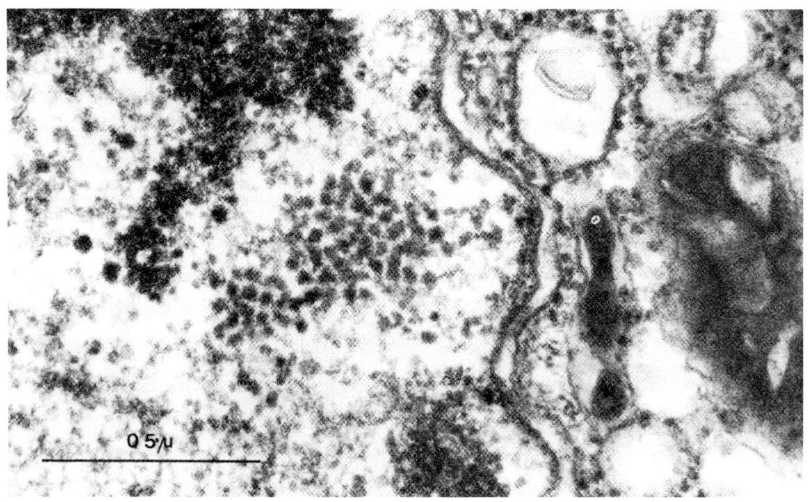

Fig. 4. Liver biopsy of δ-infected patient: group of
round particles in a nucleus.

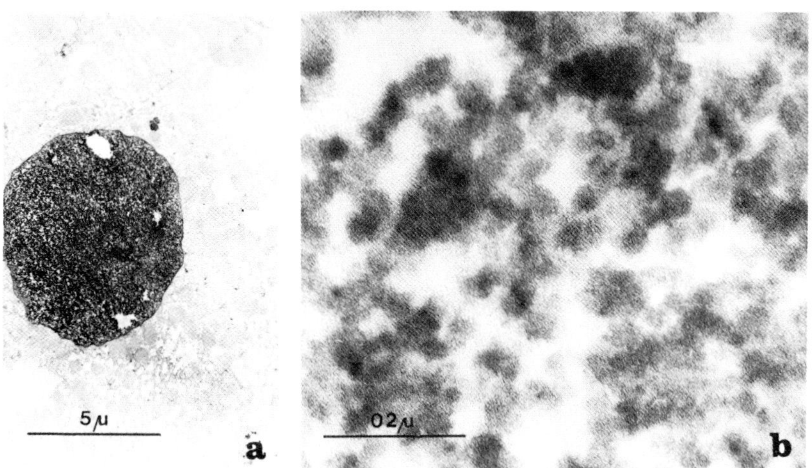

Fig. 5. Liver biopsy of a δ-infected chimpanzee stained
with HRPO labelled anti-δ. a) A nucleus intensely
stained; b) at higher magnification: granular aspects
of the reaction product.

REFERENCES

Cabral GA, Marciano-Cabral F, Patterson M, Galen EA,
    Carithers RL. (1981). Nuclear changes in
    hepatocytes of patients with non A-non B hepatitis.
    Gastroenterol 81:120.
Canese MG, Rizzetto M, Arico S, Crivelli O, Zanetti AR,
    Macchiorlatti E, Ponzetto A, Leone L, Mollo F, Verme
    G. (1979). An ultrastructural and
    immunohistochemical study on the δ antigen associated
    with the hepatitis B virus. J Pathol 128:169.
Canese MG, Rizzetto M, Novara R, London WT, Purcell RH.
    (1983). Experimental infection of chimpanzees with
    the HBsAg-associated Delta (δ) agent. An
    ultrastructural study. J Med Virol (in press).
Jackson D, Tabor E, Gerety RJ. (1979). Acute non A-non
    B hepatitis: Specific ultrastructural alterations in
    endoplasmic reticulum of infected hepatocytes.
    Lancet 1:1249.
Pfeifer U, Thomssen R, Legler K, Bottcher U, Gerlich W,
    Weinmann E, Klinge O. (1980). Experimental non

A-non B hepatitis: four types of cytoplasmic
alteration in hepatocytes of infected chimpanzees.
Virchows Arc B Cell Path 33:233.
Rizzetto M, Canese MG, Gerin JL, London WT, Sly DL ,
Purcell RH. (1980). Transmission of the hepatitis B
virus-associated Delta-antigen to chimpanzees.
J Infect Dis 141:590.
Shimizu YK, Feinstone SM, Purcell RH, Alter HJ, London
WT. (1979). Non A-non B hepatitis: Ultrastructural
evidence for two agents in experimentally infected
chimpanzees. Science 205:197.

Viral Hepatitis and Delta Infection, pages 107–112
© 1983 Alan R. Liss, Inc., 150 Fifth Avenue, New York, NY 10011

EXPERIMENTAL TRANSMISSION OF THE DELTA AGENT TO THE
EASTERN WOODCHUCK (Marmota Monax).

Antonio Ponzetto, MD[1], Robert H. Purcell,
MD[2], John L. Gerin, PhD[3]. [1]Div. of
Gastroenterology, Ospedale Molinette, Torino,
Italy; [2]Laboratory of Infectious Disease,
NIAID, NIH, Bethesda, MD; [3]Georgetown
University, Rockville, MD.

INTRODUCTION

All available evidence indicates that delta agent
depends on obligatory helper function of HBV for
biological expression (Rizzetto, 1980a, 1980b). The
discovery of viruses that have characteristics and
tissue tropism similar to HBV, and naturally infect
animal species different from primates (for review:
Summers, 1981), has posed the question of whether this
novel family (collectively named Hepadnaviruses) can
also support delta infection.

Delta infectivity studies were planned in
woodchucks chronically infected with a virus related to
HBV, the woodchuck hepatitis virus (WHV). Reasons for
selecting this animal were the availability of the full
battery of assays for serum and liver markers of WHV
infection (Wong, 1982, Cote, 1982, Mitamura, 1982), and
the demonstration that only this species (among those
infected by HBV-like viruses) mimics the range of
lesions observed in HBV-infected humans (Popper, 1981,
Summers, 1980).

TRANSMISSION STUDIES

Three woodchucks (numbers 69, 35 and 80), whose
chronic WHV carrier status were well documented by
serological and immunofluorescence studies, were
inoculated with the delta agent. All had circulating
Woodchuck hepatitis surface antigen (WHsAg) for longer
than six months and had woodchuck hepatitis core antigen

(WHcAg) in liver tissue. In each animal, the WHV-DNA
and DNA-polymerase in serum had also remained elevated
for the same period of time.

The inoculum was plasma containing delta-antigen
(δAg), taken from a chimpanzee at the peak of δ viremia
while the animal was experiencing acute hepatitis. This
inoculum contained 10^6 chimpanzee infectious doses of
HBV, and was infectious for the δ agent (in HBsAg
positive chimpanzees) at a dilution greater than 10^{-11};
plasma was injected undiluted in a 1 ml dose,
intravenously.

Evidence of delta infection was found in all three
woodchucks, and the course was similar to that described
in chimpanzees (Rizzetto, 1980a). The animals exhibited
δ-Ag in the nuclei of hepatocytes, demonstrated by
direct immunofluorescence (IF) with fluoresceinated
human antibody to δ (anti-δ) on frozen section from
liver biopsies. Delta-Ag appeared one week
post-inoculation in liver of animal N° 35, and on the
third week in the two other. In each woodchuck it could
be demonstrated in hepatic tissue for two to three weeks
(Figure 1).

At variance with the large number of positive
nuclei observed in experimental delta infection of
chimpanzees the number of hepatocytes showing δ-Ag
in woodchucks was limited: it ranged from 2 to about
10% of cells, despite the abundant presence in the same
hepatocytes of the core antigen of WHV (WHcAg) (from 30%
to 60% of cells).

Delta-Ag was shed in serum of woodchuck N° 35 and
69 beginning two weeks post-inoculation. For its
detection a standard radioimmunoassay based on human
reagents was used. Animal N° 80 did not circulate
demonstrable levels of δ-Ag. Delta antigenemia was
observed in both positive animals for two weeks, and
then abruptly disappeared from serum. Antibody to δ
appeared in serum of woodchuck N° 35 five weeks after
inoculation, and one week after clearance of δ-Ag from
circulation. Antibody to rapidly rose to a titer of
$10^{3.5}$ and this titer persisted until the animal died
with primary hepatocellular carcinoma (PHC) six months
later.

Woodchuck N° 69 had already developed a large PHC
at the time of delta infection. It was sacrificed while
still δ-Ag positive; δ-Ag was not detected in the
carcinomatous portion of the liver and transformed
hepatocytes also failed to stain for WHV antigens.

No antibody response was elicited in animal N° 80 which had not developed delta antigenemia. To determine whether the delta agent needed some form of adaptation to the new species, a second woodchuck was inoculated with serum containing agent from the first passage in woodchuck.

SECOND PASSAGE OF DELTA IN A CHRONIC WHV CARRIER WOODCHUCK

Inoculation of serum from the first passage (woodchuck N° 69) to another chronic WHV carrier (N° 86) resulted in higher levels of δ-Ag in serum, at least twice as much as that produced on first passage. There was a increase in the number of δ-Ag positive nuclei in the liver: about 40% of hepatocyte nuclei were stained in immunofluorescence by anti-δ (Figure 1).
Serum with peak δ-Ag from woodchuck N° 86 was used to demonstrate the presence of the putative virion.
Isopycnic banding of the woodchuck serum in cesium chloride was carried out in parallel with serum taken from a chimpanzee at the peak of delta antigenemia. Particles at the expected buoyant density of 1.245 gm/cm^3 were recovered from the chimpanzee serum. Woodchuck serum also generated a discrete band of δ-Ag; which was revealed only after detergent treatment (Nonidet P40). Electron microscopic examination of the δ-Ag peak showed particles similar in morphology to the delta particle of chimpanzee, but with a lower buoyant density.
Testing the gradient fractions by two sets of monoclonal antibodies (McAbs), highly specific toward HBsAg and WHsAg (Cote, 1982), demonstrated that woodchuck δ-Ag was circulating within a capsid provided by WHV. Woodchuck serum and fractions were strongly positive in the McAb WHsAg test, and negative in the McAb HBsAg test. It appears, therefore, that δ-Ag, was transcapsidated within a WHsAg coat of lower buoyant density than HBsAg, in analogy with the previous finding in chimpanzees that the surface antigen coat of the delta particle is specified by host HBV and not by HBV introduced with inoculum (Rizzetto, 1980b).

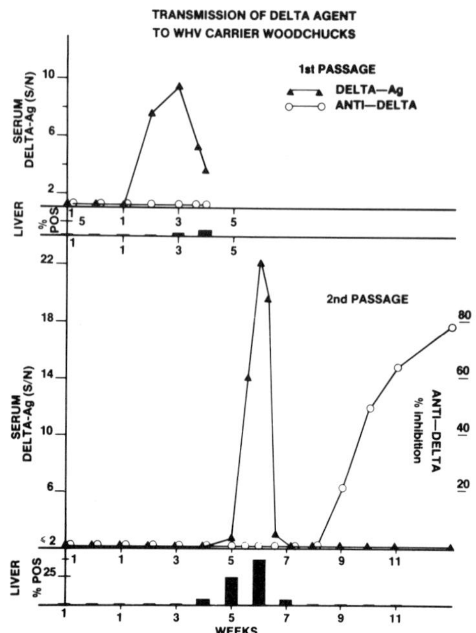

<u>Figure</u> 1

Course of delta infection in woodchuck.

<u>Top</u>: Woodchuck N° 69 inoculated with chimpanzee derived δ-Ag. At week 4 post-inoculation the animal was sacrificed, while still positive δ-Ag in liver and serum.

<u>Bottom</u>: Second passage of δ agent in woodchuck N° 86 inoculated with serum from woodchuck N° 69. Closed triangles represent δ-Ag, open circles anti-δ. Black bars stand for the amount of liver δ-Ag.

SUPPRESSION OF WHV SYNTHESIS BY DELTA INFECTION IN
WOODCHUCKS.

A further similarity of woodchuck delta infection
with the chimpanzee infection was the marked inhibition
of synthesis of the markers of WHV seen in coincidence
with appearance of δ-Ag in serum. Typically, WHsAg
levels decreased while δ-Ag was rising, and they
remained temporarily depressed thereafter. WHV-DNA in
serum fell to an almost undetectable level as soon as
delta-Ag appeared, but quickly returned to pre-delta
values once δ-Ag was cleared from the blood.

CONCLUSIONS

The host range of delta agent extends to
non-primates. The woodchuck represents a suitable model
to study the biology of the new pathogen and the
mechanism whereby it induces disease. Since WHV can
provide "helper" effect to the delta agent, it is
possible that other HBV-like viruses are able to do so.
The delta containing particle of the woodchuck has
an outer coat consisting of the woodchuck surface
antigen, borrowed from WHV. It is thus a property of
delta agent to transcapsidate, and to use surface
antigen from the hepatitis virus already infecting the
host. This peculiarity might provide delta with the
capacity of adaptation in different animal species.

REFERENCES

Cote PJ, Dapolito GM, Shih JW-K, Gerin JL (1982).
    Surface antigenic determinants of mammalian
    "Hepadnaviruses" defined by group- and class-specific
    monoclonal antibodies. J Virol 42:135.
Gerin JL, Ponzetto A, London WT, Sly DL, Purcell (1982).
    Serial passage of the delta agent in chimpanzees.
    Federation Proceedings 41:445.
Mitamura K, Hoyer BH, Ponzetto A, Nelson J, Purcell RH,
    Gerin JL (1982). Woodchuck hepatitis virus DNA in
    woodchuck liver tissues. Hepatology 2:47 (Suppl).
Popper H, Shih JW-K, Gerin JL, Wong DC, Hoyer BH, London
    WT, Sly DL, Purcell RH (1981). Woodchuck hepatitis
    and hepatocellular carcinoma: correlation of
    histologic with virologic observations. Hepatology
    1:91.

Rizzetto M, Canese MG, Gerin JL, London WT, Sly DL, Purcell RH (1980a). Transmission of the hepatitis B virus-associated delta antigen to chimpanzees. J Inf Dis. 121:590.

Rizzetto M, Hoyer BH, Canese MG, Shih JW-K, Purcell RH, Gerin JL (1980b). Delta antigen: the association of delta-antigen with hepatitis B surface antigen and ribonucleic acid in the serum of delta infected chimpanzees. Proc Natl AcaD Sci USA 77:6124.

Summers J (1981). Three recently described animal virus models for human hepatitis B virus. Hepatology 1:179.

Summers J, Smolec JM, Werner BG, Tyler GV, Snyder R (1979). Properties and distribution of woodchuck hepatitis virus. In Bianchi L, Gerok W, Sickinger K, Stalter GA (eds): Virus and the liver, Lancaster: MTP Press p. 223.

Wong DC, Shih JW-K, Purcell RH, Gerin JL, London WT (1982). Natural and experimental infection of woodchucks with woodchuck hepatitis virus, as measured by new, specific assays for woodchuck surface antigen and antibody. J Clin Immunol 15:484.

Viral Hepatitis and Delta Infection, pages 113–119
© 1983 Alan R. Liss, Inc., 150 Fifth Avenue, New York, NY 10011

EPIDEMIOLOGY OF THE DELTA AGENT: AN INTRODUCTION

R.H. Purcell, M.D.[1] and J. L. Gerin, Ph.D.[2]

[1]Laboratory of Infectious Diseases, NIAID
National Institutes of Health, Bethesda, MD. 20205

[2]Division of Molecular Virology and Immunology
Georgetown U. Medical School, Rockville, MD. 20852

In 1977 Rizzetto et al. described a "new" antigen that was detected by immunofluorescence in the nuclei of hepatocytes from Italian patients with chronic type B hepatitis (Rizzetto, 1977). The antigen resembled hepatitis B core antigen (HBcAg) and, indeed, was originally thought to be HBcAg until discrepant results obtained with different fluorescein-labelled convalescent sera revealed it to be antigenically distinct from HBcAg but related in some way to chronic infection with hepatitis B virus (HBV). The new antigen, which appeared to be associated invariably with HBV infection, rarely coexisted with HBcAg: usually one or the other antigen was present in any given liver biopsy from a patient with chronic type B hepatitis. The antigen was never found in biopsies from patients with HBsAg-negative hepatitis and only a proportion of patients with HBsAg-positive hepatitis had the antigen or antibody to it (Arico et al. 1978, Picciotto et al. 1981). The new specificities were called delta antigen and anti-delta.

In subsequent studies carried out at the National Institutes of Health and Georgetown University in the United States, Rizzetto was able to extract delta antigen from the liver of a fatal case of hepatitis and to use this partially characterized antigen for the development of a sensitive and specific radioimmunoassay for delta antigen and anti-delta (Rizzetto 1980). The human anti-delta-containing serum used in these solid-phase radioimmunoassays was selected because it contained a high titer of anti-delta but a negligible titer of anti-HBc. The resultant assays were highly specific and did not cross-react with HBsAg, HBcAg, HBeAg, or hepatitis A viral antigen (or their respective antibodies) or with human serum components or a variety of autoantibodies associated with various types of liver disease.

Inoculation of chimpanzees with serum from Italian patients with chronic type B hepatitis and delta antigen resulted in the transmission of type B hepatitis that was also associated with delta antigen in the chimpanzees (Rizzetto 1980). Inoculation of chimpanzees with HBV from other clinical sources resulted in transmission of HBV but not the appearance of delta antigen. Other transmission studies in chimpanzees confirmed that delta antigen was an internal component of a transmissible agent that was defective and required coinfection with HBV for viral replication (Rizzetto 1981).

Armed with sensitive and specific radioimmunoassays for delta antigen and anti-delta and the knowledge that the antigen was associated with a transmissible agent, Rizzetto studied the seroepidemiology of the delta agent (Rizzetto 1979, Rizzetto 1980). Anti-delta was never found in HBsAg-negative individuals, whether or not they had hepatitis (except in an occasional individual who had only recently recovered from HBsAg-positive hepatitis). Among HBsAg-positive individuals, anti-delta was found in less than 10% of patients with acute hepatitis or who were asymtomatic carriers of HBsAg but it was found in 25% of patients with chronic type B hepatitis (Rizzetto 1981). Additional studies established that the delta agent was, indeed, more likely to be associated with clinically important forms of type B hepatitis. Furthermore, cases of clinically important chronic "type B hepatitis" often lacked the markers of active HBV replication (serum hepatitis B e antigen and DNA polymerase activity and intrahepatic HBcAg) that are usually present in such patients (Arico et al 1978, Picciotto et al. 1979, Rizzetto 1980, Rizzetto 1979), suggesting that the delta agent played an active role in the pathology of type B hepatitis and that it was not simply a "passenger". The pathogenicity of the delta agent was established by transmission studies in chimpanzees (Rizzetto 1980). Recently several seroepidemiologic studies of HBsAg-positive fulminant hepatitis in Europe and the United States have revealed that between a quarter and a half of such cases have evidence of an associated infection with the delta agent (Smedile 1982, Mosley, unpublished). The association of the delta agent with other sequelae of HBV infection is less certain. A convincing association between infection with the delta agent and hepatocellular carcinoma has not been detected although extensive serologic surveys of hepatocellular

carcinoma patients from different geograpic regions have not
yet been carried out.

Other seroepidemiologic studies revealed a high prevalence
of anti-delta in individuals who received massive or repeated
exposures to blood, blood products or secretions. These
included recipients of massive blood transfusions, patients
with hemophilia or thalassemia, users of illicit parenteral
drugs and, to a lesser extent, male homosexuals (Rizzetto 1981,
Rizzetto 1979, Rizzetto 1980, Raimondo 1982).

The geographic distribution of the delta agent, based upon
studies of the prevalence of delta antigen or anti-delta in
HBsAg-positive individuals, has been particularly interesting
but confusing. Initial studies revealed that 27% of
HBsAg-positive Italians had anti-delta (Rizzetto 1980, Rizzetto
1981). When examined by region, the prevalence was found to be
73% in Southern Italy and only 16% in Northern Italy. This
high prevalence of anti-delta in Italians from the South was
confirmed (Rizzetto 1982) and the frequent association of the
delta agent with acute type B hepatitis established (Rizzetto
1982). Furthermore, most of the positive patients in the north
were found to be immigrants from the south. Analysis of sera
from other parts of Europe suggested a very spotty distribution
for the delta agent, with high prevalences detected in
Scandinavian countries but low prevalences in other Western and
Central European countries (Rizzetto 1980, Rizzetto 1981).
This unusual pattern of distribution was largely explained by
analysis of the patients tested: many of the sera from
apparent high-prevalence countries were from individuals from
high-risk populations such as hemophiliacs and illicit drug
users. More extensive seroepidemiologic surveys have confirmed
a higher prevalence of anti-delta in Southern European
countries and a lower prevalence in Northern European countries
in the general population but a high prevalence in high-risk
populations in both regions (Rizzetto 1982, Hansson 1982).

Recent seroepidemiologic studies of the delta agent,
carried out in collaboration with Drs. S. Hadler and D. Francis
of the Centers for Disease control as well as others, and using
more sensitive assays for delta antigen and antibody have
conclusively demonstrated a world-wide distribution of the
agent. Regions with particularly high prevalences of antibody
have been found in South America, Africa, the Middle East and
Southern Europe. An epidemic of severe hepatitis associated
with the delta agent was studied in Venezuela (Hadler 1983).
That outbreak occurred among an indigenous Indian population

and was characterized by a high prevalence of fulminant and
severe subacute hepatitis. A similar association with severe
hepatitis probably exists in Brazil. The ecology of the delta
agent is less clear in Africa and the Middle East but
prevalences of anti-delta as high as 50% in HBsAg-positive
individuals in some regions suggest an important pathologic
role. Interestingly, very little evidence for infection with
the delta agent has been found throughout Asia despite a
relatively high prevalence of HBsAg-positive hepatitis that
resembles dual infections of HBV and the delta agent elsewhere.
Additional testing must be carried out to determine if the
delta agent is responsible for this "delta-like" hepatitis or
if possibly another serotype of delta-like agent fills the
ecological niche that the delta agent fills elsewhere.

Transmission of the delta agent is still poorly understood.
Because of its obligatory association with HBV, its epidemiology
resembles that of the latter agent. Thus, the delta agent can
be transmitted by blood and blood products and probably by
those mechanisms of nonparenteral transmission associated with
HBV such as sexual transmission. Maternal-fetal transmission
of the delta agent was demonstrated in one case in which HBV
was similarly transmitted (Zanetti 1982). Hadler suggested
that the delta agent may have been transmitted with HBV among
Venezuelan Indians by exposure to weeping skin lesions of
scabies, by sexual exposure and by the practice of an
acupuncture-like form of folk medicine (Hadler 1983).

The high prevalence of anti-delta in HBsAg-positive
individuals from developing countries suggests that the delta
agent may be an exotic pathogen that was transplanted in
relatively recent times into developed countries. Evidence for
this has come from recent studies of drug addicts in Sweden
(Hansson 1982), where it was found that Swedish drug addicts
did not have serologic evidence of exposure to the delta agent
prior to the mid 1970's but that prevalence of anti-delta has
increased annually to approximately 70%. This introduction of
a "new" pathogen into a high risk population and its rapid
distribution is strikingly similar to the epidemiology of the
recently recognized acquired immune deficiency syndrome (AIDS),
and the delta agent, although not shown to be etiologically
associated with AIDS itself, is a model that may be useful in
better understanding the etiology of this "new" disease (Marx
1983).

Our present knowledge of the delta agent is sufficient to
give us a tantalizing glimpse of a pathogen that appears to be

unique among transmissible agents but there are currently more
questions than answers. What is the true origin of the delta
agent? How and when was it introduced into Europe and North
America? What is the spectrum of illness associated with it?
Does it play a role in hepatocellular carcinoma? What is the
relative importance of intrinsic virulence and host response in
the pathogenesis of delta-associated hepatitis? What is the
true prevalence of infection throughout the world? How is the
agent maintained and transmitted in various populations? Why
has it been found infrequently throughout Asia, a region where
the HBsAg carrier rate is among the highest in the world?

Answers to these and other questions will only be obtained
by carefully planned and executed seroepidemiologic studies in
different geographic and ecological areas throughout the world.
Attention must be paid to the clinical status of HBsAg-positive
individuals included in these studies and uniform criteria
should be applied. Such global studies can best be organized
by world bodies such as the World Health Organization. In
addition, retrospective and prospective studies of high risk
populations should be conducted to determine the incidence of
delta agent-associated hepatitis and its medical impact on
these populations. Of particular interest would be prospective
studies of recipients of blood transfusions or blood products,
illicit drug users, male homosexuals and other sexually
promiscuous individuals and indigenous populations in which HBV
is highly endemic.

The delta agent deserves intensive study. From the
standpoints of its epidemiology, virology and medical
importance, it appears to be one of the most interesting
hepatitis viruses yet discovered.

REFERENCES

Arico S, Rizzetto M, Crivelli O, Canese MG, Zanetti A,
  Ponzetto A, Ferrari G, Bonino F, Pera A, Verme G (1978).
  The clinical and immunological significance of a new antigen/
  antibody system (δ/anti-δ)in chronic carriers of the HBsAg.
  Ital J Gastroenterol 10:146.
Hadler SC <u>et al</u>. (1983). An epidemic of severe hepatitis due
  to delta virus infection in Yucpa indians in Venezuela.
  Submitted to Ann Int Med.
Hansson BG, Moestrup T, Widell A, Nordenfelt E (1982). Delta
  infection in sweden: introduction of a new hepatitis agent.

J Infect Dis 146:472.
Marx JL (1983). Spread of AIDS sparks new health concern.
    Science 219:42.
Picciotto A, Fuliano P, Mansi C, Savarino V, Testa R, Celle G,
    Bennicelli C, DeFlora S (1979). Correlation between delta,
    core, surface and e antigens in chronic hepatitis B. IRCS
    Medical Science; Pathology 7:507.
Picciotto A, Crovari P, Cuneo-Crovari P, De Flora S, Dodero M,
    Celle G. (1981). Interplay of cell and serum immunologic
    markers in chronic persistent or active hepatitis B. J Med
    Virol 8:195.
Raimondo G, Smedile A, Gallo L, Balbo A, Ponzetto A, Rizzetto
    M. (1982). Multicentre study of prevalence of HBV-Asso-
    ciated delta infection and liver disease in drug-addicts.
    Lancet 1:249.
Rizzetto M, Canese MG, Arico S, Crivelli O, Bonino F, Trepo
    CG, Verme G (1977). Immunofluorescence detection of a new
    antigen-antibody system (delta/anti-delta) associated with
    hepatitis B virus in the liver and in the serum of HBsAg
    carriers. Gut 18:997.
Rizzetto M, Shi SW-K, Gocke DJ, Purcell RH, Verme G, Gerin JL
    (1979). Incidence and significance of antibodies to delta
    antigen in hepatitis B virus infection. Lancet 2:986.
Rizzetto M, Canese MG, Gerin JL, London WT, Sly LD, Purcell RH
    (1980). Transmission of the hepatitis B virus-associated
    delta antigen to chimpanzees. J Infect Dis 141:590.
Rizzetto M, Shih, JW-K, Gerin JL (1980). The hepatitis B
    virus-associated delta antigen: isolation from liver,
    development of solid-phase radioimmunoassays for delta
    antigen and anti-delta and partial characterization of delta
    antigen. J Immunol 125:318.
Rizzetto M, Purcell RH, Gerin JL (1980). Epidemiology of
    HBV-associated delta agent: geographical distribution of
    anti-delta and prevalence in polytransfused HBsAg carriers.
    Lancet 1:1215.
Rizzetto M, Gerin J, Purcell RH (1981). Delta antigen:
    evidence for a variant of hepatitis B virus or a non-A, non-B
    hepatitis agent? In Pollard M (ed): "Perspectives in
    Virology XI", New York: Allen R. Liss, p. 195.
Rizzetto M (1982). Biology and characterization of the delta
    agent. In Szmuness W, Alter HJ, Maynard JE (eds):
    Proceedings 1981 International Symposium on Viral Hepatitis.
    Philadelphia, Franklin Institute Press, p. 355.
Rizzetto M, Morello C, Mannucci PM, Gocke DJ, Spero JA, Lewis
    JH, Van Thiel DH, Scaroni C, Peyretti F (1982). Delta
    infection and liver disease in hemophilic carriers of

hepatitis B surface antigen. J Infect Dis 145:18.
Smedile A, Farci P, Verme G et al. (1982). Influence of delta
  infection on severity of hepatitis B. Lancet ii:945.
Zanetti AR, Ferroni P, Magliano EM, Pirovano P, Lavarini C,
  Massaro AL, Gavinelli R, Fabris C, Rizzetto M (1982).
  Perinatal transmission of the hepatitis B virus and of the
  HBV-associated delta agent from mothers to offspring in
  northern italy. J Med Virol 9:139.

Viral Hepatitis and Delta Infection, pages 121–126
© 1983 Alan R. Liss, Inc., 150 Fifth Avenue, New York, NY 10011

METHODS FOR DETECTION OF THE DELTA ANTIGEN AND
ANTIBODY IN LIVER AND SERUM

O.Crivelli, J.W.K.Shih, M.Rizzetto

Molinette, Torino-Italy
National Inst.of Health , Bethesda, MD

The delta antigen and antibody to it were first detected
by immunofluorescence (Rizzetto 1977).The initial evaluation
of the new system was carried out using this technique.
Once a stable form of solubilized delta antigen became available, the currently used serological assays were developed.

Methods to detect delta antigen in liver and serum
Intrahepatic delta antigen can be detected by immunofluorescence (IFL) or immunoenzymatic techniques using gamma
globulin or IgG labeled with fluorochromes or enzymes
(Rizzetto 1977,Stoecklin 1981,Recchia 1981,Govindarajan 1983).
   The reagents are prepared from serum of HBsAg carriers that
invariably contain anti-HBc .Usually sera with high titers
of anti-delta have a low titer of anti-HBc; this is diluted
out at the working dilution of the fluorescein or enzyme
conjugate.Immunohistological interference between the delta
and the HBe antigen/antibody systems was never observed.
   The delta has many analogies with the HB core system.
Delta antigen is also found in liver while the homologous
antibody is present in serum and delta-positive nuclei are
likewise reactive with antisera to human IgG, a phenomenon
due to tissutal immunocomplexes of delta antigen (or HBcAg)
with the respective antibody (Rizzetto 1981).
   The localization of delta antigen in the liver is predominantly nuclear.The staining is granular,globular or diffuse

and thus different from the uniformely finely speckled IFL
appearance of nuclei containing HBcAg.

A discrete cytoplasmic localization can be also occasionally observed.

Delta antigen is not denatured by conventional fixatives
and can be demonstrated in ordinary histological material
fixed with formalin(Stoecklin 1981). Demonstration of the
antigen in fixed material requires preliminary digestion of
the section with pronase or trypsin. Immunoperoxidase in
fixed specimens permits the simultaneous analysis of histological features and of distribution of delta antigen; the
specimens can be stored for long.

Serum delta antigen is measured by radio- and enzyme-linked
immunoassays(RIA,ELISA)(Rizzetto 1980, Crivelli 1981)based
on binding of antigen in test sera to anti-delta fixed on a
solid phase(polyvinil tubes, balls or microtiter wells),and
subsequent development of the reaction with radioiodinated
or enzyme-labeled IgG anti-delta.

The only circulating form of delta antigen identified to
date is sequestered inside a HBsAg particle. Its detection
requires treatment with detergent that disrupts the particle
and exposes the antigen. Both in men and chimpanzees delta-
antigenemia was a transient event occurring during the early
phase of primary acute delta infection(Rizzetto,Hoyer 1980,
Bonino 1981).

We were unable to detect delta antigen in serum of HBsAg
carriers with chronic delta infection;negative results were
also obtained after removal by ultracentrifugation and gel
filtration of the homologous antibody that could interfere
with the reaction.

ELISA seems somewhat more sensitive than RIA for determining serum delta antigen;this might depend on amplification
of the reaction entailed by the enzymatic nature of this
assay(Crivelli 1981).

Sera of drug-addicts with chronic delta or non A,non B
hepatitis occasionally give a low titer reaction in the
delta-antigen ELISA(more rarely in RIA) that is equally
observed with and without detergent treatment and is not

abolished by preincubation with sera containing a high titer
of anti-delta. The nature of this reaction is uncertain. If
representing a genuine immune phenomenon, it seems distinct
from the delta antigen.

Methods to detect anti-delta in serum.
In early studies serum anti-delta was determined by IFL.
Because of the intrinsic IgG reactivity in nuclei containing
delta antigen, the indirect(sandwich) IFL technique could
not be employed as the second layer of the test(anti-human
IgG) would inevitably bind to the nuclear immunoglobulin,
resulting in false positive reactions. Attempts to elute the
IgG from tissue were unsuccessfull. The initial screening
for anti-delta was therefore carried out using a direct IFL
procedure that implied conjugation of each single test serum
with fluorochrome(Aricò 1978). The test was tedious and of
weak sensitivity;low titer antibodies,such as arised in acute delta infection,could not be detected. A more practical
IFL blocking assay was then developed,based on blocking of
tissutal delta antigen by anti-delta present in test serum
(Crivelli 1978); this test was also of low sensitivity and
often difficult to interpret.
In 1981 Stoecklin et al. reported that ordinary histologic
.fixation denatures the intrinsic IgG reactivity but does
not alter delta antigen, thus allowing the use of the indirect IFL technique on delta antigen-positive substrates
fixed with formalin.
Currently used RIA and ELISA employ delta antigen purified from human liver. The antigen was extracted using 6 M
guanidine-HCl or 8 M urea. Extraction without dissociating
agents yielded an unstable reactivity which was lost within
24-48 hours.
In initial studies the antigen was prepared from isolated
liver nuclei(Rizzetto 1980). Homogenates of whole liver
yield a greater amount of delta antigen per gram of tissue
without variation in antigen quality. The liver is homogeni-
zed in 6 M guanidine and left for 3 hours at room temperature; the homogenate is then diluted to 1.2 M guanidine
(Crivelli 1981). This represents the standard antigen which

is titered,aliquoted and stored at -80°C or lyophilized.

A better but limited source of antigen is liver of experimentally infected chimpanzees obtained at peak expression of intrahepatic delta antigen, prior to development of anti-delta. This antigen can be obtained in a stable form simply by acqueous extraction(Rizzetto 1980).

Tests for anti-delta are competitive,based on blocking by antibody in test serum of delta antigen fixed to a solid phase.The blocked antigen is not available for the subsequent reaction with the radioiodinated or the enzyme-labeled anti-delta tracer.

RIA and ELISA have a high degree of sensitivity and specificity; positive sera can be titered up to $1:10^5$-$1:10^6$ dilutions.Variations in sensitivity between published methods depend on technical details(Tedder 1982).Interference or cross-reactivity with other HBV systems have not been a problem.Anti-delta reagents are devoid of anti-HBs and anti-HBc is diluted out at the working dilution. HBcAg possibly contaminating delta antigen preparations is denatured by dissociating agents(Raimondo 1982).Serological interferences between the delta and HBe systems have not been observed.

Blocking assays do not discriminate the type of antibody, as each class binds to the insolubilized antigen. A radioimmunoassay specific for IgM anti-delta was developed (Smedile 1982), based on capture of IgM in test serum by anti-μ antiserum attached to a solid phase. If IgM anti-delta is present in test serum it fixes delta antigen subsequently introduced in the system; the reaction is revealed by the addition of radiolabeled IgG anti-delta.

This assay is useful in the diagnosis of acute delta hepatitis as in this context the serological response to the infection is often represented by a transient IgM antibody.

REFERENCES

Aricò S, Rizzetto M, Crivelli O,Canese MG, Zanetti A,
  Ponzetto A, Ferrari G, Bonino F, Pera A, Verme G(1978).
  The clinical and immunological significance of a new
  antigen/antibody system(delta/anti-delta) in chronic
  carriers of the HBsAg. Ital J Gastroenterol 10:146
Bonino F, Hoyer B, Ford E, Shih JWK, Purcell RH, Gerin JL
  (1981). The delta agent: HBsAg particles with delta antigen and RNA in the serum of an HBV carrier. Hepatology 1:
  127.
Crivelli O, Aricò S, Bonino F, Lavarini C, Rizzetto M(1978).
  Distribution of antibodies against delta antigen detected
  by a simple immunofluorescence blocking test. Acta gastro-
  ent Belg 41: 351.
Crivelli O, Rizzetto M, Lavarini C, Smedile A, Gerin JL
  (1981). Enzyme-linked immunosorbent assay for detection
  of antibody to the Hepatitis B surface Antigen-associated
  delta antigen. J Clin Microbiol 14:173.
Govindarajan S, Lim B, Peters RL(1983). Immunohistochemical
  localization of the delta antigen associated with hepatitis B virus in liver biopsy sections embedded in araldite.
  Histopathology, in press.
Raimondo G, Recchia S, Lavarini C, Crivelli O, Rizzetto M
  (1982). Dane particle associated hepatitis B e antigen in
  patients with chronic hepatitis B virus infection and
  hepatitis B e antibody. Hepatology 2: 449.
Recchia S, Rizzi R, Acquaviva F, Rizzetto M, Tison V,
  Bonino F, Verme G(1981). Immunoperoxidase staining of the
  HBV-associated delta antigen in paraffinated liver speci-
  mens. Pathologica 73:773.
Rizzetto M, Canese MG, Aricò S, Crivelli O, Trepo C,Bonino F,
  Verme G (1977). Immunofluorescence detection of a new
  antigen/antibody system(delta/anti-delta)associated with
  hepatitis B virus in liver and serum of HBsAg carriers.
  Gut 18:997.

Rizzetto M, Shih JWK, Gerin JL (1980). The hepatitis B virus associated delta antigen: isolation from liver,development of solid phase radioimmunoassays for delta and anti-delta and partial characterization of delta. J Immunol 125:318.

Rizzetto M, Hoyer B, Canese MG, Shih JWK, Purcell RH,Gerin JL (1980). Delta antigen:the association of delta antigen with hepatitis B surface antigen and ribonucleic acid in the serum of delta infected chimpanzees. Proc Natl Acad Sci USA 77:6124.

Rizzetto M, Canese MG, Purcell RH, London WT, Sly LD, Gerin JL (1981). Experimental HBV and delta infection of chimpanzees: occurrence and significance of intrahepatic immuno-complexes of hepatitis B core antigen and delta antigen. Hepatology 1:567.

Smedile A, Lavarini C, Crivelli O, raimondo G, Fassone M, Rizzetto M (1982). Radioimmunoassay detection of IgM antibodies to the HBV-associated delta antigen:clinical significance in delta infection. J Med Virol 9:131.

Stoecklin E, Gudat F, Krey G, Durmuller U, Gasser M,Schmid M,Stalder G,Bianchi L (1981). Delta antigen in hepatitis B:immunohistology of frozen and paraffin-embedded liver biopsies and relation to HBV infection. Hepatology 1:238.

Tedder RS, Briggs M, Howell DR (1982). U.K. prevalence of delta infection. Lancet 2: 764.

Viral Hepatitis and Delta Infection, pages 127–132
© 1983 Alan R. Liss, Inc., 150 Fifth Avenue, New York, NY 10011

VERTICAL TRANSMISSION OF THE HBV-ASSOCIATED DELTA AGENT

Zanetti R. Alessandro, Tanzi Elisabetta, Ferroni
Pierino, Magliano Enrico
Institute of Virology
University of Milan
Via Pascal, 38 - 20133 Milano - Italy

Available evidence indicates that delta (δ) has properti
es of a viroid-like nucleoprotein coated with HBsAg, which re
quires helper function of hepatitis B virus for its synthesis (Rizzetto 1980a). Because of the defective nature of δ
and its obligatory dependence on HBV infection, transmission
follows the routes of HBV. Since transmission of HBV from in
fected mother to offspring represents an important mechanism
mantaining the endemicity of HBV infection, we have in this
study investigated the epidemiologic relevance of vertical
route in the spreading of the HBV-associated δ agent.

Antibody to δ (anti-δ) was tested in 455 HBsAg carrier
mothers identified among 12.965 pregnant women in Northern
Italy (Zanetti 1983). Of these, 22 (4.8%) were positive for
HBeAg, 419 (92.1%) for anti-HBe and 14 (3.1%) were negative
for both HBeAg and anti-HBe.

A further 26 HBsAg carrier mothers with HBeAg, parteci
pating to a multicenter study on hepatitis B vaccine prophy
laxis of perinatal HBV infection were also examined for an-
ti-δ .

Blood specimens were taken at birth, at 1 month of age
and about every three months thereafter from all babies born
to mothers with anti-δ . HBsAg, anti-HBs, anti-HBc, HBeAg
and anti-HBe were detected by RIA using commercial kits (Ab
bott Labs. USA). Delta antigen a d anti-δ (total and of IgM
class) were assayed by RIA as previously described (Rizzetto
1980b; Smedile 1982). Titration of anti-δ was performed by
diluting test samples in normal human sera negative for HBV

markers and for rheumatoid factor. Liver function tests (LFT) were measured by standard laboratory methods.

Prevalence of anti- δ in HBsAg-carrier mothers

As reported in Table 1, anti- δ was found in 36 of the 481 (7.5%) carrier mothers examined. Each mother positive for anti- δ was asymptomatic with normal LFT and no history of past hepatitis, blood transfusion or parenteral drug abuse. Three of them had HBeAg in serum and 33 had anti-HBe.

		N.	anti- δ +	anti- δ -
HBeAg	+	48	3	45
anti-HBe	+	419	33	386
HBeAg/anti-HBe	-	14	-	14
total		481	36 (7.5%)	445 (92.5%)

Table 1. Prevalence of anti- δ in HBsAg carrier mothers according to HBeAg/anti-HBe status.

Delta Ag/anti-delta in newborns of HBsAg carrier mothers with anti-δ .

34 babies that were born to anti- δ positive mothers with anti-HBe did not exhibit serological evidence of HBV and δ infection throughout the follow-up. Passively transmitted anti- δ detectable at birth, was no longer present at three months of life. 9 of these newborns received specific immunoprophylaxis; they were injected at birth and at 1 month of age with HBIG (Biagini, Pisa, Italy; 0.2 ml/Kg i.m.; anti-HBs content 180 IU/ml). One baby who was born to an anti- δ positive mother with anti-HBe and was not given prophylaxis acquired both HBV and δ infection (Figure 1). He was found to be HBsAg and anti-HBe positive at 3 months of age. Aminotransferase (AT) increased concurrently with the appearance of HBsAg and returned to normal value in five weeks. HBsAg disappeared in one month with seroconversion to anti-HBs. The titer of anti- δ increased from $1:10^2$ to $1:10^3$ between 3 and 4 months of age.

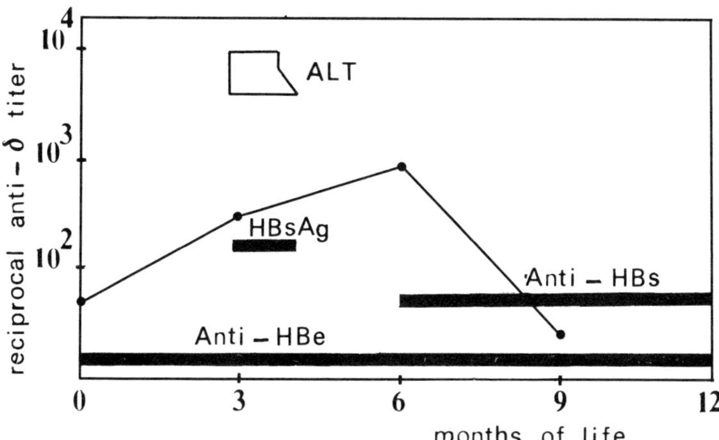

Figure 1. Serologic pattern of a baby born to anti-HBe positive mother with anti-δ who acquired acute HBV and δ infection (anti-δ •——•).

      Two babies that were born to anti-δ positive mothers
with HBeAg received gammaglobulins at birth and at 1 month
of age followed by three doses of vaccine (Merck Sharp and
Dohme, USA, 10 ug protein) at 3, 4 and 9 months of age; they
did not exhibit serological evidence of HBV and δ infection
throughout the follow-up. One baby that was born to an anti-
δ positive mother with HBeAg and was not given prophylaxis
acquired both HBV and δ infection (Figure 2). He was found

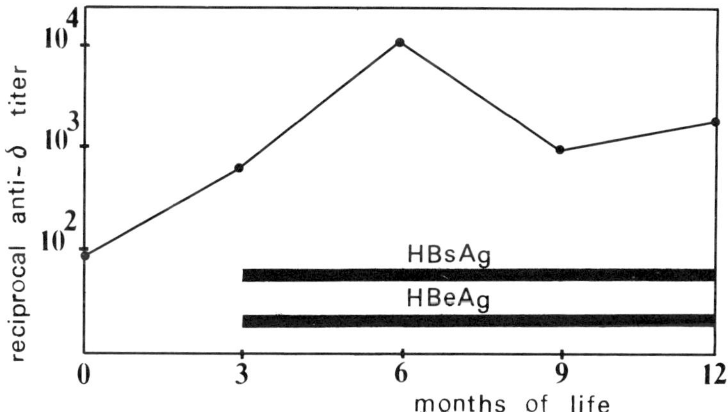

Figure 2. Serological pattern of a baby born to HBeAg positive mother with anti-δ who acquired chronic HBV and δ infection (anti-δ •——•).

to be HBsAg and HBeAg positive at the serological control performed at 3 months of age. Anti- δ increased from a titer of $1:10^3$ to $1:10^4$ between 3 and 6 months of life. Low level of IgM anti- δ was also detected. The baby remained asymptomatic with normal LFT throughout the follow-up.

Delta antigen was not detected in any of the babies.
The HBsAg subtype of infected babies (ay) was similar to that of the carrier mothers.

Conclusions

Since delta infection appears to require ongoing replication of hepatitis B virus, vertical transmission of δ agent may occur only under circumstances permitting transmission of HBV. Vertical HBV transmission is a major problem in populations with a high rate of HBV infection and a high prevalence of HBeAg among carriers (Stevens 1980). In Italy, a country where HBsAg prevalence in adults is over 3% (Zanetti 1979), the rate of HBV infection in newborns of carrier mothers (diagnosed by detection of HBs antigenemia or in its absence by appearance of IgM anti-HBc and/or anti-HBs) is approximately 20%. Nearly all babies born to HBeAg positive mothers are at risk of acquiring HBV infection and developing the HBsAg carrier state, while for those born to anti-HBe carriers the risk is significantly lower (Zanetti 1982).

The prevalence of anti- δ in the carrier mothers examined (7.5%) is significantly lower than in carriers with hepatitis from the same HBsAg populations (Rizzetto 1980c; Smedile 1983), probably due to the association of δ with severe forms of liver disease (Rizzetto 1977) that are incompatible with procreation.

Since in addition most carrier women with δ infection have anti-HBe and are thus unlikely to transmit HBV infection to the prole, vertical transmission of the δ agent from mother to newborn appears to be of minor epidemiological relevance. Despite the infrequent transmission of δ directly from mother to newborn, in areas where δ is endemic, vertical acquired HB viremia may expose the baby to the risk of contracting δ from other δ-positive relatives, or conversely, HB viremia acquired perinatally from relatives infectious for HBV, may expose the baby to the risk of maternal δ ; possibly the latter mechanism applied to the δ-infection acquired by the infant born to the anti-HBe positive mother.

Given the invariable association of δ with HBV, preven
tion of perinatal HBV infection is likely to be also useful
in preventing transmission of δ . Preliminary data are in a-
greement with this hypothesis.

<u>Acknowledgements</u>: we are greateful to Dr. C. Lavarini for
help in testing δ/anti- δ .

<u>References</u>

Rizzetto M, Canese MG, Aricò S, Crivelli O, Bonino F, Trepo
CG, Verme G (1977). Immunofluorescence detection of a new
antigen-antibody system (δ/anti- δ) associated to the hepatitis B virus in the liver and in serum of HBsAg carri-
ers. Gut 18:997.
Rizzetto M, Hoyer B, Canese MG, Shih JWK, Purcell RH, Gerin
JL (1980a). Delta antigen: the association of delta antigen
with hepatitis B surface and ribonucleic acid in the serum
of delta infected chimpanzees. Proc Natl Acad Sci 77:6124.
Rizzetto M, Canese MG, Gerin JL, London WT, Sly DL, Purcell
RH (1980b). Transmission of the hepatitis B virus associated delta antigen to chimpazees. J Infect Dis 141:590.
Rizzetto M, Purcell RH, Gerin JL (1980c). Epidemiology of
HBV associated delta antigen: geographical distribution of
anti-delta and prevalence in polytransfused HBsAg carriers.
Lancet 1:1215.
Smedile A, Lavarini C, Crivelli O,'Raimondi G, Fassone M, Riz
zettoM(1982). Radioimmunoassay detection of IgM antibodies
to the HBV-associated delta (δ) antigen: clinical signifi
cance in δ infection. J Med Virol 9:131.
Smedile A, Lavarini C, Farci P, Aricò S, Marinucci G, Dentico P, Giuliani G, Cargnel A, Del Vecchio Blanco C, Rizzetto M (1983). Epidemiologic patterns of infection with the
hepatitis B virus-associated delta agent in Italy. Am J
Epidemiol 117:223.
Stevens CE, Szmuness W (1980). Vertical transmission of hepa
titis B and neonatal hepatitis B. In Bianchi L, Gerok W,
Sickinger K, Stalder GA (eds): "Virus and the liver" Lancaster: MTP Press limited, p 285.
Zanetti AR, Ferroni P, Legnani F, Bergamini F (1979). Preva
lence of HBeAg, anti-HBe and Dane particle-associated DNA
polymerase activity in asymptomatic carriers of HBsAg. La
Ricerca Clin Lab 9:35.
Zanetti AR, Ferroni P, Magliano EM, Pirovano P, Lavarini C,
Massaro AL, Gavinelli R, Fabris C, Rizzetto M (1982). Peri

natal transmission of the hepatitis B virus and of the HBV-associated delta agent from mothers to offspring in Norhtern Italy. J Med Virol 9:139

Zanetti AR, Magliano EM, Tanzi E, Ferroni P, Pirovano G, Pizzocolo G, Pillon N, Zunin C (1982). HBIG immunoprophylaxis of babies born to HBsAg carrier mothers. In Karger S (ed): Developments in Biological Standardization, 2nd International Symposium on Viral Hepatitis (in press).

Viral Hepatitis and Delta Infection, pages 133–137
© 1983 Alan R. Liss, Inc., 150 Fifth Avenue, New York, NY 10011

FAMILIAR CLUSTERING OF DELTA INFECTION

Rocca G.,Poli G.,Gerardo P.,Ascione A.,Caporaso N.,
Craxi A.,Dentico P.,Marinucci G.,Piccinino F.,
Raimondo G.,Schiraldi O.,Valeri L.,Vinci M.
Torino,Bari,Messina,Napoli,Roma and Palermo,Italy

Familiar clustering of chronic HBsAg carriers is frequent in Italy and perinatal transmission from parents to children appears its major cause in endemic areas (Zanetti,1982).
Liver disease and Delta infection have also been described
in households of patients with chronic Delta hepatitis
(Smedile 1983).Since chronic carriers of HBV are the prefe-
rential victims of Delta Agent and clusters of these individuals might promote intrafamily spreading of δ infection we
have evaluated transmission of Delta in families of 233 carriers of HBsAg.The individuals included in the study were
chronic HBsAg carriers with liver disease examined at 7 medical centers in Turin,Bari,Messina,Napoli,Roma and Palermo.
All the households were analysed for a total of 1174 indivi-
duals.The male/female ratio was 2.4,the mean age was 32years
(range 1-70 years),2% of them were from North of Italy,6%
from Center and 91% from South.Sera from all family members
were tested for HBsAg,anti-HBs,HBeAg and anti-HBe by commercial radioimmunoassays (Abbott Lab.North Chicago,Ill.USA)and
δAg and anti-δ by SP-RIA(Rizzetto,1980).

Of the 233 carriers 82 had serum anti-δ at titers $\rangle$ 1/5000.
These individuals were considered Cases;5 of them were HBeAg
positive and 77 HBeAg negative.One hundred and fifty-one carriers were anti-δ negative.These individuals were considered
Controls;40 of them were HBeAg positive and 111 HBeAg negative.

Families of Cases and Controls were comparable for number of individuals and HBsAg carriers (Table 1).

Table 1

| | Families | |
	of Cases	of Controls
Number of individuals	458	716
Number of HBsAg carriers	165	245
(%)	(36)	(34.2)
Individuals/ families(mean)	5	5

In families of Cases the prevalence of HBsAg carriers with serum anti-∂(Delta associated Cases)was significantly higher than in families of Controls (Table 2).

Table 2
Prevalence of HBsAg carriers with serum anti-∂

	In families of Cases	In families of Controls
Number of carriers with serum anti-∂/ Number of family members (%)	45/376 (12)	2/565 (0.35)

$$p < 0.0000 \quad 95\% \text{ C.L. } 8{-}14$$

Excluding Cases and Controls from analysis 45 of 376 family members of Cases (12%) had serum HBsAg and anti-∂,as opposed to 2 of 565 family members of Controls(0.35%).These results suggest a significant clustering of Delta infection within families of Delta patients.In Delta families the over-all number of individuals with serum anti-∂ was directly pro-portional to the number of HBsAg carriers;the majority of these carriers,with or without Delta markers,had serum anti-

HBe (90%).In nineteen families 10% to 60% of the carriers
were positive for serum HBeAg;in these families the relative
prevalence of anti-δ positive to negative carriers was lower
than in families where all carriers were anti-HBe positive
(Table 3).These results may suggest a role of active HBV in-
fection(HBeAg positive)in limiting the spread of Delta.

<u>Table 3</u>

Relation between the number of carriers with serum anti-δ
(% delta/carriers) and the number of carriers within
families of Delta Cases.Families are divided according
to presence or absence of HBeAg positive carriers.

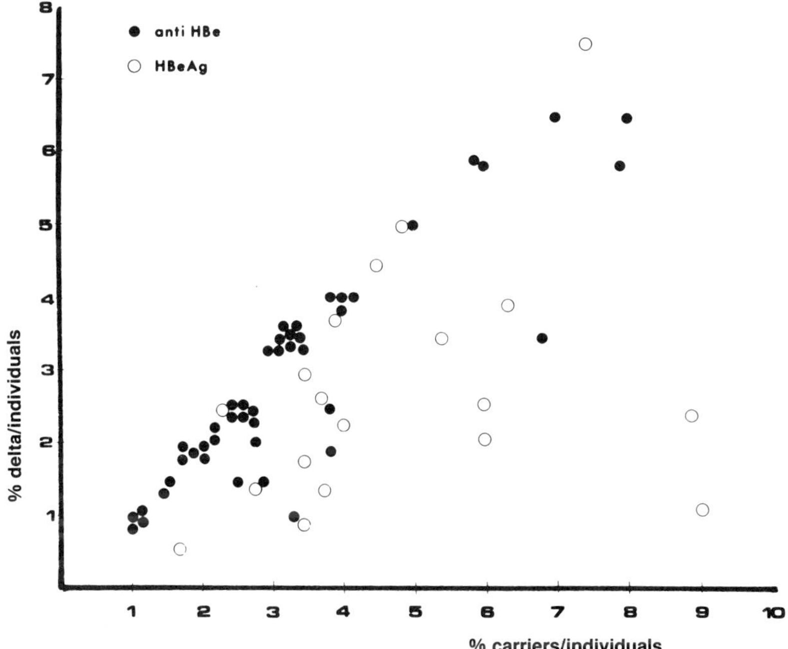

The mode of transmission of Delta was evaluated from analysis of the intrafamily relation between Delta Cases and
Delta associated Cases:in 75% (34/45)it was spouse to spouses
or sibling to siblings while only in 25%(11/45) it was parent to children (p < 0.001).In families of highly HBV infectious δ negative carriers (positive for serum HBeAg) the
intrafamily relation between Cases and HBeAg associated Cases
was as follows:in 32%(20/63) it was spouse to spouses or

sibling to siblings and in 68%(43/63) it was parent to chil-
dren(Table 4).In order to compare the mode of transmission
of Delta and of HBV the intrafamily relation of family members of Delta Cases was compared with that of family members
of HBeAg Cases.Contigency tables (Table 4) show that δ transmission was predominantly horizontal while HBV transmission
occurred predominantly from parents to children.

Table 4

Intrafamily relation between Delta Cases and Delta associated cases and between HBeAg positive Cases and HBeAg
associated Cases.Contingency Tables.

	DELTA	HBV	TOTAL
Spouse to spouses or sibling to siblings	34	20	54
Parent to children	11	43	54
TOTAL	45	63	108

$$p < 0.0001 \quad 95\% \text{ C.L. } 27\text{-}61$$

In conclusion familiar clustering of HBsAg carriers
with Delta infection occurs in families from South of Italy
where HBV and Delta infection are highly endemic.Intrafamily
transmission is horizontal and clusters of HBsAg carriers
are vehicle to spreading of this infection.

The following medical doctors partecipated in the study:
E.Sagnelli,Napoli;B.Forzani,G.Tappero and F.Bonino,Torino.

References
Zanetti A.R.,Ferroni P.,Magliano E.M.,Pirovano P.,Lavarini C.
Massaro A.L.,Gavinelli R.,Fabris C.,Rizzetto M.(1982).
 Perinatal transmission of the hepatitis B virus and of the
 HBV associated Delta agent from mothers to offsprings in
 Northern Italy.J.Med.Virol.9:139·
Rizzetto M.,Shih JW-K.,Gerin J.L.(1980)The hepatitis B virus
 associated delta antigen:isolation from liver,development of

solid phase radioimmuneassays for delta and anti-delta
and partial characterization of delta . J.Immunol.125:318
Smedile A.,Lavarini C.Aricò S.,Marinucci G.,Dentico P.,
Giuliani G.,Cargnel A.,Del Vecchio Blanco C.,Rizzetto M.(1983)
Epidemiological patterns of infection with the hepatitis B
virus-associated delta (δ) agent in Italy.Am.J.Epidemiol.
117:223

Viral Hepatitis and Delta Infection, pages 139–143
© 1983 Alan R. Liss, Inc., 150 Fifth Avenue, New York, NY 10011

DELTA INFECTION: INTRAFAMILY SPREADING

Nicola Caporaso, Camillo Del Vecchio-Blanco,
Rosalba Suozzo and Mario Coltorti
Istituto di Semeiotica Medica, I Facoltà di
Medicina e Chirurgia, Università di Napoli
II Policlinico, Via Pansini 5, 80131 Napoli,Italy

Carriers of HBsAg are frequently clustered in families
(Coltorti, 1978). To establish whether intrafamily aggregation of HBV infection determines also aggregation of δ infection, family clusters of HBsAg carriers were examined
for antibody to δ and prospectively followed up for development of this infection.

Included in this study were 118 families with one or more
members carrying HBsAg in blood, collected in Naples from
January 1979 to December 1980. The mode of identification of
the clusters and details on the family units were previously
report (Coltorti, 1983).
Clinical and serological examinations were repeated every
six months for at least one year (mean follow-up 2.5 years;
range 1-4 years). None of the subjects examined was a drug
addict or had received a blood transfusion six months prior
or during the study.
HBsAg,HBeAg,anti-HBe were tested by commercial RIA Kits
(Abbott Laboratories, Chicago, Ill. U.S.A.); anti-delta
(total and IgM) was tested using previously described RIA
methods (Rizzetto, 1979; Smedile, 1982).

The age and the prevalence of HBsAg and anti-δ among the
members of the 118 families is reported in Table 1.

Table 1 -

Family members	No.	Mean age (range) years
Total	566	23.6 (1 - 67)
HBsAg negative	340	23.3 (1 - 67)
HBsAg positive	226	23.8 (1 - 61)
- anti-δ positive	51	27.7 (7 - 55)
- anti-δ negative	175	20.1 (1 - 61)

39.9% of the family members were positive for HBsAg and 22.5% of the HBsAg-positive subjects had anti-δ. The mean age of HBsAg-positive subjects was similar to that of HBsAg-negative subjects; the mean age of anti-delta-positive subjects was older than the age of anti-delta-negative subjects.

At the initial screening, in 83 families all the members carrying HBsAg were negative for anti-delta. In 27 families all the members carrying HBsAg were positive for anti-delta. In 8 families 20.0% to 66.7% of the HBsAg components were positive for anti-delta; overall, in this group 9 of the 22 HBsAg carriers were already positive for delta at the initial examination,while the other 13 were negative. Thus 175 HBsAg carriers were still susceptible to infection by delta agent. These data are summarized in Table 2.

Table 2 -

No. of families	No. of family members	A	B	C
83	360	162	0	162
27	137	42	42	0
8	50	22	9	13
118	547	226	51	175

A = No. of members carrying HBsAg
B = No. of HBsAg carriers with delta infection in the initial examination
C = No. of HBsAg carrier susceptible to delta infection at the follow-up

Table 3 shows the frequency of chronic liver disease in carriers of HBsAg in relation to anti-delta and presence of HBeAg in serum.

Table 3 -

	anti-δ positive (No.51)	anti-δ negative (No.175)
Chronic HBsAg liver disease	48 (94.1%)	74 (42.3%)
HBeAg positive	6	47
Age (years), mean and range	27.8 (4-55)	17.5 (1-61)

Almost all anti-delta-positive subjects were diseased and only a few were HBeAg positive whereas only 42.3 % of the anti-delta-negative subjects were diseased and many of them had HBeAg. The follow-up documented that 4/13 (30.8%) of HBsAg-positive members belonging to families with at least one member positive for anti-delta, and only 2/162 (1.2%) of HBsAg-positive members belonging to the other families, acquired delta infection (p < 0.001) (Table 4).

Table 4 -

	No. of members susceptible to δ	No.of members who developed anti-δ at follow-up	%
Families negative for anti-δ at initial screening 83	162	2	1.2%
Families with one or more members positive for anti-δ at initial screening 8	13	4	30.8%

Delta superinfection caused a severe hepatitis in 3 healthy carriers: in 1 the acute hepatitis progressed to chronic active hepatitis within two years; the other two cases had not yet recovered after 7 months. In the remaining 3 subjects, with known chronic active hepatitis, infection by delta agent was documented by the appearance of IgM anti-delta and by total anti-delta.

Conclusions

Our data show that familial clusters of HBsAg carriers may represent the background for intrafamily spreading of delta agent. When a δ-infected individual is present in a family, the risk of delta for other HBsAg positive components is high, as shown by the clustering of subjects positive for anti-delta and by the higher incidence of new delta infections in families with one or more members positive for anti-delta, compared to families whose members were all anti-delta negative.

The higher prevalence of chronic liver disease in subjects with anti-delta compared to subjects without this antibody, indicates that delta-superinfection increases the risk of chronic liver disease and contributes to its familial clustering. The low number of chronic delta hepatitis with HBeAg supports the hypothesis that the liver disease of individuals with anti-delta is related to delta superinfection rather than HB virus damage. This is confirmed by our observations that superinfection by delta agent of asymptomatic carriers of HBsAg modified the healthy state of these patients, inducing first an acute hepatitis and than chronic HBsAg positive liver disease.

References

Coltorti M, Del Vecchio-Blanco C, Caporaso N, Ambrogio G, Mattera D (1978). Prevalence of HBsAg, HBsAb and CALD in families of HBsAg or Ab positive subjects. Excerpta Med Int Congr Series, p 559.

Coltorti M, Del Vecchio-Blanco C, Caporaso N, Suozzo R, Servillo F (1983). Familial clustering of HBV infection and chronic liver disease. In Gentilini P, Dianzani MU (eds): "Cirrosi epatica in Italia", Basel: Karger in press.

Rizzetto M, Shih JWK, Gocke DJ, Purcell RH, Verme G, Gerin JL (1979). Incidence and significance of antibodies to delta antigen in hepatitis B virus infection. Lancet 2:986.

Smedile A, Lavarini C, Crivelli O, Raimondo G, Fassone M, Rizzetto M (1982). Radioimmunoassay detection of IgM antibodies to HBV associated delta antigen. Clinical significance in delta infection. J Med Virol 9:131.

DELTA INFECTION AMONG HAEMOPHILIACS

P. Dentico, F. Negro, F. Peyretti, P.M. Mannucci,
G.L.Molaro, H.Thomas, W.G.Schiller, R. J.Gerety

Bari, Torino, Milano, Pordenone; Italy – London;
England – Potsdam; East Germany – Bethesda; U.S.A.

Direct parenteral inoculation, the classical mechanism
of HBV transmission, is the most efficient mode of transmitting the delta agent (Rizzetto 1980). This virus represents therefore a risk to individuals polytransfused with
blood and its constituents. To evaluate the relevance of δ
infection following transfusion, the prevalence of antibody
to δ (anti-δ) was determined in serum of different groups
of polytransfused individuals and correlated with clinical
evidence of liver disease.

Three groups of Italian patients were studied.
1) 202 patients with acquired haematological disorders
requiring the occasional transfusion of blood.
2) 414 patients with thalassemia, subjected throughout
life to a variable number of blood transfusions (from a
dozen to several hundreds).
3) 326 patients with haemophilia, who required continuous
therapy with coagulation factors.

Patients were screened for HBV markers by commercial
Radioimmunoassays and for anti-δ by a previously reported
RIA (Rizzetto 1979).

Results are shown in table 1.

TABLE 1. DELTA AND BLOOD TRANSFUSION

ANTI-δ IN MULTITRANSFUSED PATIENTS WITH CHRONIC HAEMATO-
LOGICAL DISORDERS

HBV STATUS	ACQUIRED	CONGENITAL	
		THALASSEMICS	HAEMOPHILIACS
	202	(414)	(326)
HBsAg+	0/ 22	2*/34 (6%)	14/37 (38%)
anti-HBs+	0/108	0/308	2**/233 (1%)
HBsAg− anti-HBs−	0/ 72	0/ 72	0/56

ANTI-DELTA POSITIVE / N° EXAMINED

* Positive patients received 256 and 80 transfusions
** Low titer ($<$ 1:500)

None of the 202 patients with acquired blood disorders
were found positive for anti-δ. Among the 414 patients with
thalassemia, anti-δ was detected in 2 (6%) of 34 HBsAg
chronic carriers; they had been exposed to 256 and 80 blood
transfusions, respectively. The antibody was not detected
in the 308 thalassemics positive for anti-HBs and in the 72
negative for HBsAg and anti-HBs.

Among haemophiliacs, 14 of 37 HBsAg carriers (38%) were
positive for anti-δ. The antibody was also detected at low
titers in 2 of 233 haemophiliacs positive for anti-HBs (1%)
but in none of 56 patients without serological evidence of
current or past HBV infection.

It thus appears that the risk of post-transfusion δ infection to patients given blood tested for HBsAg is negligible and the current HBsAg testing with third generation
assays provides a high degree of safety in preventing parenteral transmission of δ.

The risk of this infection, instead, is constant in
haemophiliacs receiving substitution therapy with coagulation factors. In keeping with the obligatory dependence
of δ on HBV, the prevalence of anti-δ was maximal in
haemophiliacs carrying the HBsAg; many of them circulated
the antibody in high titers, indicative of active replication of the delta agent (Rizzetto, 1979). Only two haemophiliacs without HBs antigenemia (both with anti-HBs) had
anti-δ, the titer of which was low, presumably reflecting
a recent self-limited infection or an anamnestic response
to δ re-infection.

To define the risk factors of δ infection in haemophiliacs, the prevalence of anti-δ was determined in a separate series of adult HBsAg positive haemophiliacs collected
in countries using different types of substitution therapy.
Besides the Italian series, there was a USA, an English
and an East German series. Commercial coagulation factors
are almost exclusively used in Italy and in the USA; besides commercial products, cryoprecipitates obtained from
single blood donors are also used in England, and to some
extent in the USA. Only products (cryoprecipitates and
PPSB) locally prepared and obtained from individual donors
are used in East Germany. Results are shown in table 2.

TABLE 2. ANTI-DELTA IN ADULT* HBsAg POSITIVE HAEMOPHILIACS
FROM DIFFERENT COUNTRIES

I T A L Y		U S A	ENGLAND	EAST GERMANY
Milano Torino	Bari	Maryland	London	Potsdam
5/10 (50%)	6/12 (50%)	10/21 (48%)	2/11 (18%)	0/5 –

ANTI-DELTA POSITIVE / N° EXAMINED

* = age $\geq$ 15

The prevalence of anti-δ in Italian HBsAg-positive haemophiliacs was 50% both in Northern Italy and Southern Italy.

A similar prevalence (48%) was observed in haemophiliacs
from Maryland (USA). A distinctly lower prevalence (18%)
was observed in haemophiliacs from Great Britain and none
of the five HBsAg carrier haemophiliacs from East Germany
was found infected with δ.

Thus, the risk of δ infection to HBsAg-positive haemophiliacs seems to be primarily determined by type and
source of substitution therapy. Commercial products prepared from pools of thousands of blood donors were associated with the highest rate of δ infection. The lower prevalence of anti-δ in English haemophiliacs is probably due to
the use, together with commercial products, of products
prepared locally by the National Health Service from single
plasma donors, that account for about 40% of the substitution therapy used in this country. The exclusive administration of products from single or mini-pool donors, as
in the use in East Germany, would appear the best way to
limit δ infection among HBsAg-positive haemophiliacs.
Extent of therapy, however,is also important and may not
have been equal in each country; all δ-positive USA and
Italian haemophiliacs had severe clotting deficiency and
were treated with concentrate for years.

To evaluate the clinical relevance of δ infection in the
liver disease of the haemophiliac, the prevalence of anti-δ
and chronic hepatitis was determined in 187 Italian haemophiliacs including 37 carriers of HBsAg. The diagnosis of
chronic hepatitis was based on the finding of persistently
abnormal serum aminotransferase values and on increases in
the gamma-globulin fraction of serum.

Biochemical evidence of chronic liver disease was found
in 12 of 37 haemophiliacs with HBsAg (32.4%) and in 6 of
150 without HBV infection (4%). Nine of 12 (75%) haemophiliacs with chronic HBsAg hepatitis were also positive
for anti-δ at high titers; a liver biopsy, available from
3 of these patients demonstrated cirrhosis in two and a
chronic active hepatitis in one (table 3). Two of these

patients has intrahepatic δ-Ag.

TABLE 3. CHRONIC LIVER DISEASE IN ITALIAN HAEMOPHILIACS

HBsAg+	12*/37	(32.4%)
HBsAg−	6/150	(4.0%)

n° chronic liver disease/n° examined;
* 9 of them with anti-δ

Comparison of clinical data and liver chemistry showed
that the liver disease was significantly more severe in δ-
positive than δ-negative haemophilic carriers of HBsAg.

These data confirm the conclusion (Rizzetto et al. 1982)
that δ infection is a major cause of severe liver disease
of the haemophiliac.

The following participated in this study:
L. Baldi, G. Pastore, F. Trotta, O. Schiraldi (Bari);
M. Colombo, S. Fargion, C. Scaroni (Milano).

References

Rizzetto M, Shih JW-K, Gocke DJ, Purcell RH, Verme G,
  Gerin JL (1979). Incidence and significance of antibodies
  to delta antigen in hepatitis B virus infection. Lancet
  2: 986.
Rizzetto M, Purcell RH, Gerin JL (1980). Epidemiology of
  HBV-associated delta agent: geographical distribution of
  anti-delta and prevalence in polytransfused HBs-Ag
  carriers. Lancet 1: 1215.
Rizzetto M, Morello C, Mannucci PM, Gocke DJ, Spero JA,
  Lewis JH, Thiel DH, Scaroni C, Peyretti F (1982). Delta
  infection and liver disease in hemophilic carriers of
  hepatitis B surface antigen. J Infect Dis 145: 18.

Viral Hepatitis and Delta Infection, pages 151–154
© 1983 Alan R. Liss, Inc., 150 Fifth Avenue, New York, NY 10011

SPREAD OF DELTA (δ) INFECTION IN A GROUP OF HAEMODIALYSIS CARRIERS OF HBsAg

G. Marinucci, L. Valeri, C. Di Giacomo, D. Morganti

Ospedale San Giacomo,
Via Canova 29, 00186 Roma, Italia

The high frequency of hepatitis B virus (HBV) infection in dialysis patients is well known (London 1969; Garibaldi 1973). Dialysis patients are immune deficient, expecially at cellular immunity levels (London 1969; Blumberg 1970), and subject to very high rates of HB viral replication; they are often positive for HBeAg and HBV-specific DNA-polymerase activity in serum and for HB core antigen in liver. (Miller 1978; Bianchi 1979). Though some develop typical viral hepatitis, most have only a subclinical infection without apparent manifestations of liver damage.

Over the last 3years we have carried out periodical follow-up checking for delta infection on 63 HBsAg-positive patients undergoing haemodialysis in four centers in Rome. Patients were screened for anti-δ by Radioimmuneassay (Rizzetto 1980) Since results were consistently negative, we concluded that either no patient with delta infection had ever utilised the machinery shared by the members of the groups studied or haemodialysis patients were resistent to delta infection, possibly because of the high level of HBV replication characteristic of these individuals. (Marinucci 1982).

The serological features of the 63 HBsAg-positive patients from 4 centers in Rome, followed up during the years 1979-1982 are shown in the table:

HBeAg +	anti HBe +	anti Delta +
40	23	–
(63,5%)	(36,5%)	(0%)

It is only during the past 8 months that we noticed the spread of δ infection in a group of 5 haemodialysis patients from another center in Rome, all chronic HBsAg carriers for at least five years and all using the same artificial kidney. Two of them had an acute viral hepatitis type B (AVH) that progressed to chronicity and the other three had a chronic active hepatitis (CAH). The five patients had HBeAg and anti-δ in serum and were negative for the antibody of IgM class to the HB core antigen. Their serum pattern appears therefore different from that observed in ordinary carriers with δ infection who usually have anti-HBe in serum and lack markers of active HBV synthesis (Smedile 1981).

Backlog led to the hypothesis that the probable source of infection was a drug addict suffering from anti-δ positive CAH, added to the group in 1980. The other two patients with CAH were admitted to the group in 1981; shortly after they experienced a clinical episode of AVH. The two patients who suffered from anti-δ positive AVH which is now progressing to chronicity were admitted to the group in 1982. These data are summarized in the figure number one.

Family studies have shown that the son of one of these patients (5) had AVH positive for anti-δ and his brother-in-law was positive for anti-δ with no signs of liver damage. Both family members have been chronic HBsAg carriers for many years. The haemodialysis facilities nurse of the group, who was also a known carrier of HBsAg, is now positive for anti-delta without apparent liver damage.

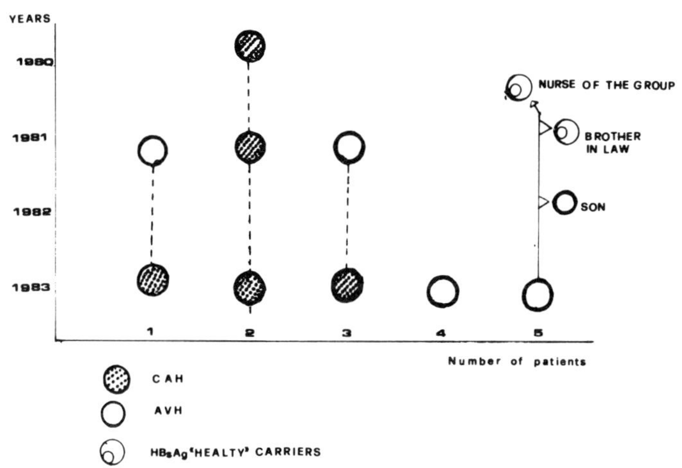

Fig. 1.

In conclusion, haemodialysis patients appear to be susceptible to delta infection just as non dialysis patients, despite the high rate of HBV replication characteristic of these individuals. Since the pathogenic effect of delta is maximal in carriers of HBsAg, our results stress the danger of HBsAg carriers sharing contaminated machinery, thus exposing the δ-negative carrier to superinfection with δ co-infecting other carriers in the same dialysis unit.

REFERENCES

Bianchi L., Gudat F (1979). Immunopathology of hepatitis B. In : Progress in Liver disease.Vol 6. Popper and Schaffner Eds. Grune and Stratton . New York.

Blumberg BS, Sutnick AI, London WT (1970).Australia antigen as a hepatitis virus. Variation in host response. AM. J. Med. 48:I

Garibaldi RA, Forrest JN, Bryan JA (1973). Haemo-
dialyisis associated hepatitis. Jama 225:384.

London WT, Di Figlia M, Sutnick AI, Blumberg BS
(1969). An epidemic of hepatitis in a chronic
haemodialysis Unit. Australia antigen and diffe
rences in host response. N. Engl. J. Med.281:571

Marinucci G,, Muglia M, Di Giacomo C. (1982) Con-
siderazioni epidemiologiche sul sistema δ/anti δ
in epatopatie croniche nella città di Roma. Fo-
lia Allergol. Immunol. Clin. 29:316.

Miller DJ, Alan EW, Le Bouvier G., Dwyer J.M.,
Grant J, Klitskin G. (1978). Hepatitis B in hae
modialysis patients: significance of HBeAg.
Gastroenterology 74: 1208

Rizzetto M, Purcell RH, Gerin JC, (1980). Epidemiology of HBV⊤ associated delta agent: geographical distribution of anti delta and prevalence in polytransfused HBsAg carriers.
Lancet i: 1215

Smedile A, Dentico P, Zanetti A, Sagnelli E,
Nordfelt E, Actis GC, Rizzetto M (1981). Infec-
tion with delta agent in chronic HBsAg carriers.
Gastroenterology 81:992

EPIDEMIOLOGY OF DELTA INFECTION IN SCANDINAVIA

B.G. Hansson*, G. Norkrans, M. Weibull,
O. Weiland, J. Nielsen, P. Leinikki, P. Ukkonen,
O. Jensson and J.-C. Siebke
*Department of Clinical Virology, University of
Lund, Malmö General Hospital, Malmö, Sweden

Epidemiological studies have shown the delta agent to
be world wide distributed. Delta infection has been found to
be especially prevalent in HBsAg-carriers from southern
Italy and in patients who have received multiple transfu-
sions of blood or blood products, such as hemophiliacs
(Rizzetto et al 1980). In western Europe, Scandinavia and
USA intravenous drug addicts seem to be a main reservoar for
the delta agent (Raimondo et al 1982; Hansson et al 1982).
In the present study a survey of delta infections in
Scandinavia including Iceland and Finland has been made.

Table 1 shows the prevalence of anti-delta in chronic
HBsAg-carriers collected from various regions and from
different patient categories. Anti-delta was found in high
frequency among drug addicts in Denmark, Norway and Sweden.
No HBsAg-positive sera from drug addicts in Finland were
available for analysis. One out of 10 HBsAg-carrier hemophilia patients had anti-delta. The delta infection had been
acquired simultaneous with hepatitis B infection by a factor
VIII preparation.

One homosexual man from Copenhagen and one from
Stockholm were found positive for anti-delta. However, at
least the patient from Stockholm also had a history of drug
addiction.

Altogether 12 non-Scandinavians, one from West Germany,
one from East Europe, the others from Turkey, Syria or
Africa, were positive for anti-delta.

Table 1. Anti-delta in chronic HBsAg-carriers

	Drug addicts	Hemo- philiacs	Homo- sexuals	Immi- grants	Unknown exposure
Denmark					
Copenhagen	3		1/17		
Finland					
Helsinki					0/100
Tampere					0/62
Iceland				0/1	0/7
Norway	21/64	0/2	0/4		0/105
Sweden					
Falun	1/6		0/1	1/5	1/10
Gothenburg	11/16			0/9	0/21
Malmö	41/80	1/8	0/15	2/53	0/137
Stockholm	9/14		1*/15	9/19	1/13

*Also a drug addict

Analysis of consecutive serum samples from the HBsAg-positive drug addicts of Norway and the city of Malmö showed the first anti-delta positive patients to appear in 1975 and 1973, respectively (Fig 1). The prevalence of anti-delta in these populations increased from year to year. By 1981 87 % of the HBsAg-carrier drug addicts of Malmö had anti-delta. In Norway 40 % had turned positive for anti-delta by 1982.

Patients with acute, self-limited hepatitis were analysed for simultaneous delta infection. From Copenhagen 79 patients, about half of them drug addicts, with hepatitis B in 1973, 1976, 1979 and 1982 and from Norway 94 drug addicts with type B hepatitis between 1973 and 1982 were tested. All of the patients registered with acute hepatitis B in Malmö between 1970 and 1981 were also included. The delta diagnosis were made by the detection of delta antigen in early sera and/or development of anti-delta in convalescent sera. Cases of simultaneous B and delta hepatitis were found in Denmark already in 1973 (Table 2). Among the Norwegian patients one case from each of the years 1978, 1981 and 1982 was seen.

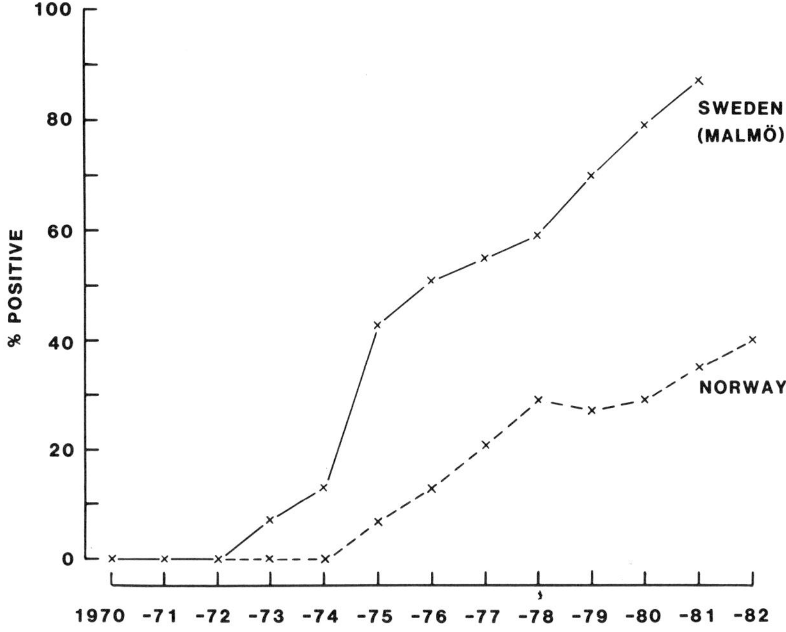

Fig 1. Prevalence of anti-delta in chronic HBsAg-carrier
drug addicts.

Relative to the many cases of delta infection among the
HBsAg-carriers in Norway the incidence of simultaneous delta
infection in the cases of acute hepatitis B seems low. However, in many of these patients the convalescent sera were
collected in rather early stage of the disease, before anti-
delta could have developed. When all the 623 patients with
acute hepatitis B seen in Malmö were analysed for delta
markers, the first positive case occurred in 1973 in a patient who four months previously had received blood transfusions in Spain. Beginning in 1975 between 18 and 50 % of
the drug addicts with acute hepatitis B were also delta infected. During the study period five cases appeared among
non-addicts. However, two of these persons had probably been
infected through sexual intercourse with drug addicts and
the other three by non-sexual contacts with friends who were
drug addicts.

Table 2. Delta infection in patients with acute, self-limited hepatitis B.

| | Denmark (Copenhagen) | Norway | Sweden (Malmö) | |
	All patients	Drug addicts	Drug addicts	Non-addicts
1970			0/17	0/41
1971			0/40	0/34
1972			0/40	0/29
1973	3/18	0/4	0/51	1/31
1974		0/5	0/15	0/27
1975		0/12	6/16	0/36
1976	5/25	0/10	5/11	2/27
1977		0/11	20/45	1/23
1978		1/11	12/30	0/24
1979	2/19	0/10	3/17	1/23
1980		0/14	4/9	0/13
1981		1/11	3/11	1/13
1982	3/17	1/6		

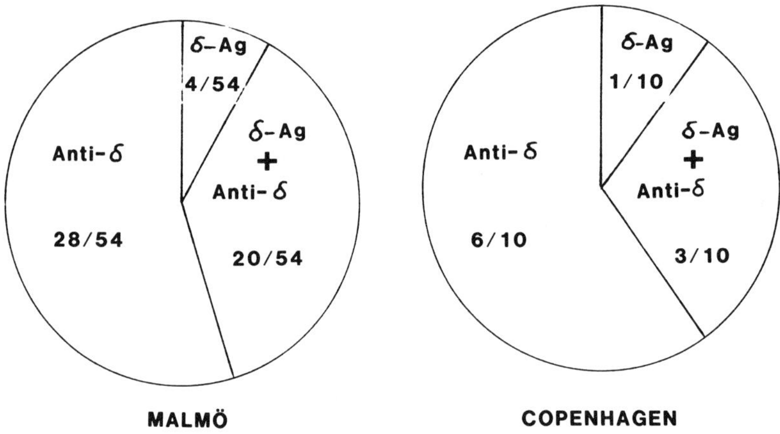

Fig 2. Delta markers in acute, simultaneous HBV and delta hepatitis.

Delta antigen was detected in early sera in almost half

of the diagnosed simultaneous type B and delta hepatitis cases (Fig 2). Actually, in four of 54 patients from Malmö and one of ten from Copenhagen delta antigen was the only marker of the infection because convalescent-phase sera had not been collected. In half of the patients only the development of anti-delta could be detected. In many cases early acute phase sera were not available making the possibility of finding delta antigen low.

According to our experience, anti-delta persists for many years after an acute type B and delta hepatitis. Not in a single case we have found anti-delta to disappear.

The results of this study have shown the delta agent to be a newly introduced hepatitis agent in Scandinavia. Probably, the first cases appeared in Denmark followed by spreading to Sweden and Norway. So far, the delta infection has almost exclusively been found among intravenous drug addicts. Drug addicts from Finland and Iceland are awaiting to be analysed.

Hansson BG, Moestrup T, Widell A, Nordenfelt E (1982). Infection with delta agent in Sweden: introduction of a new hepatitis agent. J Infect Dis 146:472.
Raimondo G, Smedile A, Gallo L, Balbo A, Ponzetto A, Rizzetto M (1982). Multicentre study of prevalence of HBV-associated delta infection and liver disease in drug-addicts. Lancet 1:249.

Rizzetto M, Purcell RH, Gerin JL (1980). Epidemiology of HBV-associated delta agent: geographical distribution of anti-delta and prevalence in polytransfused HBsAg carriers. Lancet 1:1215.

Viral Hepatitis and Delta Infection, pages 161–165
© 1983 Alan R. Liss, Inc., 150 Fifth Avenue, New York, NY 10011

ASPECTS ON THE EPIDEMIOLOGY OF DELTA-AGENT AMONG ARABS

Erik Nordenfelt, Bengt Göran Hansson, Basil
Al-Nakib, Saleh Al-Kandari and Widad Al-Nakib
Department of Microbiology,
Faculty of Medicine, Kuwait University,
P.O. Box 24923, Safat, Kuwait

The epidemiology of infection with delta-agent has been
studied through the prevalence of its antibody (anti-delta).
Anti-delta has been found among all populations studies so
far. The prevalence is high, 40-47 %, in chronic HBsAg
carriers in Southern Italy. In other parts of the world, the
prevalence has been found to be low, < 5 %, except among
polytransfused haemophiliacs and drug addicts in Europe and
USA where 30-75 % have anti-delta (Rizzetto, 1982).

Kuwait presents a unique opportunity to study the
epidemiology of the delta agent among Arabs, since most Arab
nationa ities are well represented in its population. Kuwait
is situated at the top of the Arabian Gulf, bordering Iraq
and Saudi Arabia. It has a population of 1.5 million of whom
about 45 % are Kuwaitis, the rest are mainly from other Arab
countries and from the Asian subcontinent. There is a high
movement rate of foreign population from various countries
especially those from neighbouring Arab countries. Thus in
the present study, the prevalence of anti-delta in Kuwait
has been investigated.

<u>MATERIAL:</u>

144 hepatitis B surface antigen (HBsAg) positive sera
from different patients diagnosed among samples received for
HBsAg testing at the Department of Microbiology, Faculty of
Medicine, Kuwait University. All sera have been stored at
-20°C after primary testing.

<u>METHODS</u>:

Presence of HBsAg was investigated by radioimmunoassay
(RIA) (Ausria, Abbott, Chicago, USA).

Tests for presence of delta-antigen and anti-delta were
done at the Department of Clinical Virology, University of
Lund, Sweden by a solid phase RIA as earlier described
(Hansson et al, 1982).

<u>RESULTS</u>:

In none of the 144 HBsAg positive sera, could the
delta antigen be found. However, 58 or (40%) were found to be
anti-delta positive. Full information regarding diagnosis,
age, sex, and nationality was available from 80 of the
patients investigated. Among those 32 or 40% were positive
for anti-delta. In Table 1 the results are presented in
relation to diagnosis.

Table 1.   <u>Antibodies to delta-agent in relation to diagnosis.</u>

Diagnoses	Total	Positive	Negative	%Positive
Chronic liver disease	38	25	13	66
Acute hepatitis	30	4	26	13
Others	12	3	9	25
	80	32	48	40

The highest number of anti-delta positives was thus
found among those patients with chronic liver disease where
25 of 38 or 66% were found to be positive. These cases
included 16 with cirrhosis, 7 with Bilharzia, 7 with chronic
active hepatitis, 3 with hepatoma and 5 with unspecified
cause of chronic liver disease. One of the cases of acute
hepatitis was fatal and this patient had anti-delta.
"Other" included diagnosis without correlation to liver
disease i.e. diabetes, cerebral stroke, malignancies and
infections. The frequency of anti-delta in relation to
nationality is presented in Table 2.

Table 2. <u>Antibodies to delta-agent in relation to nationality.</u>

	Total	Positive	Negative	% Positive
Gulf Arabs	43	15	28	35
Mediterranean Arabs	26	15	11	58
Others	11	2	9	18
	80	32	48	40

Gulf Arabs are those coming from the Arabian peninsula
i.e. Kuwait, Iraq, Oman, UAE, Yemen and Saudi Arabia.
Mediterranean Arabs represent those from Egypt, Syria,
Jordanian and "others" include Iranians, Indians, Pakistanis
and Philipinos. As can be seen all except two of the anti-
delta positive are either Gulf or Mediterranean Arabs.

Thirty-five of the cases with chronic liver disease are
Arabs and these are presented according to country of origin
in Table 3.

Table 3. <u>Cases with chronic liver disease in relation to
Arab country of origin and anti-delta frequency</u>

		Positive	Negative	Total
Gulf Arabs	Kuwait	4	3	7
	Iraq	2	–	2
	Oman	1	1	2
	Yemen	1	3	4
	Saudi Arabia	1	1	2
Mediterranean Arabs	Egypt	11	2	13
	Jordan	2	2	4
	Syria	1	–	1
		23	12	35

Most of these patients come from Egypt and among them
are included all the 7 cases of Bilharzia. The percentage of
positive cases among the Egyptians was 85%.
Of the 7 anti-delta positive Arab patients there were 4 with
the diagnosis acute hepatitis and 3 with "others". Five were

Kuwaitis and one case respectively was from Yemen and Syria.
Of the 80 patients, 70 were male and 10 female. Only
one of the anti-delta positive patients was female. She was
of Philipino origin with a diagnosis of chronic active
hepatitis. The mean age of the anti-delta negatives was 30.4
years and anti-delta positives 39.4 years.

DISCUSSION:

A very high prevalence of anti-delta, 66% was found
among the patients with chronic liver disease. When cases
were grouped according to their countries of origin, it was
found that patients of Egyptian origin were the most predominate group and had a very high frequency of delta
infection. However, the numbers were small and therefore
conclusions must await the results of further studies.

Thus, infection with the delta-agent clearly is an
important co-factor in the pathogenesis of chronic liver
disease in this region, as delta-infection in HBsAg carriers
is known to become chronic (Smedile et al, 1981).

It has not been possible to differentiate between
chronic and transient HBsAg carriers among the patients.
However, patients with a diagnosis of chronic liver disease
and "others" are probably all chronic carriers. Some of the
patients with acute hepatitis are probably also chronic
HBsAg carriers with a superimposed delta-infection. The
carriership in Kuwait is between 2.8 - 4% (Al-Nakib et al,
1982, Al-Nakib in press). It is noteworthy that the only
fatal case reported in this study was found among the anti-
delta positive patients.

This investigation therefore, has shown that delta
infections is endemic in this region and has about the same
or even higher frequency than that found in Southern Italy.
Historically, of course, there have been many connections
between these areas, and possibly both belong to perhaps one
larger region with an endemic presence of delta agent where
Egypt could be an important link.

If the results of the present investigation is representative for the Arab nations, the Arab world could be an
important reservoir for the delta agent.

Al-Nakib B, Al-Nakib W, Bayoumi A, Al-Liddawi H, Aziz Bashir A (1982). Hepatitis B virus (HBV) markers among patients with chronic liver disease in Kuwait. Trans Roy Soc Trop Med Hyg 76:348.

Hansson BG, Moestrup T, Widell A, Nordenfelt E (1982). Infection with Delta agent in Sweden. Introduction of a new Hepatitis agent. J Inf Dis 146:472.

Rizzetto M (1982). Biology and characterization of the Delta agent. In Szmunness W, Alter HJ, Maynard JE (eds): "Proceedings of the Third International Symposium on Viral Hepatitis New York City, "Philadelphia: Franklin Institute Press, p 355.

Smedile A, Dentico P, Zanetti A, Sagnelli E, Nordenfelt E, Actis GC, Rizzetto M (1981). Infection with the Delta agent in chronic HBsAg carriers. Gastroenterology 81:992.

DELTA INFECTION: PATHOLOGICAL AND CLINICAL ASPECTS

HISTOPATHOLOGY OF CHRONIC DELTA HEPATITIS

Verme G.,Rocca G.,Rizzi R.,Mollo F.,David E.,
Solcia E.,Sessa F.
Gastroenterology Dept.and Epidemiology Service,
San Giovanni Hospital,Turin;Institutes of Morbid
Anatomy,Universities of Turin and Pavia,Italy.

Intrahepatic expression of delta antigen has been invariably associated with liver damage.This encompasses the
whole spectrum of hepatitis from an acute self limited or
fulminant illness to chronic active liver disease with cirrhosis (Rizzetto 1977,1983;Stöcklin 1981;Smedile 1982;Govin-
darajan 1983;Farci 1983;Weller 1983).
There have been reports in recent years of histological
aspects characteristic of A,B and NANB hepatitis,both in experimentally infected chimpanzees and in naturally infected
humans(Popper 1980;Dienes 1982;Purcell 1982).To determine
whether Delta hepatitis exhibits also characteristic histological features,in this study the independent association of
different histological parameters was evaluated in chronic
HBsAg hepatitis accompanied by delta infection and compared
with chronic type B hepatitis without delta infection and
with NANB hepatitis.
The study is based on a series of 110 liver biopsies
from patients collected during the years 1979-1983 in Turin.
Slides were routinely stained for ordinary histology by
Hematoxylin-Eosin and Van Gieson;delta-Ag was demonstrated
by immunofluorescence and immunoperoxidase using IgG anti-
delta labeled with fluorescein or horseradish peroxidase
(Rizzetto 1977;Recchia 1981).
The diagnosis of type B hepatitis was based on the presence of HBsAg in the serum and HBcAg in the liver.The diagnosis of Delta hepatitis was based on the presence of

delta-Ag in the liver and/or anti-delta at high titer in the serum.NANB hepatitis was diagnosed on the absence of HBV markers ,negative serology for known hepatitis viruses and clinical evidence suggestive of viral disease.The three aetiological types of hepatitis considered were adequately distributed in the different diagnostic categories examined,i.e. nonspecific reactive (NSRH),acute (AH),chronic persistent (CPH), chronic lobular (CLH),chronic active hepatitis (CAH) with or without cirrhosis.(Figure 1).

<u>Figure 1</u>

Histological Diagnosis

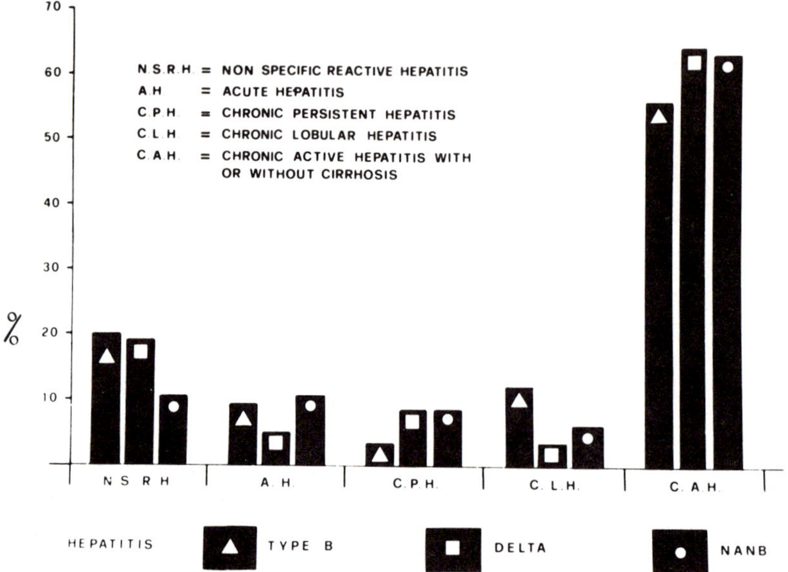

All three types,however,were prevalent in the last group (CAH).

The slides were evaluated according to the observation of three anatomical areas of the liver (portal tract,limiting plate and lobule).Forty-one histological items were first analysed blindly and from their grouping six histological levels (inflammation,fibrosis,necrosis,degeneration,regeneration,immunofluorescence)were defined and quantitated (Fleiss 1981).

Contingency tables with X^2 analysis were used to study the statistical associations of all histological characteristics with the three groups of hepatitis.Log linear model analysis was performed with BMPD statistical program on a IBM 370 computer.

Among the features considered ,five resulted significantly associated with one or the other of the three groups of hepatitis (Table 1).

Table 1

Histological features characteristic of Delta,B and NANB hepatitis*.

	DELTA	B	NANB
Inflammation	0.0228	NS	NS
Sinusoidal cell diffuse activation	NS	0.00024	NS
Degeneration without peripolesis	0.0000	NS	NS
Cytoplasmic eosinophilia	0.006	NS	NS

* Log linear model analysis.

General inflammation,sinusoidal cell activation,topographic association between degeneration and cellular inflammation (peripolesis) and cytoplasmic eosinophilia were asymmetrically distributed in the three groups of hepatitis.In particular the level of lobular inflammation was consistently higher in Delta than in B or NANB cases.The sinusoidal cell diffuse activation was prevalent in hepatitis B.The level of degeneration was evenly distributed in the three types of hepatitis,but in Delta hepatitis the degeneration of the hepatocytes was topographically independent from cellular inflammation.

Though the other types of degenerative lesions were equally distributed in the three groups of hepatitis,hepatocyte eosinophilia was prevalent in Delta cases (Figure 2).

Figure 2

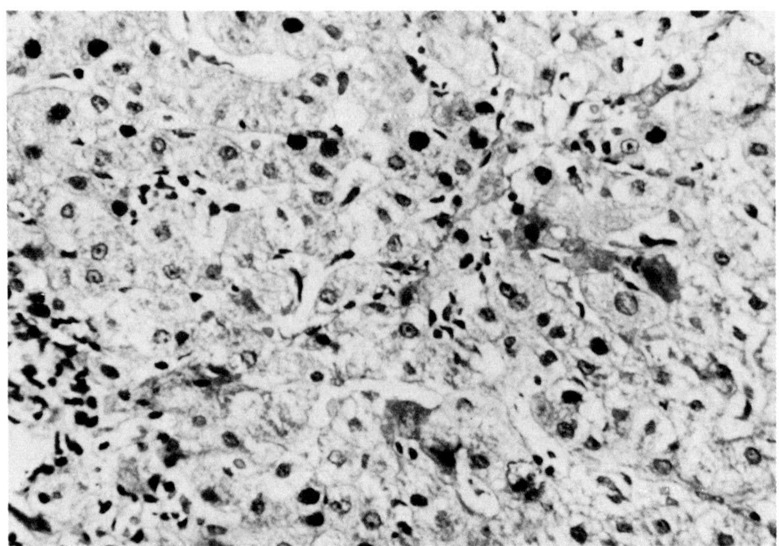

   A typical feature of chronic Delta hepatitis:hepatocytes
with cytoplasmic eosinophilia and other types of degeneration not surrounded by inflammatory cells.Delta positive nuclei stained by immunoperoxidase (500X).

In Delta hepatitis the eosinophilic hepatocytes (and hepatocytes with other degenerative aspects)were also topographically independent from cellular inflammation.These histological features are summarized in Figure 3.

   Besides the blind histological assessment,slides were
also examined for a correlation between morphology and presence and distribution of Delta,Core and Surface antigens,
demonstrated by immunoistochemistry.HBsAg and delta antigen
were identified by immunoperoxidase in the same slide used
for histologic analysis after counterstaining with Hematoxy-
lin-Eosin.Because of denaturation of HBcAg by fixation this
antigen was identified in frozen blocks adjacent to fixed
blocks used for ordinary histology.Evaluation of the relationship between delta antigen and HBcAg was performed in
frozen material.The findings of this analysis were:

 1)Delta antigen was always nuclear with the exception of
few acute cases in which Delta appeared also in cytoplasms.

2)The nuclei containing delta-antigen were equally contained in apparently normal,degenerated and eosinophilic hepatocytes.They were distributed randomly throughout the lobule.

4)Eosinophilic hepatocytes containing or not nuclear Delta antigen were equally located close to bridges of connective tissue (Figure 4).

5)In all except three cases delta-antigen was mutually exclusive with HBcAg.No relationship instead emerged between the expression of HBsAg and presence or absence of delta-Ag. In the three cases with Delta and Core antigens in the same biopsy,the antigens were expressed together in the same hepatocytes in one case and in different hepatocytes in two cases.

Figure 3

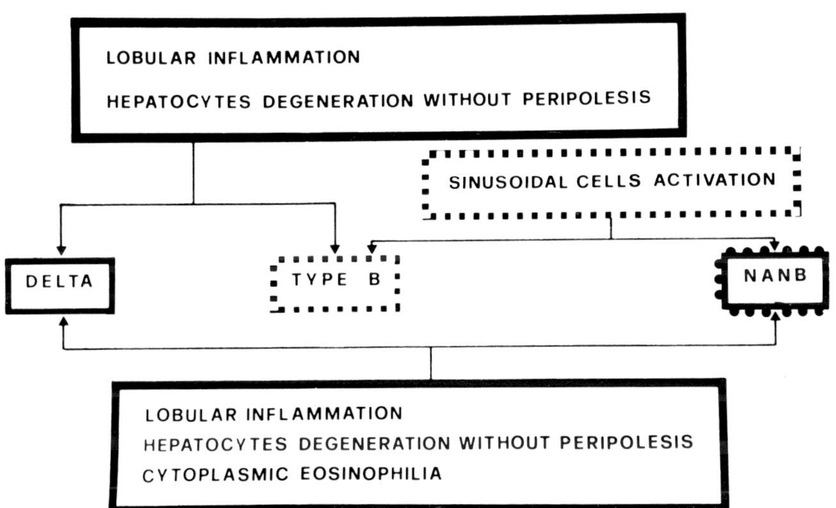

Figure 4

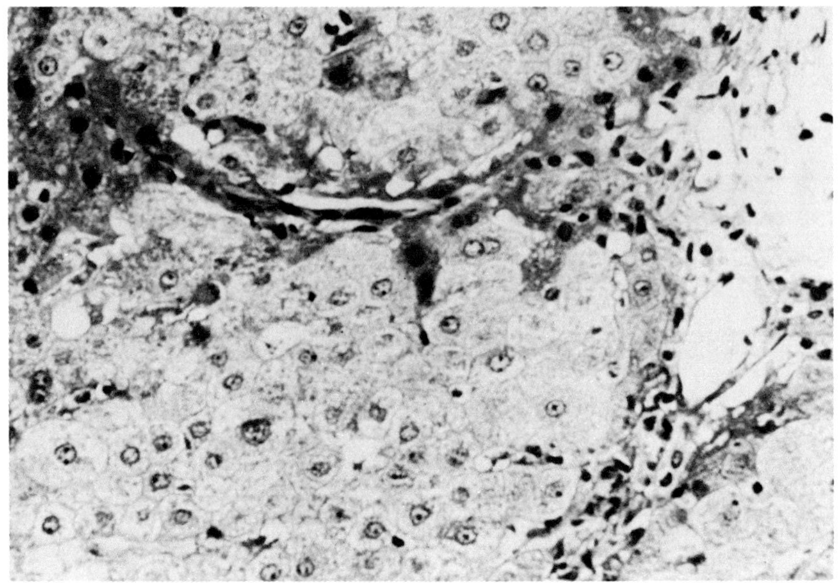

Delta chronic hepatitis.Portal to central bridging associated with cytoplasmic eosinophilia.(500X).

Conclusions.No histological feature appears to be specific of delta hepatitis.The demonstration of this entity re-
lies upon serological and immunohistologic detection of the
delta-Ag/anti-delta system.Nevertheless a few histologic
characters occur frequently in Delta hepatitis and their
combination may therefore be helpful in addressing to this
diagnosis.They are:
 1)a marked degree of inflammation with active bridging.
 2)degeneration of hepatocytes dissociated from inflammation
and without diffuse sinusoidal cell activation.
The eosinophilic degeneration in the lobule is common;
this is also dissociated from inflammation and often strictly connected with direct interlaminar fibrillogenesis.Cyto-
plasmic eosinophilia seems to lead often to eosinophilic
bodies (acidophilic)and therefore to hepatocyte necrosis and

assigned to this stage; the serum contained delta antibodies.
4. Transition to cirrhosis (four autopsy specimens, disease
duration 3 1/2 to 22 months): Extensive areas of collapse
alternated with partly fat-containing regenerative nodules
separated by connective tissue septa. Abundant delta antigen
was demonstrated in nuclei of some nodules. Three biopsy
specimens (disease duration 2 to 7 months), one associated
with delta antibodies, were assigned to this stage, with one
of them showing a chronic active hepatitis with cytopathic
changes. In none of the autopsy specimens could hepatitis B
surface or core antigens be demonstrated by immunoperoxidase
staining.

The demonstration of delta antigen confirms its role in
the causation of the epidemic, supplementing the presence of
delta antibodies in ill persons. During the massive-necrotic
stage, when barely any hepatocytes are present, little or no
delta antigen is found and several months seem to be required
until large amounts of delta antigen are seen. The tissue
reaction is characterized by mainly cytopathic hepatocellular
lesions, reflected in small-droplet steatosis and predominance of macrophages over lymphocytes in the lobular
parenchyma, seemingly in contrast to fatal lesions induced by
hepatitis B infection alone. The observations prove occurrence of delta agent infections independent of Italian ethnic
origin, drug addiction or other factors conventionally associated with this infection. This raises the possibility
that delta agent infection may be responsible for epidemics
of severe hepatitis in various parts of the world. Preliminary support for this assumption was obtained by the
study of two cases of LaBrea fever, common in the northern
part of South America, particularly around the Amazon river,
from the files of the Armed Forces Institute of Pathology,
Washington, D.C. These showed the same changes as stage 1 or
2 of the Venezuelan material; in one of them, delta antigen
was found in the liver nuclei.

(in press, Ann Int Med)

Viral Hepatitis and Delta Infection, pages 181–189
© 1983 Alan R. Liss, Inc., 150 Fifth Avenue, New York, NY 10011

ELECTRON MICROSCOPIC STUDIES OF DELTA INFECTION

Fred Gudat, MD, Hans-Peter Spichtin, MD,
Elisabeth Stöcklin, MD, Gunthild Krey,
Josef Altorfer, MD, Martin Schmid, MD,
Leonardo Bianchi, MD
Department of Pathology, University of Basel
CH-4056 Basel (Switzerland)

Following the hypothesis of Rizzetto et al (1980) that
the superinfection with the delta agent might modify the
presentation and natural course of hepatitis B (HB), we studied the ultrastructure of the liver cell in 13 patients with
delta infection as compared to histologically matched cases
of uncomplicated HB. Our working hypothesis was that the
delta agent enhances cellular reactions in response to the
additional viral insult. Therefore, special attention was
paid (1) to (em)peripolesis as a possible sign of increased
immune surveillance due to virus-induced neo-antigens, (2)
to bleb formation as a possible mechanism of shedding cell
constituents bearing such antigens, and (3) to the formation
of intranuclear inclusions of the "non-A, non-B (NANB) type"
as a possible nonspecific sign of altered nuclear metabolism
(Cervera et al 1983) rather than as an indication of the
synthesis of a NANB agent (Shimizu et al 1979).

MATERIAL AND METHODS

Delta-Positive Patients

13 consecutive patients of the current bioptic series
(8 with acute lobular hepatitis (ALH), 5 with chronic active
hepatitis (CAH)) were identified by the immunofluorescent
(IF) demonstration of intranuclear delta antigen on cryostat
sections of liver biopsies. The immunohistological and serological procedures for the determination of HB and delta

markers as well as the electron microscopic methods have
been described in detail elsewhere (Stöcklin et al 1981,
Gudat et al 1975).

With the exception of one homosexual and one hepatitis
contact, all patients were drug users. Ten patients had
anti-delta as determined by indirect immunofluorescence, 2
with ALH had not. Two other patients were negative for HBsAg
by commercial radioimmunoassay and immune electron microscopy (EM) but one was positive for IgM-anti-HBc and the
other had both anti-HBc and anti-HBs. HBcAg was not detectable
in any liver biopsy but circulating Dane particles were found
in 3 of 5 patients with CAH and in 2 of 7 patients with ALH.

Delta-Negative Patients

For comparison, 7 patients with ALH and 8 patients with
CAH were randomly selected from the same bioptic series. All
had ongoing HBV infection by serological and histological
criteria.

RESULTS

1. Bleb Formation

This was seen as broad-based or pedunculated protrusions of liver cells bulging from the sinusoidal pole into
the sinus (Fig. 1). These protrusions were void of the major cell organelles and contained mainly free ribosomes,
glycogen rosettes, and occasionally short pieces of endoplasmic reticulum or vacuoles.

Affected cells usually showed no alterations of their
cell organelles, especially no condensation of the cytoplasm
or of the nucleus. Occasionally, however, there was also
ballooning of bleb-forming cells suggesting a possible
transition to lytic necrosis.

In an advanced stage, blebs were seen as vesicles apparently freely floating in the sinusoids, with loss of

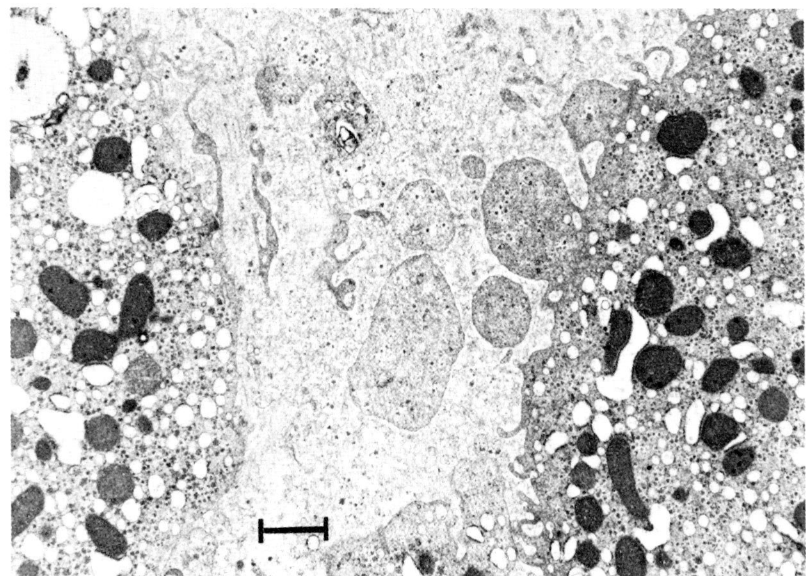

Fig. 1. Bleb formation of a hepatocyte. Note the similarity
of the contents of blebs and "free" vesicles. Delta-
positive CAH. (bar = 1 micron)

electron density supposedly due to dissolution of the content
and/or influx of water. Occasionally, strings of almost empty
vesicles plugged the sinusoidal lumen. This went together with
various stages of phagocytosis by Kupffer cells (Fig. 2).
Occasionally, there was also a severe swelling of endothelial cells with shedding of vesicles making it often impossible to classify vesicle formation as hepatocytic or endothelial in origin.

In ALH, true bleb formation by hepatocytes was demonstrated in 6 of 8 delta-positive patients but in only 2 biopsies of the 7 controls with uncomplicated HB. However, in-
trasinusoidal vesicles were seen in 6 patients of either
group. This tended to be more marked, however, in delta-positive ALH. It was not a significant finding, however, in
2 patients.

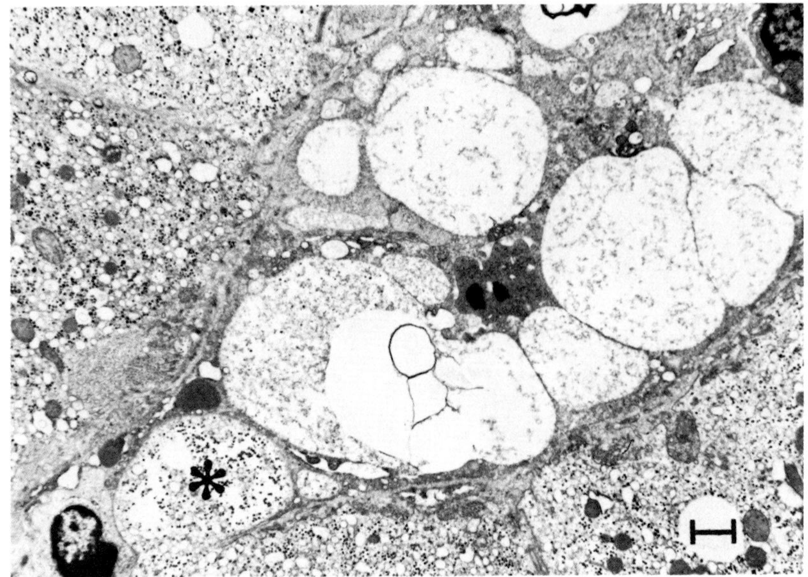

Fig. 2. Plugging of sinusoid by large ballooned vesicles,
one of them (*) in the process of protruding from a
hepatocyte. Delta-negative CAH. (bar = 1 micron)

Between the two groups of CAH no significant differences with respect to bleb formation (3 patients each group)
and appearance of vesicles (4 patients each group) could be
verified. The severity of vesicle formation appeared rather
correlated to the degree of the inflammatory activity than
to co-infection with the delta agent.

2. Peripolesis

A typical example of peripolesis is shown in Fig. 3,
demonstrating a conspicuous flattening of the liver cell
surface at the present and probably former zone of contact.
Peripolesis was readily seen in ultrathin sections of delta-
positive livers (11of 13patients) but less prominent in the
delta-negative control group (5 of 12 patients).

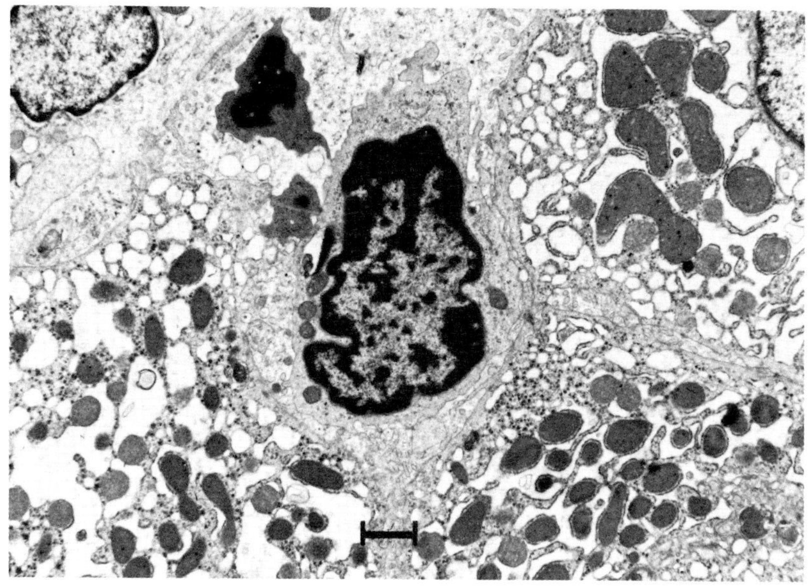

Fig. 3. Peripolesis with direct attachment of a lymphocyte
to liver cells. Note flattening of the villous hepatocyte surface in the contact area. Delta-positive ALH.
(bar = 1 micron)

3. Nuclear Particles of the "NANB Type"

Intranuclear aggregates of spherical and filamentous
particles (Fig. 4), identical to those demonstrated in experimental NANB hepatitis of chimpanzees (Shimizu et al 1979)
were seen in low numbers (2 per 150-200 nuclei) in both
acute and chronic HB, irrespective of co-infection with the
delta agent. Among delta-positive patients 5 of 8 patients
with ALH and 4 of 5 patients with CAH had intranuclear particles. The frequency for delta-negative patients was 4 of
7 and 2 of 5, respectively.

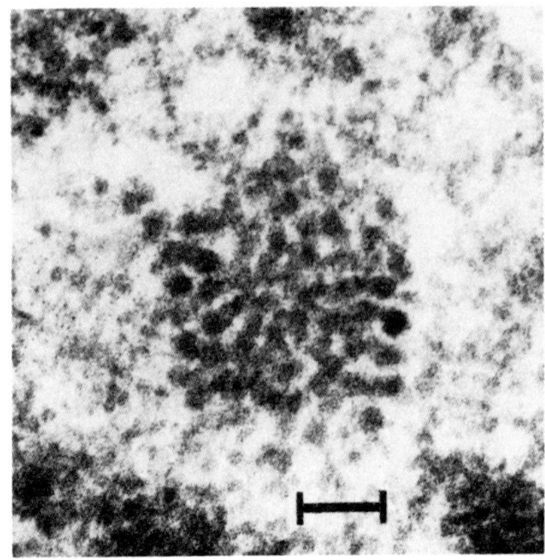

Fig. 4. Intranuclear aggregates of spherical and tubular virus-like particles as seen in NANB hepatitis. Delta-negative CAH.
(bar = 0.1 micron)

DISCUSSION

In the present study we were unable to define a specific ultrastructural marker of delta infection. Bleb formation, nuclear inclusions and peripolesis were seen in biopsies with or without delta co-infection. This is plausible because it is even uncertain whether all three alterations are virus-specific at all and nonspecific instead. Nevertheless, it appears that these alterations were more pronounced in delta infection although not in a diagnostic way. Certainly, further studies are needed to substantiate morphological differences induced by the delta agent.

Bleb formation is a well known feature of cell damage (Trump et al 1978), particularly in viral hepatitis (Schaffner 1966). It has also been seen with cultured cells including normal human liver cells brought into suspension (Trevisan et al 1983). The relation of bleb formation to early stages of apoptosis as defined by Kerr et al (1979) is not clear. Typical apoptosis implies, indeed, protrusions of cell surfaces but condensation of both nucleus and cytoplasm at the same time as a particular mode of single cell destruction (for review see Searle et al 1982). This was not observed in bleb-forming cells which showed a rather preserved cytoplasm and rarely ballooning as a possible sign of early lytic necrosis. Therefore, the phenomenon described here might not lead to cell death but might be a cellular defense

mechanism of shedding altered external cell membranes allowing survival of the affected cell. Our notion that this
process is more pronounced in delta co-infection would therefore indicate a more intense cellular damage by delta co-
infection. Whether this is due to enhanced antigen expression and increased immunologically mediated cell damage cannot be substantiated at present.

The pronounced peripolesis seen in these patients would
be compatible with this hypothesis. However, a direct cytopathic effect of the delta agent (Smedile et al 1982) cannot
be excluded on the basis of the presented EM alterations.

There is increasing evidence that nuclear aggregates of
virus-like particles originally described to be specific for
experimental NANB hepatitis of the chimpanzee (Shimizu et al
1978) are not specific for human NANB infection. This change
of view comes mainly from the observation of a high incidence
ce of such inclusions in HB and other hepatopathies (De Vos
et al 1983) and even in healthy human volunteers (Spichtin
et al 1983). In the present series the occurrence of this
alteration in HB has been confirmed. There is no significant
prevalence of such inclusions for delta infected biopsies
militating against the view that the delta agent specifically behaves like a NANB agent.

Recent experiments on nuclear alterations induced by
canavanine and cadmium in HeLa cells strongly suggest that
such aggregates represent a deficient assembling of constituents of perichromatin granules (Cervera et al 1983) and
may, therefore, be regarded as a nonspecific perturbation of
the nuclear nucleoprotein metabolism.

In summary, we conclude that there is no firm ultrastructural marker to recognize delta co-infection of HB.
We cannot exclude, however, that nonspecific reactions of
liver cells such as the formation of blebs, intrasinusoi-
dal vesicles of both hepatocytic and endothelial origin,
as well as nuclear inclusions are more readily induced in
double-infected cells.

Acknowledgment

Supported by grant No 3.849-0.81 from the Swiss National Science Foundation.

REFERENCES

Cervera J, Alamar M, Martinez A, Renau-Piqueras J (1983). Nuclear alterations induced by cadmium chloride and L-canavanine in HeLa S3 cells. Accumulation of perichromatin granules. J Ultrastruct Res 82: 241

De Vos R, Vanstapel MJ, Desmyter J, De Wolf-Peeters C, De Groote G, Colaert J, Mortelmans J, De Groote J, Fevery J, Desmet V (1983). Are nuclear particles specific for non-A, non-B hepatitis ? Hepatology (in press)

Gudat F, Bianchi L, Sonnabend W, Thiel G, Aenishaenslin W, Stalder GA (1975). Pattern of core and surface expression in liver tissue reflects state of specific immune response in hepatitis B. Lab Invest 32: 1

Kerr JFR, Cooksley WGE, Searle J, Halliday JW, Halliday WJ, Holder L, Roberts I, Burnett W, Powell LW (1979). The nature of piecemeal necrosis in chronic active hepatitis. Lancet ii: 827

Rizzetto M, Canese MG, Gerin JL, London WT, Sly DL, Purcell RH (1980). Transmission of the hepatitis B virus-associated delta antigen to chimpanzees. J infect Dis 141: 590

Schaffner F (1966). Intralobular changes in hepatocytes and the electron microscopic mesenchymal response in acute viral hepatitis. Medicine 45: 547

Searle J, Kerr JFR, Bishop CJ (1982). Necrosis and apoptosis: Distinct modes of cell death with fundamentally different significance. In Sommers SC, Rosen PP (eds): "Pathology Annual, part 2, vol. 17". Norwalk, Connecticut: Appleton-Century-Crofts, p. 229

Shimizu YK, Feinstone SM, Purcell RH, Alter HJ, London WT (1979). Non-A, non-B hepatitis: Ultrastructural evidence for two agents in experimentally infected chimpanzees. Science 205: 197

Smedile A, Farci P, Verme G, Caredda F, Cargnel A, Caporaso N, Dentico P, Trepo C, Opolon P, Gimson A, Vergani D, Williams R, Rizzetto M (1982). Influence of delta infection on severity of hepatitis B. Lancet ii: 945

Spichtin HP, Gudat F, Berthold H, Krey G, Schmid M, Piro-
vino M, Altorfer J, Stalder G, Eder G, Bianchi L (1983).
Nuclear particles of non-A, non-B type in healthy volun-
teers and patients with hepatitis B (in preparation)
Stöcklin E, Gudat F, Krey G, Dürmüller U, Gasser M, Schmid
M, Stalder G, Bianchi L (1981). δ antigen in hepatitis B:
Immunohistology of frozen and paraffin-embedded liver
biopsies and relation to HBV infection. Hepatology 1: 238
Trevisan A, Gudat F, Guggenheim R (1983). Electron microscopy
of isolated human hepatocytes: Micromethods for scanning
and transmission electron microscopy. La Ricerca (in press)
Trump BF, Jesudason ML, Jones RT (1978). Ultrastructural
features of diseased cells. In Trump BF, Jones RT (eds):
"Diagnostic Electron Microscopy, vol 1". New York: John
Wiley & Sons, p. 1

Viral Hepatitis and Delta Infection, pages 191–194
© 1983 Alan R. Liss, Inc., 150 Fifth Avenue, New York, NY 10011

DELTA INFECTION IN MAN:
ULTRASTRUCTURAL OBSERVATIONS

C.A. Busachi, P. Landi,L. Badiali De Giorgi, F.B.
Bianchi, A. Stacchiotti, S. Ferrari, M. Colombo,
A.Alberti, G.Realdi, R.Laschi, E. Pisi.
Patologia Medica I, Microscopia Elettronica,
Università di Bologna. Medicina Clinica, Univer-
sità di Padova.

To analyze by Electron Microscopy (E.M.) the
hepatic alterations during the course of human
delta hepatitis we studied three groups of liver
biopsies for the presence of viral tissue markers
by immunohistochemical and ultrastructural techniques. Serological markers of HBV and delta agent
were measured by RIA (Serology for delta system
was tested in the laboratory of Dr.Rizzetto).
The first group was composed by liver biopsies
from 8 patients positive for HBsAg and anti-delta
and negative for delta Ag in serum.
A second group of 41 biopsies from patients with
non A, non B viral hepatitis (acute, chronic,spo-
radic,high risk, post transfusion) and a third
group of 20 liver biopsies from HBsAg positive,
delta-negative chronic hepatitis were examined as
controls.
In the first group all the biopsies were positive
for delta agent on tissue when tested by immunohi
stochemical methods (immunofluorescence:IFL, or
immunoperoxidase:IPX) on 4µ and 1µ sections. The
mean nuclear positivity ranged from 1 to 50%.
In three of these cases (two drug addicts and a
patient transfused after surgery) we found, as
previously reported (Busachi,1983),intranuclear
aggregates of particles similar in morphology and

size (15-27 nm) to those described by Shimizu in chimpanzees (Shimizu,1979) and by other authors in humans with non A,non B hepatitis (Busachi, 1980; Busachi, 1981; Grimaud, 1980; Gmelin,1980; Cabral, 1981.). Since these patients were at high risk of acquiring viral infections, the hypothesis of multiple viral hepatitis must be considered. In the other delta-positive cases there were no intranuclear alterations resembling the Shimizu-like particles (table 1). The results in control groups, summarized in table 2, show a strict association between aggregates of intranuclear particles and non A,non B hepatitis, whereas these alterations were never observed in HBsAg positive viral hepatitis.

   Recently intranuclear round dense particles (25-30 nm) have been described in liver biopsies from chimpanzees experimentally infected with delta-positive inocula (Canese,1982). In our experience on human material, we have not found a correlation between Shimizu-like particles and HBsAg carriership, whether or not accompained by delta co-infection. We found Shimizu-like particles in cases of non A,non B viral hepatitis and in the three high risk patients with delta infection in whom a multiple viral exposure was highly probable. We therefore consider these particles as a reliable marker of non A,non B hepatitis. The E.M. expression of delta infection in human beings is still to be defined.

Table 1

| | | delta-positive cases | | | | | | | |
Case		1	2	3	4	5	6	7	8
delta (IPX IFL)	*	3	4	30	1	3	50	1	1
NANB intranuclear particles (E.M.)	*	30	8	–	8	–	–	–	–
risk factors		+	+	+	+	–	–	–	–

* Number (%) of affected cells.

Table 2

| Controls | n° | NANB particles E.M. | |
		acute	chronic
NANB transfused	19	5/9	8/10
" high risk	7	–	4/7
" sporadic	15	1/2	4/13
HBsAg CPH	6	–	–
" CAH	12	–	–
" CAH-C	2	–	–

REFERENCES

Busachi C.A., Patrizia Landi, F.B.Bianchi,A.Alberti, F.Tremolada,Lucilla Badiali De Giorgi,G.Realdi, R.Laschi and E.Pisi (1983). Non-A,non-B intranuclear particles inHBsAg and delta positive patients with chronic active hepatitis. Ital J Gastroenterol, 15;23.
Busachi C.A.,Realdi G.,Alberti A.,Badiali De Giorgi L., Tremolada F. (1981). Ultrastructural changes in the liver of patients with chronic non-A, non-B hepatitis. J Med Virol,7; 205.

Busachi C.A.,Realdi G.,Badiali De Giorgi L.,Alberti A. (1980). Hepatocellular ultrastructural changes in patients with acute and chronic non-A,non-B hepatitis. J Submicrosc Cytol,12;681.
Cabral G.A.,Marciano-Cabral F.,Patterson M.,Galen E.A.,Carither R.L. (1981). Nuclear-changes in hepatocytes of patients with non-A,non-B hepatitis. Gastroenterology, 81; 120.
Canese M.G.,Novara S., Rizzetto M.,Purcell R.H. Delta-infection in chimpanzee: an ultrastructural study. 17th Meeting of the European Association for the Study of the Liver. Goteborg 1982, September 9-11. Abstract n.122.
Gmelin K., Kommerell B.,Waldherr F.,Ehrlich B.V. (1980). Intranuclear virus-like particles in a case of sporadic non-A, non-B hepatitis. J Med Virol, 5; 317.
Grimaud J.A.,Peyrol S.,Vitvitski L.,Chevallier-Queyron P.,Trepo C.(1980). Hepatic intranuclear particles in patients with non-A,non-B hepatitis. N Engl J Med, 303; 818.
Shimizu Y.K.,Feinstone S.M.,Purcell R.H.,Alter H.J.,LondonW.T. (1979). Non-A,non-B hepatitis. Ultrastructural evidence for the agents in experimentally infected chimpanzees. Science, 205; 197.

Viral Hepatitis and Delta Infection, pages 195–202
© **1983 Alan R. Liss, Inc., 150 Fifth Avenue, New York, NY 10011**

CLINICAL ASPECTS OF DELTA AGENT INFECTION IN SOUTHERN ITALY

Evangelista Sagnelli,M.D. and Giuseppe Manzillo,
M.D.
Clinic of Infectious Diseases,1st Sch.Med.
University of Naples and "D.Cotugno" Hospital
Via D.Cotugno 1 (Osp.Gesù e Maria) Naples,Italy

Delta agent is a pathogenic and transmissible agent which
requires the helper function of HBV for its replication
(Rizzetto 1980).
Epidemiological studies have shown that delta agent infection is distributed World-wide with higher prevalence in
the South of Italy (Rizzetto,1978; Rizzetto,1980). It has
also been suggested that delta agent infection may have
clinical relevance. In HBsAg asymptomatic carriers it may
be followed by the development of chronic active hepatitis
(CAH) (Smedile,1981).

This paper deals with the clinical aspects of delta agent
infection observed in two series of patients with HBsAg
positive acute viral hepatitis (AVH) and in 142 patients
with HBsAg positive CAH either treated with immunosuppressive drugs or untreated and observed from 4 to 8 years.

We searched delta agent infection in two series of patients with HBsAg positive AVH in 1977 and in 1981-82 and in
142 patients with biopsy proven HBsAg positive CAH.
The 1st series of AVH patients (1977) was composed of 35
consecutive patients with HBsAg positive icteric AVH observed until they recovered or progressed to chronicity.None
of these patients was drug-user.
The 2nd series (1981-82) is composed of 213 patients with

HBsAg positive icteric AVH of whom 45 were drug addicts
One-hundred twenty-two patients of the 2nd series were observed from 1 to 2 years; patients who showed clinical and/
or biochemical features suggesting progression to chronicity underwent a liver biopsy after a period varying from
9 to 18 months of observation.

We have also examined 142 consecutive patients with
HBsAg positive CAH who were observed from 4 to 8 years with
liver biopsies performed every two years. These patients
were consecutively left untreated or treated with one of
the following regimens: prednisolone 20 mg daily; an association of 20 mg of prednisolone and 50 mg of azathioprine given daily and referred as "combination therapy".
The outcome was evaluated on the basis of clinical, biochemical and histological parameters. In particular, the
criteria for deterioration were a development of histologically proven cirrhosis or an increase of the histologic lesions characteristic of CAH associated with one
of the following changes: 100% increase of bilirubin above
the initial level and in any case above 2.5 mg per deci-
liter; 100% increase of aminotransferases above the initial
value;physical deterioration with incapacity to have the
previous occupations. Liver histology was independently
evaluated by two observers and lesions were graduated with
the Knodell's scores (Knodell 1981). The results of the two
observers were almost always similar.

Markers of HBV, HAV and delta agent in serum were determined by RIA. Delta antigen was determined on formalin-
fixed and paraffin-embedded liver biopsies by the direct
IF using an antiserum kindly given by Dr. Rizzetto. Statistical analysis: for data not normally distributed (ALT
and IgG) the Wilcoxon signed rank test and the Kruskal-
Wallis test were used; contingency table analysis was performed by the chi square test with Yate's correction and by
the Fisher's exact test; data normally distributed were
analyzed by the Student's test and variance analysis.

DELTA INFECTION IN AVH

In AVH of the 1st series (1977) anti-δ of IgM class was detected in 91% of the patients. All patients but one (anti-δ negative) recovered.

Among the patients of the 2nd series (1981-82) anti-δ was found in 6% of non drug-users and in 36% of drug addicts. Considering that in 1980 in the same geographic area anti-δ was found in 27% of 87 non-drug using patients with HBsAg-positive AVH (Smedile, 1983) it may by hypothesized that an epidemic of delta agent infection occurred in Naples around or before 1977 and that subsequently the infection rate dramatically decreased. Out of the 213 patients of the 2nd series 132 were observed until they recovered or progression to chronicity was documented by liver histology. The remaining 81 patients lacked to cooperate and were considered dropouts. At admission (within a week from the onset of jaundice), 43% of these 132 patients were HBeAg positive, 30% circulated anti-HBe and 27% lacked both HBeAg and anti-HBe. Compared to drug-addicts, non-addict patients showed less frequently anti-δ in serum and progression to chronicity (Table 1).

		DRUG USERS		NON DRUG-USERS	
		No.of patients	Progression to chronicity (%)	No.of patients	Progression to chronicity (%)
Anti-HBe positive	Anti-δ+	6	100	2	0
	Anti-δ-	7	57	24	29
Anti-HBe negative	Anti-δ+	9	78	4	0
	Anti-δ-	11	0	69	6

Table 1. Progression to chronicity in 132 patients with HBsAg positive AVH in relation to drug addiction,delta agent infection and HBeAg/anti-HBe status.

DELTA INFECTION IN CAH

Delta agent infection, demonstrated by presence of δ-Ag in hepatocytic nuclei, was observed in 58% of patients with HBsAg positive CAH, at the time of the 1st liver biopsy. Subsequently clearance of δ-Ag or a marked reduction of prevalence of δ-Ag positive nuclei were observed in 28% of the 43 treated and in 57% of the 27 untreated patients. Among the patients lacking δ-Ag in the 1st liver biopsy this antigen became detectable in 50% of the 37 treated and in 31% of the 14 untreated.

At the time of the 1st liver biopsy 29% of the patients were HBeAg positive, 60% circulated anti-HBe and the remaining 11% lacked both HBeAg and anti-HBe. HBeAg positive patients were δ-Ag positive less frequently than those showing anti-HBe (34% vs. 71%, respectively). The data regarding the course of the disease are separately reported for the "δ-Ag positive group" and for the "δ-Ag negative group" in table 2. The δ-Ag positive group is composed of 50 patients who displayed δ-Ag in all liver biopsies and 22 patients who became positive for δ-Ag in the 2nd biopsy and remained positive in subsequent biopsies. The δ-Ag negative group is composed of 31 patients who were always negative and 18 patients who became negative in the 2nd biopsy and remained negative in subsequent biopsies. The patients in the δ-Ag negative group infrequently deteriorated regardless of treatment and HBeAg/anti-HBe status; no patient in this group had died at the end of the study (Table 2). In the δ-Ag positive group, HBeAg positive patients frequently showed an unfavourable course of the disease in all the three groups of treatment. Instead, among anti-HBe positive patients, those treated with combination therapy deteriorates or died less frequently than patients untreated or receiving prednisolone. These differences are significant to statistical analysis with a P value lower than 0.001 (Table 2). At the end of the study only 5 patients had died, all untreated in the δ-Ag positive group.

	Prednisolone		Combination		No treatment	
	No.of		No.of		No.of	
	pat.	%det.	pag.	%det.	pat.	%det.
"δ-Ag negative group"						
HBeAg+	7	14	8	16	8	24
anti-HBe+	7	14	6	0	8	16
HBeAg/anti-HBe neg.	2	50	1	0	2	0
"δ-Ag positive group"						
HBeAg+	4	75	5	80	4	50
anti-HBe+	17	82	18	17	17	65
HBeAg/anti-HBe neg.	2	50	3	67	2	50

Pat.=patients; det.=deteriorated or died

Table 2. Course of the disease in 121 patients with HBsAg positive CAH.

CONCLUSIONS

In our geographic area the rate of delta infection in HBsAg positive AVH dramatically decreased from 1977 to 1982. The rate remains high in drug-users who represent a reservoir of the delta agent. Progression to chronicity of HBsAg positive AVH was more frequent in drug addicts, especially those anti-δ positive, and in patients circulating anti-HBe in the early stage of the disease. These observations may suggest that some patients who showed progression to chronicity were already chronic carriers of HBsAg before the acute illness. AVH in this case could represent the clinical expression of delta agent superinfection or ot Non A/Non B hepatitis.

In patients with HBsAg positive CAH, persistence of δ-Ag in the liver may be considered a sign of an unfavourable course of the disease since more patients deteriorated or died and rapidly developed cirrhosis in the δ-Ag positive

than in the negative group. However, it is not clear whether
delta infection may accelerate the progression to an unfavourable outcome or this depends on other unknown factors
inherent in the natural clinical course of chronic hepatitis
B. δ-Ag negative patients infrequently deteriorated regardless of treatment and immunosuppressive therapy is therefore not indicated. Prednisolone did not modify favourably
the prognosis in any of the subgroups of patients in the
δ-Ag positive group, whereas combination therapy was helpful
only for patients who showed anti-HBe in serum. It is still
unknown whether immunosuppressive treatments may influence
delta agent biology. We observed a tendency of δ-Ag positive
untreated patients to clear this antigen during the study,
whereas δ-Ag positive patients under immunosuppressive
therapy infrequently cleared δ-Ag. Thus, prednisolone possibly may enhance the expression of δ-Ag in the liver. This
phenomenon may be due to a direct action of immunosuppressive drugs on the synthesis of delta agent or to more
complex mechanisms. Since delta agent needs the presence
of HBV in the hepatocytes for its replication it might be
hypothesized that an enhanced synthesis of this virus due
to immunosuppressive treatment (Sagnelli, 1980; Scullard,
1981) may allow an increased expression of δ-Ag in the
liver. Patients who became δ-Ag positive during the study
frequently had an unfavourable outcome. This observation
indicates that delta agent superinfection occurring in patients with HBsAg positive CAH correlates with aggravation
on the disease. Delta agent coinfection or superinfection
may have different effects in HBsAg positive AVH. HBsAg
positive, anti-δ positive AVH in non drug-users generally
represents the epiphenomenon of HBV and δ agent coinfection; this is a benign self limited illness since all
our patients recovered. In a proportion of drug addicts
HBsAg positive, anti-δ positive AVH is possibly the clinical manifestation of delta agent or Non A/Non B viruses
superinfection in patients who were already chronically
infected by HBV before the onset of illness. It is doubtful whether HBsAg positive CAH should be treated. Our
observations indicate that immunosuppressive therapy should

not be considered for patients showing HBeAg in serum or
lacking δ-Ag in the liver. Instead, for anti-HBe positive,
δ-Ag positive patients, combination therapy is the only
treatment modifying favourably the course of the disease.

REFERENCES

Knodell RG,Ishak KG,Blak WC,Chen TS,Kraig R,Kalpowitz N,
   Kierman TW,Wollman J (1981). Formulation and application
   of a numerical scoring system for assessing histological
   activity in asymptomatic chronic active hepatitis. Hepatol.
   1:431.
Rizzetto M,Shih JW-K, Cocke DJ,Purcell RH,Verme G,Gerin JL
   (1978). Incidence and significance of antibodies to delta
   antigen in hepatitis B virus infection. Lancet 2:986.
Rizzetto M,Canese MG,Gerin JL,London WT,Sley LD,Purcell RH
   (1980). Transmission of the hepatitis B virus associated
   delta antigen to chimpanzees. J Infect Dis 141:590.
Rizzetto M,Purcell RH,Gerin JL (1980). Epidemiology of HBV
   associated delta agent: geographic distribution of anti-
   delta and prevalence in polytransfused HBsAg carriers.
   Lancet 1:1215.
Sagnelli E,Manzillo G,Maio G,Pasquale G,Felaco FM,Filippini
   P,Izzo CM,Piccinino F (1980). Serum levels of hepatitis B
   surface and core antigen during immunosuppressive treatment
   of HBsAg positive chronic hepatitis infection.Lancet 2:395.
Scullard GH,Smith CD,Merrigan TC,Robinson WS,Gregory PB(1981)
   Effect of immunosuppressive therapy on viral markers in
   chronic active hepatitis B. Gastroenterology 81:987.
Smedile A,Dentico P,Zanetti A,Sagnelli E,Nordenfelt E,Actis
   GC,Rizzetto M (1981). Infection with delta (δ) agent in
   chronic HBsAg carriers. Gastroenterology 81:992.
Smedile A,Lavarini C,Farci P,Aricò S,Marinucci G,Dentico P,
   Giuliani G;Cargnel A,Del Vecchio Blanco C,and Rizzetto M
   (1983). Epidemiologic patterns of infection with the
   hepatitis B virus-associated delta agent in Italy. Am. J.
   Epidemiol. 117:223

DELTA INFECTION IN THE COURSE OF CHRONIC HEPATITIS B

M. Colombo M.D. , M. G. Rumi M. D. , M. F. Donato M. D. ,
A. Rossi, M. D. , N. Dioguardi M. D.
Scuola di Specializzazione in Malattie del Fegato ,
Clinica Medica III, University of Milan, Italy .

To assess the prevalence and clinical significance of delta infection in patients with chronic hepatitis B, we examined 249 liver biopsies from 101 retrospectively selected patients by immunofluorescence. Delta antigen (δAg) was detected in 87 specimens from 35 carriers (35%) with peak prevalence in patients with cirrhosis (55%), and generally in close association with progressive liver disease (85%). Patients with intrahepatic δAg had more severe liver disease than those without it, but the rates of worsening of the liver disease were similar in δAg positive and δAg negative patients. 51% of δ positive patients had past histories of acute hepatitis as compared to 26% of δ negative individuals ($p < .01$). Therefore, δ superinfection might play a role in worsening the histologic picture of HBsAg positive CAH, possibly by liver injury induced acutely at the moment of infection.

The recent demonstration that the antigenic reactivity of the δ agent is well preserved in routine biopsy material (Stoecklin et al., 1981) has enabled us to study δ infection in chronic HBsAg carriers retrospectively. We determined the prevalence of intrahepatic δAg in 101 patients with HBsAg positive chronic hepatitis. The correlation between δAg positivity and the severity of liver disease was calculated. In 249 follow-up liver biopsies, the relationship between δAg positivity and the course of the disease was also studied.

249 formalin-fixed hepatic sections from 101 patients
(M:F ratio : 158/54; mean age 37 years; range 8-72) with
HBsAg positive chronic hepatitis were examined by direct
immunofluorescence (IF) for the presence of δAg. 63% ori-
ginated in Northern Italy, 5% were haemophiliacs or drug
users. 35 δAg positive and 66 δAg negative patients were
followed-up for 1 to 5 years, with serial liver biopsies
(mean : 2.9 biopsies per patient). Initially, 62 patients (11
δAg positive) were on steroid therapy (10-20 mg of methyl
prednisone/day); in the follow-up, the same treatment was
given to 20 additional patients with CAH or AC. The therapeutic criteria for these patients were not related to study
protocol for δ infection. All liver specimens were obtained
with Tru-Cut (Travenol) or Menghini needles (Jamshidi),
and were more than 1.5 cm in lenght. In all cases, the liver disease was diagnosed following established criteria
(Leevy et al., 1976) and the histological activity was assessed blind by one of us, using a numerical scoring system
(HAI) (Knodell et al., 1981). The IF staining of δ Ag in de-
paraffinized sections was performed as previously reported (Colombo et al., 1983). Radioimmunoassay (RIA) for
HBsAg, HBs antibody (anti-HBs), core antibody (anti-HBc),
HBe antigen and antibody (HBeAg and anti-HBe) were car-
ried out with commercial kits (Abbott, North Chicago, ill.).
Data were analyzed by the Spearman-Kendall, Kruskall-
Wallis and Wilcoxon tests.

δ Ag was detected in 87 liver biopsies from 35 chronic
HBsAg carriers (35%), with a peak prevalence in the patients with AC (55%) (Table 1). δ Ag was localized within
the liver cell nuclei in all but one patient. δAg positive liver cells ranged between 2 and 50% (mean : 11%) and were
preferentially located in the periportal or paraseptal zones
of the parenchima. δAg positive carriers with CAH and or
AC had higher HAI scores than age-matched δ Ag negative
patients ($p < .01$). In these patients, however, the intrahepatic expression of δ Ag was unrelated to any of the para-

Table 1. Correlation between intrahepatic δAg and hepatic lesions

Liver Histology	Number of patients	Age (yrs)	Intrahepatic δAg N.	%
Chronic persistent hepatitis (CPH)	16	36+ 6	3	19
Chronic active hepatitis (CAH)	63	36+ 6	20	32
Active Cirrhosis (AC)	22	43+12	12	55
Total	101	37+14	35	35

meters of histologic activity scored in the HAI index. 18 of 35 (51%) δAg positive carriers had past histories of acute hepatitis, as compared to 17 of 66 (25. 7%) δAg negative patients ($p < .01$). In both δAg positive and δAg negative patients, the histological parameters of activity (HAI scores) remained unchanged during follow-up, whether or not the patients was treated with steroids (Table 2).

Table 2. Correlation between delta infection and evolution of chronic hepatitis. The histological activity was scored by the Knodell index (HAI)

HBsAg pos CAH	Number of patients	HAI scores during follow-up (1–5 years, mean : 2.9 years)	
		Initial	Final
delta pos.	35	13.5 ± 4.5 [1,2]	13.6 ± 4.7 [1]
delta neg.	66	11 ± 3.3 [2]	10.9 ± 3.8

1. Delta pos. vs delta ng. : $P < .01$
2. Initial vs final : not significant

The same was true for the pattern of immunofluorescence in δAg positive carriers. Nevertheless, in some of the patients, the histological diagnoses of follow-up biopsies did change from those of the initial biopsy (Table 3). In δAg positive patients, the follow-up biopsies did not change in 77%, showed deterioration in 14% and slight improve-

Table 3. Histologic evolution in 101 patients with HBsAg positive chronic liver disease, according to intra hepatic δ Ag status

Histologic Evolution	Initial Diagnosis	Last follow-up	Intrahepatic δ Ag status			
			δ +(n=35)		δ -(n=66)	
Unchanged	AC	AC	12		10	
	CAH	CAH	13	77. 1%	23	62. 1 %
	CPH	CPH	2		8	
Deteriorated	CAH	AC	4	14. 3%	13	25. 8%
	CPH	CAH	1		4	
Improved	CAH	CPH	3	8. 6%	8	12. 1%

ment in 8%. In δ Ag negative patients, the follow-up biopsied did not change in 60%, showed deterioration in 27% and improvement in 12%. The differences in this respect between δ Ag positive and δ Ag negative patients were not statistically significant.

This study showed a high prevalence of δ superinfection among patients with chronic hepatitis B and confirmed previous reports of a strong association between the δ agent and progressive liver disease (Rizzetto et al, 1977; Rizzetto et al. 1979, Rizzetto et al. 1983). This association constitues an additional evidence of direct delta pathogenicity in HBV-related liver disease. However, the effects of delta superinfection on the course of HBV-related chronic hepatitis remain to be clarified. If continuing intrahepatic replication of the delta agent has a damaging effect, one would expect delta positive carriers to show more rapid progression of the liver lesions. Only 14% of δ Ag positive patients, followed-up for 1-5 yr, progressed from CAH to cirrhosis or from CPH to CAH. In addition, the rates of deterioration were similar in δ Ag positive and δ Ag negative cases. This goes against the hypothesis that continuing intrahepatic replication of the δ agent has an unfavorable effect on the course of HBV-related chronic hepatitis (Rizzetto et al.,

1983). A clue to interpretation of the pathogenic role of the δ agent in HBV-related chronic hepatitis might be derived from the observation that δ Ag positive patients had histories of a previous episode of acute hepatitis much more frequently than δAg negative patients (51% versus 25.7%; p < 0.01). Possibly, the episode of acute hepatitis was the moment of superinfection with delta. One might thus speculate that delta superinfection results in acute liver damage, worsening preexisting chronic hepatitis (Smedile et al., 1982), with the further course of the disease being independent of the presence or absence of intrahepatic delta agent. It may be argued that the population in our follow-up study is skewed toward the patients with more severe inflammatory lesions, since it does not include follow-up biopsies from HBsAg carriers with normal liver histology. However, none of these latter subjects had intrahepatic delta Ag as also stated in literature (Aricò et al., 1978).

References

Aricò S, Rizzetto M, Crivelli O et al (1978). The clinical and immunological significance of a new antigen/antibody system (delta/anti-delta) in chronic carriers of the HBsAg. Ital J Gastroenterol 10 : 146-151.

Colombo M, Cambieri R, Rumi MG, Ronchi G, Del Ninno E, de Franchis R . Long-term delta superinfection in hepatitis B surface antigen carriers and its relationship to the course of chronic hepatitis. Gastroenterology 85:235 .

Knodell RG, Ishak KG, Block WC et al (1981). Formulation and application of a numerical scoring system for assessing histological activity in asymptomatic chronic active hepatitis. Hepatology 5 : 431-435.

Leevy CM, Popper H, Sherlock S (1976). Disease of the liver and biliary tract : standardization of nomenclature, diagnostic criteria and diagnostic methodology. Year Book Medical Publishers Inc. Chicago 9-21.

Rizzetto M, Canese MG, Aricò S et al. (1977). Immunofluo_
    rescence detection of a new antigen/antibody system
    (delta/anti-delta) associated with hepatitis B virus in
    liver and serum of HBsAg carriers. Gut 18 : 997-1003.
Rizzetto M, Shih JWK, Gocke DJ, et al. (1979) Incidence
    and significance of antibodies to delta antigen in hepa-
    titis B virus infection. Lancet 11 : 986-980.
Rizzetto M, Verme G, Recchia S et al. (1983). Chronic
    HBsAg hepatitis with intrahepatic expression of the
    delta antigen. An active and progressive disease un-
    responsive to immunosuppressive treatment. Ann
    Intern Med, 98: 437-444.
Smedile A, Farci P, Verme G et al. (1982). Influence of
    delta infection on severity of hepatitis B. Lancet ii :
    945-947.
Stoecklin E, Gudat F, Krey G et al. (1981). Delta-antigen
    in hepatitis B : Immunohistology of frozen and paraffin-
    embedded liver biopsies and relation to HBV-infection.
    Hepatology 1 : 238-242.

Hadziyannis SJ (1980). Hepatocellular carcinoma and type B
    hepatitis. Clinics Gastroent 9:117.
Moestrup T, Hansson BC, Widell A, Nordenfelt E (1983). Cli-
    nical aspects of delta infection. Brit Med J 286:87.
Raimondo G, Smedile A, Gallo L, Balbo A, Ponzetto A, Rizzet-
    to M (1982). Multicentre study of prevalence of HBV-asso-
    ciated delta infection and liver disease in drug-addicts.
    Lancet 1:249.
Rizzetto M, Purcell RH, Gerin JL (1980). Epidemiology of
    HBV-associated delta agent, geographical distribution
    of anti-delta and prevalence in polytransfused HBsAg car-
    riers. Lancet 1:1215.
Rizzetto M, Verme G, Recchia S, Bonino F, Farci P, Arico S,
    Calzia R, Picciotto A, Colombo M, Popper H (1983). Chro-
    nic hepatitis in carriers of hepatitis B surface antigen,
    with intrahepatic expression of the delta antigen. Ann
    Intern Med 98:437.
Smedile A, Dentico P, Zanetti A, Sagnelli E, Nordenfelt E,
    Actis GC, Rizzetto M (1981). Infection with the delta (δ)
    agent in chronic HBsAg carriers. Gastroenterology 81;992.
Theodoropoulos G, Papaevangelou G, Tzivra M, Tzivras M, Kal-
    liakmanis N, Koumaditis A (1982). The incidence of anti-δ
    in the serum of Greek patients with hepatic diseases. Hip-
    pocrates 10:9.
Wright R (1980). Type B hepatitis Progression to chronic
    hepatitis. Clinics Gastroent 9:97.

EPIDEMIOLOGY AND CLINICAL COURSE OF DELTA INFECTION IN
BRITAIN

ASF LOK MBBS MRCP, P FARCI MD, HC THOMAS BSc
PhD FRCP

Academic Department of Medicine, Royal Free
Hospital and School of Medicine, London

Delta agent is a defective virus which requires the
presence of hepatitis B virus (HBV) for its replication
(Rizzetto et al, 1980). Delta antigen was first described
in an Italian HBsAg carrier (Rizzetto et al, 1977) but
epidemiological studies have now shown that this infection
is world-wide in distribution with a predominance in
Mediterranean, Middle Eastern, South American and African
countries. In Northern Europe and USA, the prevalence of
delta markers is still low and is mainly confined to
intravenous drug abusers and polytransfused subjects
(Rizzetto et al, 1980; Hansson et al, 1982; Weller et al,
1983).

To investigate the epidemiology and clinical course
of delta infection in Britain, sera from 332 consecutive
HBsAg positive British patients, collected from 1976–1982
at the Royal Free Hospital London, were tested for delta
antigen (δAg) and antibody (anti-δ), and the characteristics
of the delta positive patients were analysed.

Serum markers of delta infection were detected in 40
patients. 33 were male and 7 female (M=F 4.7 : 1). The
mean age was 27 years (range 11–59 years). The annual
prevalence of delta infection from 1976–1982 is listed in
Table 1. Serological evidence of delta infection was
already present in 1976.

Table 1   Prevalence of delta-markers in serum of British
HBsAg +ve patients.

Year	No of Patients tested	+ve delta serology	
		Number	% of total
1976*	20	4	20
1977	41	13	32
1978	42	9	21
1979	40	5	13
1980	48	5	10
1981	66	2	3
1982	75	2	3
TOTAL	332	40	11

*Oct - Dec 1976

The prevalence was higher in the earlier years with
a gradual decline to 3% in 1981-1982. This marked difference
could be attributed to the occurrence of an epidemic around
1976-1978. An alternative explanation could lie in a
changing pattern of patient referral. In recent years,
there has been a growing interest in antiviral therapy
resulting in an increased referral of young HBeAg positive
patients - predominantly homosexual men - in whom delta
infection is still infrequent.

Delta markers were present in 30/219 (13.7%) patients
presenting with acute hepatitis, 10/86 (11.6%) patients
with chronic liver disease (CLD) but none of the 27
asymptomatic carriers. This observation is consistent
with other studies in which delta markers have usually
been associated with liver damage and rarely present in
healthy carriers (Rizzetto et al, 1979).

In 30 patients, information on the possible modes
of transmission was recorded in the clinical notes. 19 of
these were parenteral drug abusers, 5 had close contact with
drug abusers and 2 were haemophiliacs. There was no
identifiable source of infection in the remaining 4 patients.

Acute hepatitis:-   Of the 30 delta positive patients who
presented with acute hepatitis, serum δAg was transiently
detectable in 8 (27%), and anti-δ (low titre) in the remaining

22 (73%). The clinical outcome of these patients is listed in
in Table II. 4 progressed to chronic liver disease with an
increasing titer of anti-δ in serum : 3 were drug abusers
and 1 a haemophiliac. 2 of these 4 patients were positive
for IgM anti-HBc when they presented with acute hepatitis.
It is likely that they acquired both HBV and δ agent
simultaneously. Liver biopsy performed 9 months after the
acute hepatitis showed active cirrhosis in 1 patient who
died 6 months later with variceal haemorrhage and encephalopathy. The other patient also had active cirrhosis on
liver biopsy 12 months after the acute hepatitis and
suffered 2 episodes of variceal haemorrhage at 15 and 18
months. The remaining 2 patients were negative for IgM
anti-HBc· and were probably chronic HBV carriers with acute
hepatitis due to superimposed δ infection.

Table II   Clinical Outcome of acute hepatitis patients
with delta markers in serum (14 were lost to follow-up)

Clinical Features	δ Ag (8)	Anti-δ(22)
Fulminant Course	2	2
Recovery with clearance of HBsAg	2	6
Progression to CLD	0	4

Chronic hepatitis: All 10 delta positive patients who
presented with chronic liver disease had high titer anti-δ
but none had detectable δAg in their serum. 7 of these
patients had liver biopsies : 2 showed chronic active
hepatitis (CAH) and 5 cirrhosis. 2 of the latter died,
1 with hepatocellular carcinoma and the other of hepatic
failure. Of the 76 delta negative patients with chronic
liver disease, 56 had liver biopsies ranging from chronic
lobular hepatitis to cirrhosis (Table III). These results
are similar to those of other studies which show that delta
infection is usually associated with more severe liver
disease (CAH and cirrhosis) but uncommon amongst patients
with milder liver damage, CPH and normal histology
(Rizzetto et al, 1983).

TABLE III   Histological Diagnosis of HBsAg +ve CLD patients with and without delta markers.

Histology	δ+ (7 cases)	δ- (56 cases)
CLH	0	7
CPH	0	10
CAH	2	27
Cirrhosis	5	12

<u>Summary</u>:

This study demonstrates the presence of serological markers of delta infection in HBsAg positive patients throughout the years 1976-1982. As in other Northern European countries, delta infection in Britain is predominantly found in drug addicts and haemophiliacs. δAg was detected transiently in serum in a minority of patients presenting with acute hepatitis. In the others and those presenting with chronic liver disease, anti-δ was the only serological evidence of delta infection. Our findings also confirm that delta infection is associated with a more severe and rapidly progressive liver disease.

<u>Acknowledgements</u>:-

The authors would like to thank Dr M Rizzetto for kindly providing the reagents for δAg anti-δ assay.

ASF Lok is supported by the University of Hong Kong. HCT is a Senior Wellcome Fellow in Clinical Science.

<u>References</u>

Rizzetto M, Canese MG, Gerin JL, London WT, Sly DL & Purcell RH (1980). Transmission of Hepatitis B virus-associated delta antigen to chimpanzees. J of Infectious Diseases. 141 : 590-602.

Rizzetto M, Canese MG,. AricoS, Crivelli O, Trepo C, Bonino F Verme G (1977). Immunofluorescence detection of new antigen antibody system (δ/anti-δ) associated to hepatitis B virus in liver and in serum of HBsAg carriers. Gut 18 : 997-1003.

Rizzetto M, Purcell RH, Gerin JL. (1980) Epidemiology of HBV-associated delta agent : geographical distribution of anti-delta and prevalence in polytransfused HBsAg carriers. Lancet ii, 1215-1218.

Hansson BG, Moestrup T, Widell A, & Nordenfelt E. (1982) Infection with delta agent in Sweden. Introduction of a new hepatitis agent. J of Infect Dis. 146, 472-478.

Weller IVD, Karayiannis P, Lok ASF, Montano L, Bamber M Thomas HC and Sherlock S (1983). The significance of delta infection in chronic hepatitis B viral infection in Great Britain. Gut (in press).

Rizzetto M, Shih JWK, Gocke DJ, Purcell RH, Verme G, and Gerin JL (1979). Incidence and significance of antibodies to delta antigen in hepatitis B virus infection. Lancet ii 986-990.

Rizzetto M, Verme G, Reechia S, Bonino F, Farci P, Arico S. Calzia R, Picciotto A, Colombo M, Popper H (1983). Chronic hepatitis in carriers of hepatitis B surface antigen, with intrahepatic expression of delta antigen. An active and progressive disease unresponsive to immunosuppressive treatment. Annals of Int Medicine 98 : 437-441

DELTA INFECTION IN CHILDREN

P. Farci, R. Calzia, C. Barbera, N. Caporaso,
F. Bortolotti, P. Vajro, A. Vegnente
Molinette,Torino - University of Genova, Torino,
Napoli, Padova.

To establish the prevalence and pathogenic role of δ infection in liver disease of infancy, 270 pediatric patients with chronic HBsAg-positive hepatitis collected in Italy during the years 1975-1982 were retrospectively examined for serological evidence of chronic δ infection, and the clinical features of δ-infected were compared with the features of ordinary (δ-negative) chronic hepatitis B of infancy.

The children were carriers of HBsAg who underwent a diagnostic liver biopsy for clinical evidence of chronic hepatitis. There were 182 males and 88 females of age varying between 1 and 14 years (mean 7.4). Ninety-eight of the patients were of North Italian heritage, 172 were of South Italian heritage. All were followed-up for 2 to 7 years (mean 3.6) with periodical examinations and biochemical tests. Follow-up liver biopsies were performed only when clinically indicated. Liver histology was interpreted according to the criteria of De Groote et al. (De Groote, 1968). Chronic δ infection was diagnosed on the finding of serum antibody to δ (anti-δ) in high titers ($\geq$ 1:5.000) (Rizzetto, 1979). Treatment was given according to protocols unrelated to presence or absence of δ infection and consisted of combination of steroids and azathioprine. HBsAg, HBeAg and anti-HBe were measured with commercial

radioimmunoassays. Anti-δ was measured with a competitive
radioimmunoassay (Rizzetto, 1979).

Histological diagnosis and prevalence of δ infection

A form of chronic hepatitis was observed at histology in
all the initial liver biopsies obtained from the 270
children. It was a chronic lobular hepatitis (CLH) in 3, a
chronic persistent hepatitis (CPH) in 100, a chronic active
hepatitis (CAH) in 158, a cirrhosis (CIR) in 9.

Anti-δ in high titers was found in 34 of the 270 children
(12.5%). It persisted in the blood specimens collected
thereafter from each positive patient. The antibody was not
found in 236 children. The prevalence of anti-δ in the
different varieties of chronic HBsAg-hepatitis is shown in
the following table.

Histological diagnosis and delta infection

Histological diagnosis

	CLH	CPH	CAH	CIR
	3	100	158	9
delta +	0	6 (6%)	24 (15%)	4 (44%)

p= <.001

p= <.01

The antibody prevalence in CIR or in CIR plus CAH was
significantly higher than in the other histological forms.
The increase of anti-δ in parallel with the activity of the
disease and its maximal prevalence in cirrhosis confirms
the association of δ infection with important liver mor-
bidity that has emerged from studies in adults (Govindarajan, 1983; Rizzetto, 1983; Weller, 1983).

Delta infection and the HBe antigen-antibody system

Serum HBeAg was found in 181 children, anti-HBe in 73 children; 16 patients were negative for both reactivities. The prevalence of anti-δ in relation to HBe status is shown in the following table.

HBeAg/anti-HBe and delta infection

	n° of children positive for	
	HBeAg	anti-HBe
	181	73
delta +	10 (5.5%)	21 (29%)

p= <.001

The prevalence of anti-δ was significantly higher in children with anti-HBe than in children with HBeAg. Because anti-HBe identifies a late phase of HBV infection (Hoofnagle, 1983) it might be argued that the severe liver disease in children with δ depended on a long duration of HBV infection rather than on the pathogenic effect of δ; the course of the hepatitis, however, was benign in almost all of our infants with anti-HBe but without δ, and the variability of duration of HBV infection prior to clinical presentation is minimized in children.

Follow-up

Improvement of the liver disease was determined from amelioration of liver biopsy findings and/or from persistent decrease or normalization of aminotransferase values (AT) with no increase or with normalization of IgG values. Deterioration was determined on worsening of follow-up biopsy findings and/or from persistent increase of AT, accompanied or not by increase in the IgG level.

The histological and/or biochemical features of the liver

disease deteriorated in a consistent proportion of the children with δ infection (38%) and improved only in a minority of these patients (9%). The course of the hepatitis, instead, was usually mild in children without δ infection, with remission in a high percentage (55%) and worsening only in a few (7%). The follow-up is summarized in the following table.

<u>Follow-up</u>

	Improved	Unvaried	Worsened
delta −			
n° of patients			
236	129 (55%)	91 (38.5%)	16 (7%)
delta +			
n° of patients			
34	3 (9%)	18 (53%)	13 (38%)

The outcome of chronic hepatitis with δ infection (next table) was not influenced by treatment, which was of no benefit in preventing progression of the disease.

<u>Outcome of chronic delta hepatitis in treated* and untreated children</u>

	Improved	Unvaried	Worsened
treated			
21	2 (9%)	10 (48%)	9 (43%)
untreated			
13	1 (8%)	8 (61%)	4 (31%)

* steroids and azathioprine

In conclusion, chronic δ infection in children carrying HBsAg is accompanied by liver disease that is usually more

important and progressive than ordinary chronic hepatitis B
in pediatric age. In contrast to predominance of HBeAg in
ordinary HBsAg liver disease of children, chronic δ hepatitis in pediatric age correlates with anti-HBe. This form
is unresponsive to conventional immunosuppressive treatment.

The following have collaborated in this study:
C.Navone, B.Ciravegna, M.G.Marazzi, P.Tolentino, GENOVA
C.Sacchetti, N.Ansaldi, A.Moiraghi, TORINO
R.Di Toro,C.Del Vecchio Blanco, M.Coltorti, M.R.D'Armiento,
G.Orso, G.Loffredo, V.Nuzzo, P.Toscano, NAPOLI
P.Cadrobbi, C.Crivellaro, A.Bertaggia, G.Realdi, PADOVA

References

De Groote J, Desmet VJ, Gedick P, Korb G, Popper H, Poulsen
   H, Schmid M, Thaler H, Uehlinger E, Wepler W (1968). A
   classification of chronic hepatitis. Lancet 2: 626.
Govindarajan S, Kanel GC, Peters RL (1983). Prevalence of δ
   antibody among chronic hepatitis B virus infected patients
   in the Los Angeles area: its correlation with liver biopsy
   diagnosis. Gastroenterology 85:160
Hoofnagle JH (1983). Chronic type B hepatitis. Gastroenterology 84: 422.
Rizzetto M, Shih JW-K, Gocke DJ, Purcell RH, Verme G, Gerin
   JL (1979). Incidence and significance of antibodies to
   delta antigen in hepatitis B virus infection. Lancet 2:
   986.
Rizzetto M, Verme G, Recchia S, Bonino F, Farci P, Aricò S,
   Calzia R, Picciotto A, Colombo M, Popper H (1983). Chronic
   HBsAg hepatitis with intrahepatic expression of delta antigen. An active and progressive disease unresponsive to
   immunosuppressive treatment. Ann Intern Med 98: 437.
Weller IVD, Karayiannis P, Lok ASF, Bamber M, Thomas HC,
   Sherlock S (1983). The significance of delta agent in
   chronic Hepatitis B Virus infection in Great Britain. Gut,
   in press.

DELTA AGENT AND HEPATOCELLULAR CARCINOMA

A.Craxì*,G.Raimondo°,G.Giannuoli*,G.Longo°,
M.Caltagirone *,M.Aragona°,G.Squadrito°,L.Pagliaro*
*Patologia Medica R,Ospedale V.Cervello-Palermo
°Clinica Medica II,Policlinico-Messina   ITALY

INTRODUCTION

Chronic Hepatitis B virus (HBV) infection plays a major
role in the etiology of hepatocellular carcinoma (HCC)(Beasley, 1981). In Southern Italy, wherein chronic HBsAg carri
age has an intermediate prevalence between high and low risk
areas (Giusti, 1981; Szmuness, 1978), HBV has been confirmed
as the main risk factor for HCC (Pagliaro, 1983). Among 1074
patients with newly diagnosed cirrhosis HCC was present at
the first observation or developed during a 5 year follow-up
in 1.3% of 178 HBsAg positive patients and in 0.6% of 896
HBsAg negative patients (D'Amico, personal communication).
In the same population superinfection of HBsAg carriers with
the δ agent is widespread and closely associated with the mo
re active stages of chronic liver disease (Craxì, 1983).

The aim of our study is to investigate the occurrence of
markers of δ infection (δAg/Anti-δ in serum, δAg in liver
tissue) in all consecutive patients with HBsAg positive HCC
observed in our Depts. since 1977. As many patients with HCC
are HBsAg negative but show features of HBV infection (serum
anti-HBc and/or anti-HBs, viral markers in the liver)(Craxì,
1983) we also assessed the prevalence of δ infection in HBsAg
negative patients with HCC.

MATERIALS AND METHODS

Patients: two hundred and sixteen patients admitted to
our Depts.between January 1977 and April 1983 were studied.

The diagnosis of HCC was based:
a) in 101 patients on a diagnostic liver biopsy
b) in 115 patients on alfafetoprotein levels consistently
above 500 ng/ml by RIA plus compatible liver US and/or scin-
tiscan. Among the 101 biopsied cases the biopsy was considered suitable for immunohistology, on the grounds of good em-
bedding and presence of non-neoplastic tissue in sufficient
amounts, in 58 cases, 52 of whom with clearcut evidence of
cirrhosis.

Methods: sera were tested for HBV markers by commercial
RIAs (ABBOTT) and for the δ/anti-δ system by RIA (Rizzetto,
1980). ^{125}I-anti-δ was a gift of Dr.Rizzetto. Anti-δ positive sera were titrated and tested for anti-δ of IgM class
(Smedile , 1982). Paraffin embedded liver biopsies were tested after trypsin digestion for HBsAg by a monoclonal anti-
HBs (RF-HBs 1) and for HBcAg and δAg by FITC-conjugated human antisera. Specificity of staining was always confirmed
by blocking.

RESULTS AND DISCUSSION

The overall prevalence of HBV markers was high, 168 of
216 patients (77.8%) having features of present (HBsAg positive, 79 patients, 36.6%) or previous (anti-HBc $\pm$ anti-HBs
positive, 89 patients, 41.2%) HBV infection. Forty-eight
subjects (22.2%) were negative for all markers. Of the 79
HBsAg positive patients, 8 (10.1%) had HBeAg. None of the patients had circulating δAg. Anti-δ was present in 8/79(10.1%)
HBsAg positive patients, all of whom HBeAg negative, but also in 13/89 (14.6%) of the HBsAg negative, anti-HBc $\pm$ anti-
HBs positive cases. It was never found in patients without
features of HBV infection. Anti-δ positive sera did never
have titres above 10^3, nor a specific antibody activity of
IgM class. The behaviour of tissue markers of HBV and δ is
shown in Table 1. Even when HBsAg and/or HBcAg were found in
non-neoplastic tissue surrounding foci of HCC, δAg was always
absent, regardless of anti-δ seropositivity.

Table 1: Tissue markers of HBV and δ in HCC

	Tissue markers		
	HBsAg	HBcAg	δAg
Serum HBV markers			
HBsAg + (18 pts)°	10	1	0
Anti-HBc + (23 pts)°°	3	2	0
All markers - (17 pts)	0	0	0

° 4 pts were anti-δ positive
°°3 pts were anti-δ positive

By comparison with the prevalence of anti-δ previously observed by us (Craxì, 1983) in chronic HBsAg carriers with and without liver disease in the same population (Table 2) it is evident that the frequency of δ superinfection in HBsAg positive HCC is grossly similar to that of healthy carriers, but substantially lower than in cirrhosis.

Table 2: Prevalence of anti-δ in chronic HBsAg carriers and HBsAg + HCC

	% anti-δ+	95% confidence limits
Healthy carriers (94 pts)	6.4	(2.4 - 13.4)
Active cirrhosis (72 pts)	56.0	(43.4 - 67.3)
Inactive cirrhosis (188 pts)	38.8	(32.0 - 46.3)
HCC (79 pts)	10.1	(4.5 - 19.0)

On the other hand if patients with HBsAg negative, anti-HBc ± anti-HBs positive HCC are compared to serologically similar subjects with active or inactive cirrhosis (Table 3) a similar prevalence of low-titered anti-δ of IgG class is found.

Table 3: Prevalence of anti-δ in HBsAg negative, anti-HBc positive CLD and HCC

	% anti-δ+	95% confidence limits
Active cirrhosis (39 pts)	10.2	(2.9 - 24.2)
Inactive cirrhosis (47 pts)	14.8	(6.2 - 28.3)
HCC (89 pts)	14.6	(8.0 - 23.7)

The low frequency of features of δ infection in patients with HCC indicates that δ agent is not involved in the neoplastic transformation of HBV-related cirrhosis. The low titer of anti-δ, the absence of a specific IgM response and the lack of δAg in the liver suggest that in both HBsAg positive and anti-HBc positive cases anti-δ is only a marker of resolved δ superinfection.

The lower prevalence of anti-δ in HBsAg positive patien
ts with HCC associated to cirrhosis than in those with cirrhosis alone might be due to an alteration of the natural
history of HBsAg positive chronic liver disease induced by
the δ agent; δ infection might in fact cause active disease
and premature death of patients, while subjects who are
uninfected (or who clear the δ agent and possibly the HBV)
proceed to HCC. Alternatively, markers of δ infection in patients with HCC could have disappeared because of the longer time elapsed since infection.

Beasley R, Hwang LY, Lin CC, Chien CS (1981). Hepatocellular
    carcinoma and Hepatitis B Virus. Lancet, II: 1129.
Craxì A, Pasqua P, Giannuoli G, Di Franco C, Simonetti RG,
    Pagliaro L (1983). Tissue markers of Hepatitis B Virus
    infection in hepatocellular carcinoma. Hepato-Gastroentero
    logy, in press.
Craxì A, Raimondo G, Longo G, Giuannuoli G, De Pasquale R,
    Caltagirone M, Squadrito G, Pagliaro L (1983). Delta agent
    superinfection in acute hepatitis B and chronic HBsAg car-
    riers with and without liver disease. Lancet, in press.
Giusti G (1981). Rapporti virus-ospite e dimensioni del pro-
    blema. In: Il portatore di HBsAg. Bologna, Editrice Compo
    sitori, p.7.
Pagliaro L, Simonetti RG, Craxì A (1983). Alcohol and HBV
    infection as risk factors for hepatocellular carcinoma in
    Italy: a multicentric, controlled study. Hepato-Gastroente
    rology, 30: 48.
Rizzetto M, Shih JWK, Gerin JL (1980). The hepatitis B virus
    associated δ antigen: isolation from liver, development
    of solidphase radioimmunoassays for δ antigen and anti-δ
    and partial characterization of δ antigen. J Immunol, 125:
    318.
Smedile A, Lavarini C, Crivelli O, Raimondo G, Fassone M,
    Rizzetto M.(1982). Radioimmunoassay detection of IgM anti-
    bodies to the HBV-associated δ antigen: clinical signifi-
    cance in δ infection. J Med Virol, 9:131;
Szmuness W, Harley EJ, Ikram H, Stevens CE (1978). Sociode-
    mographic aspects of the epidemiology of hepatitis B. In
    Vyas GN, Cohen SN, Schmid E (eds): Viral Hepatitis, Abacus
    Press, p.297.

Viral Hepatitis and Delta Infection, pages 235–236
© 1983 Alan R. Liss, Inc., 150 Fifth Avenue, New York, NY 10011

ROLE OF DELTA AGENT IN FULMINANT HEPATITIS IN THE LOS
ANGELES AREA

Sugantha Govindarajan, Kenneth P. Chin, Allan G.
Redeker and Robert L. Peters
USC Liver Unit, Rancho Los Amigos Hospital

7705 Golondrinas Street, 1200 Building
Downey, California 90242

Recent studies from Italy, France and England have
shown a significantly high prevalence (39%) of delta
markers among patients with fulminant hepatitis (FH).
[Smidile, 1982] About one half of the patients with FH
who had delta markers were presumed to have been
asymptomatic hepatitis B virus (HBV) carriers presenting
a   fulminant   course   associated   with   the   acute
superinfection with delta agent.

We have reviewed seventy–one HBsAg positive
patients with a fulminant clinical course and studied the
serological markers that reflected whether or not the
hepatitis B as well as delta infection was acute or
chronic. We found 33.8% of the 71 patients to have
evidence of acute delta infection.   In contrast, the
prevalence of acute delta markers was only 3.3% among 91
patients with ordinary acute (non–fulminant) B viral
hepatitis. Of the 24 patients with FH and acute delta
markers, 19 had evidence of simultaneous acute B and
acute delta infection and 5 had chronic HBV with
superimposed acute delta infection.   Forty–six patients
had acute HBV markers alone without delta, and one
patient had chronic HBV with superimposed acute infection
of an unknown agent.

In order to evaluate the mortality rates, the
patients were divided into three subgroups: I. Acute B
without delta markers; II.   Acute B with acute delta
markers; and III. Chronic B with acute delta markers.
Nine of the 19 (47.3%) in group I, 33 of the 46 (71.7%)

patients in group II, and 4 of the 5 in group III died.
However, when age related mortality was compared for
these groups, there was no significant difference.

The prevalence of delta markers was similar among
the Caucasians, Blacks, and the Hispanics, with FH.
There was no significant number of patients of Oriental
origin in this group of FH. The majority (75%), but not
all of the patients with delta markers were intravenous
drug addicts and the prevalence rate of delta markers
through the period of 1969 to 1983 showed no significant
change. Although the agent has been only recently
recognized, it has apparently been an infecting agent in
the Los Angeles area at the same prevalence rate since at
least 1969.

In summary, our study confirms the significant role
of delta agent in FH, and unlike the data from Sweden
[Hansson, 1982], delta is not a recently introduced
agent, but has been present at least since 1969 in the
Los Angeles area.

References:
Hansson BG, Moestrup T, Widell A, and Nordenfelt E
   (1982). Infection with delta agent in Sweden:
   Introduction of a new hepatitis agent. J Infect Dis
   146:472.
Smidile A, Farci P, Verme G, Caredda F, Cargnel A,
   Caporaso N, Dentico P, Trepo C, Opolon P, Gimson A,
   Vergani D, Williams R, and Rizzetto M. Influence of
   delta infection on severity of hepatitis B. Lancet
   1982; ii 945-947.

patients expressing serum delta-Ag in fulminant delta hepatitis (25%) was significantly higher than in uncomplicated hepatitis B with delta (2%), suggesting that delta antigenemia correlates with extensive liver necrosis and represents a prognostic marker of severe, potentially fulminant hepatitis. Interestingly, the 10 patients with serum delta Ag had serological evidence of recent HBV infection (all were positive for IgM anti-HBc), that was active in 7 of the cases, as shown by the presence in their serum of HBeAg. Possibly, the degree of delta viremia during primary infection is modulated by HBV replication and increases in parallel with the level of HB virion synthesis.

In conclusion, fulminant delta hepatitis may result from co-infection of delta with HBV or superinfection with delta of carriers of HBsAg. In co-infection the fulminant illness probably results from the cumulative pathogenic effect of HBV and delta on the hepatocytes. Suvivors are not predisposed to chronic delta hepatitis, as clearance of HBV implies clearance of the defective agent. One factor of virulence in this context may be the enhanced synthesis of the delta agent induced by an unusually prolonged or massive replication of HBV. In superinfection of long term carriers of HBsAg, delta antigenemia is not usually detectable and the factor of virulence may be represented by an increased susceptibility to the pathogenic effect of delta inherent in the HBsAg state. Survivors are predisposed to chronic delta hepatitis.

Since the hypothetical factors influencing fulminant delta hepatitis, i.e. HBsAg state and high level of HBV replication combine in the short-term carrier of HBsAg, whose HBV infection was acquired in the recent past, this type of individual may be at highest risk of developing fulminant hepatitis when exposed to the delta agent.

With the collaboration of: O.Schiraldi,G.Pastore,BARI
A.D'Arminio, M.Moroni, P.Viganò, M.Vigevani, M.Almaviva,MILANO
F.De Lalla, E.Rinaldi, COMO   R.Williams,Y.White,LONDON
C.Del Vecchio Blanco, M.Coltorti, NAPOLI   J.Shorey,DALLAS
B.Hansson,E.Nordenfelt,MALMO

References

Banninger P, Altorfer J, Frosner GG, Pirovino M, Gudat F, Bianchi L, Schmid M (1983). Prevalence and significance of antiHBc IgM (RIA) in acute and chronic hepatitis B and in blood donors. Hepatology 3:337

Chau KH, Hargie MP, Deker RH, Mushawar IK, Overby LR (1983). Serodiagnosis of recent hepatitis B infection by IgM class anti-HBc. Hepatology 3:142.

Lavarini C, Crivelli O, Smedile A, Farci P, Marinucci G, Muglie M, Rizzetto M (1982). Radioimmunoassay detection of IgM antibodies to hepatitis B core antigen in HBsAg liver disease. Boll. Ist. Sieroter. Mil. 61:210.

Wright R, Alberti KGMM, Karran S, Millard-Sadler GH (1979). Liver and Biliary Disease. W.B. Saunders Ltd. London, Philadelphia, Toronto, pag. 621.

Miyakawa Y, Mayumi M (1978). Characterization and clinical significance of HBeAg. In Vyas GN, Cohen SN, Schmid R (eds) "Viral hepatitis", Philadelphia: The Franklin Institute Press, p 192.

Raimondo G, Smedile A, Gallo L, Balbo A, Ponzetto A, Rizzetto M (1982). Multicentre study of prevalence of HBV-associated delta infection and liver disease in drug-addicts. Lancet, 1:245.

Rizzetto M, Shih JW-K, Gocke DJ, Purcell RH, Verme G, Gerin JL (1979). Incidence and significance of antibodies to delta antigen in hepatitis B virus infection. Lancet 2:986.

Rizzetto M, Shih JW-K, Gerin JL (1980). The hepatitis B virus associated delta antigen (δ): isolation from liver, development of solid phase radioimmunoassay for delta and anti-delta and partial characterization of delta. J Immunol 125:318.

Rizzetto M, Purcell RH, Gerin JL (1980). Epidemiology of HBV associated delta antigen: geographical distribution and prevalence in polytransfused HBsAg carriers. Lancet 1:1215.

Smedile A, Farci P, Verme G, Caredda F, Cargnel A, Caporaso N, Dentico P, Trepo C, Opolon P, Gimson A, Vergani D, Williams R, Rizzetto M (1982). Influence of delta infection on severity of hepatitis B. Lancet 2:945.

Smedile A, Lavarini C, Crivelli O, Raimondo G, Fassone M, Rizzetto M (1982). Radioimmunoassay detection of IgM antibodies to the HBV-associated delta (δ) antigen, clinical significance in delta infection. J Med Virol 9:131.

Smedile A, Lavarini C, Aricò S, Farci P, Marinucci G, Dentico P, Giuliani G, Cargnel A, Del Vecchio Blanco C, Rizzetto M, (1983). Epidemiological patterns of infection with the hepatitis B virus associated delta agent in Italy. Am J Epidemiol 117:223.

Viral Hepatitis and Delta Infection, pages 245–250
© 1983 Alan R. Liss, Inc., 150 Fifth Avenue, New York, NY 10011

PROSPECTIVE STUDY OF EPIDEMIC DELTA INFECTION IN DRUG ADDICTS

F. Caredda, A. d'Arminio Monforte, E. Rossi, P. Farci, A. Smedile, G. Tappero, M. Moroni
Infect.Dis.Clinic, Univ. of Milan, Osp. L.Sacco, and Div.of Gastroenterology, Osp.Molinette,Turin

Parenteral drug-addicts (PDA) are known to be at high risk of developing HBsAg-associated delta (δ) hepatitis (Ra imondo 1982). During the years 1979–81, an outbreak of δ in the drug-using community of Milan has reached epidemic proportions (Caredda 1982), with 78% of susceptibles (HBV infected) positive for δ markers. This outbreak has provided the opportunity for a prospective study of the clinical and serological characteristics of acute δ infection.

We have studied prospectively 69 PDA (56 males and 13 females; mean age: 20±3 years; range 14–35 years) admitted to the Infectious Diseases Clinic in Milan between January 1979 and December 1981 for acute HBsAg-positive hepatitis with δ infection. Patients had been using heroin for 2 to 48 months (mean: 11±9 months). A group of 150 patients without history of drug addiction, hospitalized for acute hepatitis B in the same period, were studied for comparison. Serum samples were collected within 24 hours from admission, weekly thereafter during hospitalization, and monthly after discharge for a period of 6–12 months. Sera were stored at –20 °C.

The diagnosis of acute hepatitis B was based on history and symptoms suggestive of acute liver damage, with aminotransferase (ALT) levels 10 times or more higher than nor

mal and presence in serum of HBsAg. Acute and convalescent
sera from all the patients were negative for hepatitis A vi
rus (HAV) specific IgM, Cytomegalovirus specific IgM (Enzy-
gnost-Cytomegalie; Behringwerke), and for anti-Epstein Barr
virus heterophil antibodies (Paul Bunnell reaction; and Mo-
nosticon, Organon). Hepatitis was considered severe in patients with a prothrombin activity < 50%. Resolution of hepatitis was shown by normal liver chemistry 6 months after
discharge from hospital and seroconversion to anti-HBs. Pro
gression of the acute episode to chronicity was diagnosed
on persistence of abnormal serum ALT 6 months after the onset of illness. A percutaneous liver biopsy was obtained
in these patients. The criteria for the histological diagnosis of chronic hepatitis were those of Scheuer (1973).

HBsAg, anti-HBs, HBeAg, anti-HBe, IgM anti-HAV were me
asured by commercial RIA (Abbott). Serum δAg, total anti-
δ, and IgM anti-δ were assayed by RIA according to techniques described elsewhere (Bonino 1981; Rizzetto 1980; Smedi
le 1982). Statistical analysis of the results was carried
out by the Chi-square test with Yates correction.

In serial sera taken during the acute hepatitic episode (mean hospitalization period: 32±11 days) δ markers were
detected in 65.1% of 106 addicts and in 8% of non-addicts
(table 1).

Delta system	Addicts	non-addicts
δAg positive[†]	19 (18%)	–
anti-δ positive[††]	50 (47%)	12 (8%)
δAg/anti-δ negative	37 (35%)	138 (92%)

Table 1. Incidence of delta (δ) markers in 106 addicts and
150 non-addicts with HBsAg-positive acute hepatitis. [†]:fol
lowed by seroconversion to anti-δ. [††]:without prior δ antigenemia.

All addicts (including those with serum δAg) developed
early IgM anti-δ followed by secondary sustained IgG anti-
δ. Anti-δ persisted at 6th month of follow-up in all these

patients, regardless of clearance or persistence of HBsAg in serum. Titres of the antibody at 6th month of follow-up varied between $1/10^3$ and $1/5x10^3$. This pattern was distinctly different from that of patients with sporadic δ infection examined in the present and a previous study (Rizzetto 1979); none had serum δAg and the majority developed only brief anti-δ of the IgM class.

Serum δAg and the sustained secondary IgG response, which presumably requires a stronger antigenic stimulus than the isolated primary IgM response, suggest that epidemic acute infection in addicts is comparatively more virulent than the sporadic form in non-addicts. Correspondingly, whereas the acute illness was uncomplicated in all the 50 addicts exhibiting anti-δ without δ antigenemia, hepatitis was severe in 31.5% of patients with serum δAg, with a fatal outcome in two of these individuals. Virulence of δ in addicts might depend on the large amount of the infectious agent that can be transmitted parenterally, or on adaptation of the virus to host through the multiple rapid transfers in the epidemic setting, in analogy with the progressively more severe liver disease in chimpanzees serially inoculated with delta (Gerin 1982).

The clinical context of acute δ infection in addicts was classical hepatitis type B (71%) or biphasic hepatitis (20%) with two peaks of aminotransferase a few weeks apart. In 9% it was a relapsing hepatitis occurring in individuals who had experienced acute type B hepatitis 2 to 4 months previously and had remained carriers of HBsAg. Biphasic hepatitis is possibly due to the sequential expression of HBV and δ (Raimondo 1982). A similar course was observed in δ infected addicts in Sweeden (Moestrup 1983) and seems therefore characteristic of the illness in the narcotic dependent.

The disease resolved uneventfully in the 17 addicts with δ antigenemia (all HBeAg-positive on admission) that survived the acute illness, and in 98.3% of the patients without δ markers. 18% (9/50) of the addicts exhibiting anti-δ without δ antigenemia remained chronic HBsAg carriers. 8 of these patients developed chronic active hepatitis. Acute hepatitis accompained by δ markers resolved uneventfully in the 12 non-addicts patients, none had biphasic hepatitis (table 2).

Acute phase		At six months' follow-up	
Delta system	no	HBsAg-pos.	CAH
δAg positive	17	–	–
anti-δ positive	50	9	8
δAg/anti-δ negative	37	1	1

Table 2. Correlation between delta infection and the outcome of acute type B hepatitis in addicts. CAH : chronic active hepatitis.

Within the anti-δ positive group there was a positive correlation between the development of HBsAg carriership (and chronic liver disease) and the presence of anti-HBe in serum: 46.2% (6/13) of the anti-HBe positive addicts became chronic carriers of HBsAg versus 8.1% (3/37) of the HBeAg-positive (p < 0.01). A point emerging from this prospective study is that the HBe status is most important in determining chronicity of δ, as interplays of HBe antigen/antibody system with δ were associated with different outcomes of the infection. Despite the severity of the acute illness in HBeAg-positive addicts with δ antigenemia, none developed chronic liver disease and all cleared HBsAg from serum. Anti-HBe predominated in a significant majority of patients with δ infection destined to chronicity, suggesting that this characteristic determines an increased susceptibility to persistence of the defective virus and that carriers with inactive HBV infection are more likely to became also carriers of δ than the HBeAg-positive individuals replicating complete HBV. Possibly, the mechanism inducing chronicity of δ depends on, or is enhanced by, integration of HBV-DNA sequences in the host genome, a feature of HBV infection associated with anti-HBe (Brechot 1981).

Viral Hepatitis and Delta Infection, pages 253–254
© 1983 Alan R. Liss, Inc., 150 Fifth Avenue, New York, NY 10011

HBsAg-POSITIVE CHRONIC HEPATITIS: ASSOCIATION
WITH HLA ANTIGENS IN DELTA-NEGATIVE INFECTIONS

A AMOROSO,I BORELLI,A PULEJO,B FORZANI,GA TOUSCOZ,ES CURTONI
Istituto di Genetica Medica, Università di Torino, Italy
Dpt. Gastroenterology, Molinette, Torino, Italy

Attempts to correlate chronic hepatitis (CH) and HLA markers
have brought forth an association with HLA-A1, B8 and DR3
antigens in the idiopathic non viral form whereas no
correlation emerged with HBsAg-positive CH. In previous
studies,however,HBsAg-positive patients were not subdivided
according to presence or absence of δ infection, as the new
pathogen was unknow at the time. This variable was considered in the present study.
HLA markers were investigated in 45 HBsAg carriers with
immunofluorescence and/or serological markers of δ infection
and 44 HBsAg carriers without δ markers. All the patients
were unrelated individuals of Italian origin. The male to
female ratio was 2.5 in δ-positive and 3.9 in δ-negative.
Controls included 526 healthy Italian adults. HLA-A,B,C
typing was performed according to the standard NIH lymphocytotoxicity technique. All the officially defined specific
ities (Histocompatitibility Testing 80) were tested. HLA-DR
typing (from DR1 to DRw8) was carried out on B lymphocyte-
-enriched suspensions using the NIH long incubation technique. B cell were separated from peripheral blood by ro-
sette formation of T lymphocyte with AET-treated sheep
erythrocytes. The association of HLA markers with HBsAg-pos
itive CH was estimated for each specificity calculating the
Relative Risk (RR) from phenotype frequencies in patients
and controls using Woolf or Haldane formula. The significance of the association was evaluated by Fisher's exact
test. The probability level (p) was corrected for the number
of comparisons made for each locus.
Comparisons with the control group showed no significant
difference (after correction) in incidence of HLA-A,B,C
antigens between δ-positive and δ-negative carriers and
controls. The results of HLA-DR testing are summarized in
Table 1 and Table 2. DR2 was significantly more frequent
among the δ+ CH, DR3 was significantly more frequent in δ-
CH and the frequency of DR4 was slightly lower (not signifi
cant after correction) in δ+ CH patients and significantly
lower in the δ- group.

Table 1: ANTIGEN FREQUENCIES OF HLA-DR MARKERS

Antigen	Patients HBsAg+ CH δ+ n:45	δ− n:44	Controls n:526
DR2	.378	.136	.194
DR3	.200	.364	.171
DR4	.111	.000	.185

Table 2: STATISTICAL SIGNIFICANCE IN HLA-DR FREQUENCIES

Comparisons between controls and the following groups:	HBsAg-positive chronic hepatitis					
	delta-positive			delta-negative		
HLA-DR Antigen:	DR2	DR3	DR4	DR2	DR3	DR4
p (uncorrected):	<.005	n.s.	<.025	n.s.	<.005	<.005
p (corrected):	<.035	n.s.	n.s.	n.s.	<.035	<.035
RR	2.52	−	−	−	2.77	.05
confidence limits:	4.8/1.3	−	−	−	5.3/1.4	.07/.02

This study indicates that in the absence of superimposed δ infection carriers of HBsAg are more likely to develop chronic hepatitis if DR3, a marker associated with autoimmune disease, is present in their phenotype. This would imply that there is some genetic predisposition to ordinary HBsAg liver disease. DR3 frequency, instead, was not different between controls and carriers with chronic δ hepatitis, implying that no genetic autoimmune background assists the development of δ disease and this may be related to a direct cytopathic action of δ agent, invariably effective whenever it establishes infection. The increased frequency of DR2 points to a correlation between this antigen and higher susceptibility to δ infection. Lack of DR4 in δ-negative CH may be a consequence of the increased frequency of another allele (DR3) at the same locus or it may suggest protection from chronic hepatitis in the absence of δ agent infection.

Viral Hepatitis and Delta Infection, pages 255–256
© **1983 Alan R. Liss, Inc., 150 Fifth Avenue, New York, NY 10011**

MICROSOMAL AUTOANTIBODIES IN CHRONIC DELTA INFECTION

O. Crivelli, M. Rizzetto, S.J. Hadziyannis,F.Caredda, G. Marinucci,P.L. Meroni,C. Lavarini, E. Chiaberge, Molinette
Hospital Torino,L. Sacco Hospital Milano, S. Giacomo Hospital Roma Italy and Hippokration Gen. Hospital Athens Greece

A non species-specific autoantibody reacting distinctly
with human liver and kidney cytoplasms and weakly with
human thyroid, adrenal and pancreatic cells, was found by
immunofluorescence in 13% and 30%, respectively,of 135 and
20 carriers of HBsAg with chronic delta hepatitis collected
in Italy(Torino,Milano and Roma) and in Greece.
This autoantibody was not found in 1000 patients including
HBsAg-positive subjects with acute delta infection, acute or
chronic HBsAg-positive/delta-negative hepatitis,type A or
nonA,nonB hepatitis and autoimmune or non-immune chronic
liver diseases unrelated to HBsAg and delta.
The autoantibody is of IgG class and complement fixing;
the fluorescence pattern on human liver and kidney(Figs.1
and 2) is identical to that exhibited by the liver-kidney
microsomal antibody(LKM)(1), characteristic of a subgroup
of chronic juvenile hepatitis of unknown etiology.
Cross-blocking experiments,however, failed to demonstrate
an immunological identity between the two antibodies.
Complement fixation and immunofluorescence absorption studies have shown that the homologous antigen is localized
in the microsomal membranes of human liver(2).
The organ specificity of the new autoantibody is wider
than that of LKM; the species-specificity seems more restricted since fluorescence was best observed in human liver
and kidney but decreased progressively in the corresponding
tissues of other mammals;it was borderline or often negative in the liver and kidney of rat which are instead the
best substrates to detect LKM antibodies(2).
In analogy with subjects with LKM,patients with the delta-
associated microsomal antibody were all young,often males
and generally lacked other autoantibodies or markers of

autoallergy.
The apparently exclusive occurrence of this autoantibody
in patients with advanced liver disease and chronic delta
infection suggests that its expression is induced by this
viral event.

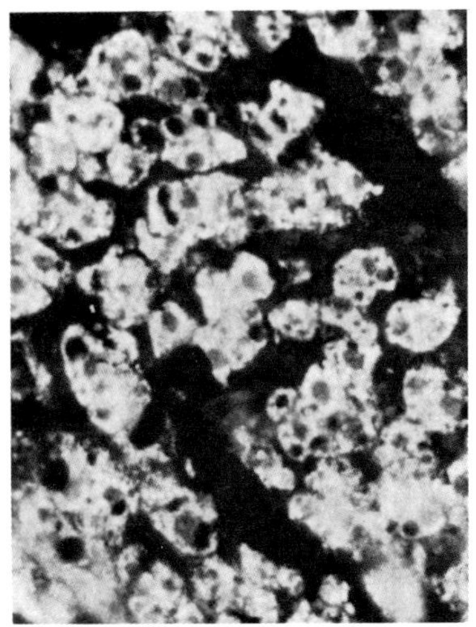

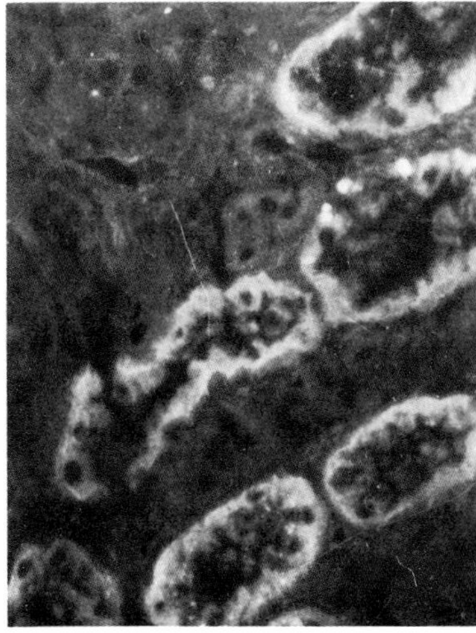

Fig. 1   Fig. 2

Human cirrhotic liver(Fig. 1) and normal kidney(Fig. 2)
stained by indirect immunofluorescence with the delta-associated microsomal antibody(x 250). Microsomal antiserum
diluted 1/20.

(1) Rizzetto M. et al. Clin. Exp. Immunol. 15, 331, 1973
(2) Crivelli O. et al. Clin. Exp. Immunol. 53, 1983,in press

PREVALENCE OF DELTA INFECTION IN HAEMODIALYSIS UNITS OF
SOUTHERN-ITALY

Pietro Dentico, Lucia Baldi, Rosalba Buongiorno, Giuseppe
Pastore, Fabrizio Trotta, Oronzo Schiraldi
Institute of Infectious Diseases, University of Bari, Italy

Blood and its constituents represent vehicles of trans
mission of the δ agent and haemodialysis patients should the
refore be frequent victims of this infection. To assess the
epidemiology of δ infection in dialysis units, 864 patients
undergoing haemodialytic treatment collected in Apulia and
Basilicata, areas of Southern Italy where δ is highly endemic (Rizzetto 1980), were examined for serum markers of HBV
and δ infection by radioimmunoassays. In each dialysis cen
ter, HBsAg-positive patients were conveyed to an HBsAg-conta
minated area and machine, that were separate from HBsAg-nega
tive patients. The results are shown in the table.

PREVALENCE OF ANTI-δ IN 864 HAEMODIALYSIS PATIENTS

HBV status		n° with anti-δ/n° examined	
		Apulia	Basilicata
HBsAg	anti-HBs		
+	−	6*/111 (5.4%)	1/ 8 (12.5%)
−	+	5 /512 (1.0%)	1/30 (3.3%)
−	−	0 /180 −	0/23 −

* 2 patients with chronic hepatitis (persistently elevated aminotransferase and gamma-globulin levels)

The prevalence of δ infection in our haemodialyzed patients (5.4%) was distinctly lower than in asymptomatic carriers (17%) and in carriers with liver disease (54%) from
the same HBsAg population (Smedile 1983). Our data suggest
that dialysis patients carrying HBsAg are less susceptible
than other categories of HBsAg carriers to infection with δ,
possibly for immunological or other causes, non yet known,
characteristic of individuals undergoing dialysis.
References:
Rizzetto et al.(1980). Lancet 1:1215
Smedile et al. (1983). American Journal of Epid. 117:223

LYMPHOCYTE SUBSETS IN BLOOD AND LIVER FROM PATIENTS WITH DELTA INFECTION

M.A.Freni, B.Forzani, M.L.Resta, A.Smedile, G.F.Tappero, G.A.Touscoz
Clinica Medica 1a, Università di Messina
Divisione di Gastroenterologia, Molinette, Torino

Immune reactions seem important in the pathogenesis of virus B related liver disease while a direct cytopathic effect has been suggested for δ Agent (1), cause of persisting liver damage in humans (2).

We studied the circulating lymphoid populations and the composition of the hepatic mononuclear infiltrate in 21 chronic patients with intrahepatic δ-Ag and in 18 with HBsAg+ chronic liver disease lacking markers for δ-Ag.

Monoclonal antibodies OKT3 (pan T), OKT4 (inducer/helper), OKT8 (cytotoxic/suppressor), OKIa (B, activated T, monocytes), OKM1 (monocytes null), Leu10 (B) were used to label in immunofluorescence and immunoperoxidase mononuclear cells isolated from blood and on frozen liver biopsies.

Most results were similar in both groups (marked histological prevalence of T3+ cells with reduced T4/T8 ratio especially in the areas of piecemeal necrosis; few T4+ cells localized in the inner portal zone; isolated groups of T8+ in contact with hepatocytes within the lobule) but δ+ patients had a conspicuous infiltration of Ia+ cells with the same localization of T8+. These cells were considered as activated T since only a limited number of Leu10+ cells could be demonstrated. In all the patients the prominence of T8+ cells in the inflammatory areas was reflected by a significant decrease of T3+ and T8+ cell concentrations in the peripheral blood while all the other subsets were within the normal range. A more marked infiltration of T8+ lymphocytes which express the Ia antigen seems therefore to be the only feature discriminating the lymphocytic settlement in patients with and without δ infection.

(1) Ann. Int. Med. 98: 437, 1983.
(2) Ital. J. Gastroenterol. 10: 146, 1978.

Viral Hepatitis and Delta Infection, page 261
© 1983 Alan R. Liss, Inc., 150 Fifth Avenue, New York, NY 10011

PRESENCE OF ANTI-DELTA IN DIFFERENT POPULATION GROUPS OF
SOUTHERN GERMANY

G.G. Frösner, E. Franco
Max von Pettenkofer-Institut, University of Munich, FRG.

Anti-Delta was determined by radioimmunoassay in 55 HBsAg
positive blood donors, in 20 anti-HBs positive but HBsAg
negative blood donors, in 40 adult hemophilic patients with
serological markers of past hepatitis B infection and in 16
patients developing non-A, non-B hepatitis after open heart
surgery. Anti-Delta was only found (in high titer) in one
hemophilic patient. From these results we can conclude that
Delta-infection is probably not frequent in the Federal Republic of Germany.

AN ELISA FOR DELTA MARKERS IN HEPATITIS B INFECTION

R.Heijtink, J.Kruining, L.Kuijpers, A.Jacobs, C.Geudens, and G.Wolters. Department of Virology, Erasmus University Rotterdam and Organon Diagnostics Res. Labs, Oss, Holland

Liver delta-antigen and serum anti-delta, kindly provided by Dr.M.Rizzetto, Torino, Italy, were used for an ELISA on delta-antigen and antibody. Microtitre plates coated with anti-delta were incubated for 2 h, 37º C with patient serum that had been preincubated either with 3 g/l NP40 (1h, 20º C) to detect delta-antigen or with a fixed amount of liver delta-antigen (16 h, 20º C) to detect delta-antibody. After washing, incubation with peroxidase-labeled anti-delta (2 h, 37º C), renewed washing and incubation with substrate (0.5 h, 20º C), the absorbance was measured. The ELISA for delta-antigen and delta-antibody did not react with HBcAg, HBeAg and HBsAg, and with anti-HBc, anti-HBe and anti-HBs, respectively. Twenty normal human sera and 4 rheumatoid-factor positive human sera were found negative for delta-antigen and antibody. Dilution series of four anti-delta positive sera were tested in both RIA (competitive sandwich test; Dr. A. Ponzetto, Torino, Italy) and ELISA. Titres in ELISA were 4 times higher than in RIA in all cases. Among sera from patients living in The Netherlands anti-delta was found in 10/ 130 chronic hepatitis B patients (1 asymptomatic carrier, 1 CPH, 5 CAH and 3 cirrhosis patients) including 2 cases from the medical profession without any other risk, in 3/30 acute HBV infections, in 4/43 anti-HBs$^+$ drug-users, in 3/40 HBsAg$^+$ drug-users and in 6/33 pregnant women born outside The Netherlands. The latter two groups of sera were kindly provided by Dr.J.Bänffer, GG & GD, Rotterdam. In 2 acute hepatitis B patients delta-agent seroconversion was observed. Surprisingly, samples taken before the peak ALT also showed elevated absorbance in the anti-delta test indicating the presence of delta-antigen. Since the patients' sera in the anti-delta test are not pretreated with detergent, this observation suggests the existence of free delta-antigen (HBeAg-like?). In conclusion, the ELISA for delta-antibody is specific and highly sensitive. The presence of delta-antigen or delta-antibody in the serum can be detected by the same test.

Viral Hepatitis and Delta Infection, pages 265–266
© 1983 Alan R. Liss, Inc., 150 Fifth Avenue, New York, NY 10011

DELTA (δ) INFECTION IN A HUMAN LIVER TRANSPLANT

G.Marinucci, L.Valeri, C.Di Giacomo, D.Morganti,
D. Alfani, P. Farci, R. Cortesini. Osp. S.Giacomo
II Pat.Chir.- Roma; Osp. Maggiore - Torino - Italia

New infection with the δ agent of a transplan ted liver was observed in the first case of liver transplantation carried out in Italy. The patient was a 33 years old female with HBsAg-positive post-hepatitic cirrhosis. She had anti-HBe, anti-HBc at low titres, anti-δ consistently positive at high titres, HBsAg in the cytoplasm of numerous hepatocytes and delta antigen in 50-60% of liver cell nuceli. HBcAg was not found in any of the liver tissue samples examined. During transplan - tation 5 doses of specific hyperimmune gamma glo- bulins were administred. Cyclosporine A was admi- nistred (10 mg/Kg pro die) as immunosuppressive therapy. The behaviour of HBV and δ markers follo wing transplantation was as follows: 1) HBsAg re- mained positive at decreasing titres for only 5 days; therefore it became negative to the moment of death; 2) approximately 3 weeks after transplan tation, anti- HBs appeared in increasing titres and was interpreted as an active response linked to the disappearance of HBsAg; 3) HBV–specific DNA polymerase activity, HBeAg, IgM anti-HBc antibody and serum δ antigen were negative during the en- tire period of survival; 4) anti-δ and anti - HBc were consistently positive at varying titres.- 60 days after transplantation the patient died from heart failure.

The transplanted liver showed no signs of re jection nor of hepatic infection. Immunofluore- scence study of the liver revealed neither HBsAg nor HBcAg whereas δ antigen was present in 5- 6% of hepatocytic nuclei. A plausible hypothesis is

that very small amounts of HBsAg undetectable by
RIA, expression of an early HBV infection in the
transplant, permitted the δ agent to enter and re
plicate in nuclei of the hepatocytes of the new
liver.

Viral Hepatitis and Delta Infection, page 267
© 1983 Alan R. Liss, Inc., 150 Fifth Avenue, New York, NY 10011

DELTA ANTIGEN AND ANTI-DELTA IN PATIENTS WITH LIVER DISEASES

Rainer Müller,Mario Rizzetto,Div.of Gastroenterology,Dept.of Medicine,Hannover Medical School,Germany and Dept.Gastroenterology,Molinette,Torino,Italy

176 randomly sampled sera and 56 liver biopsies of 122 patients with heterogenous liver diseases were investigated for presence of anti-delta and hepatitis B virus (HBV) markers in serum, HBcAg and delta-Ag in liver tissue. HBsAg, anti-HBc, anti-HBs and anti-delta were determined by RIA.Tests for HBeAg were done by EIA .HBcAg and delta-Ag were demonstrated in cryostat sections of liver biopsies by FITC labelled human anti-HBc-IgG or anti-delta-IgG

Anti-delta was detected in only 14 patients showing serological features of an ongoing or past HBV-infection(tab.1). Patients lacking HBV-markers were found negative for anti-delta.
Histological and delta-Ag /anti-delta findings are shown in tabl.2

tab.1: HBV markers and anti-delta in 122 patient with liver diseases

Anti-delta	HBsAg+ HBeAg+	HBsAg HBeAgn.t.	HBsAg+ HBeAg-	HBsAg- Anti-HBc+	Anti-HBc+ Anti-HBs+	no HBV-markers
−	45	6	26	11	15	5
+	4	1	6	1	2	0

tab.2: Anti-delta findings in 122 patients with liver diseases

HBsAg carrier	0/1	cirrhosis	1/9
viral hepatitis B	1⁺/26	unspecific lesion	1/1
chron.persist.hepatitis	0/6	miscellaneous	1/1
chron.active hepatitis	10/72	+ = deltaAg pos.	

Our data confirm that the delta-Ag/anti-delta system is observed but rarely in a population bearing a low HBsAg carrier rate.

PREVALENCE OF ANTI DELTA IN VARIOUS HBsAg-POSITIVE POPULA-
TIONS

I. K. Mushahwar and R. H. Decker
Abbott Laboratories, North Chicago, Illinois USA

Solid phase enzyme-linked immunoassays were developed for
the detection of delta (δ) antigen and its antibodies. The
assays for anti-δ were used to assess their prevalence and
relationship to the HBeAg-anti-HBe system among different
HBsAg carrier groups. The results are summarized below:

HBsAg Carrier Population	Total No.	Anti-δ and Anti-HBe	Anti-δ and HBeAg	Anti-δ, Total
California	210	4	0	4
W. Germany	32	0	0	0
Taiwan	200	2	7	9
Volunteer Donors	1008	32	7	39
Paid Donors	74	3	4	7
Drug Addicts	29	7	6	13

Of the 1553 carriers studied, 4.6% were positive for
anti-δ. Of the anti-δ positive population, 33.3% were
HBeAg positive, and 66.7% were anti-HBe positive.

Sera from 16 drug addicts which were positive for anti-HBs
were also found to be positive for anti-δ, indicating that
they had recovered from prior infections with HBV and
Delta antigen.

EPIDEMIOLOGIC CHARACTERISTICS OF DELTA INFECTION IN GREECE

George Papaevangelou
National Center for Viral Hepatitis. Athens 618, Greece.

The high prevalence of acute and chronic hepatitis B virus
(HBV) infections in Greece and its geographic vicinity to
Southern Italy provide the necessary environment for extensive spread of δ-infection. The main epidemiologic
characteristics of δ-infection were studied in a sample
of acute (144) and chronic (96) HBsAg positive liver
patients. Radioimmunoassays were used for the detection of
HBV markers as well as for δ-agent and anti-δ-antibodies
(total and IgM class).
In chronic B liver patients the prevalence of chronic δ-
infection was very high in haemophiliacs (2/6 or 33.3 %),
relatively rare in chronically active HBsAg positive liver
disease (3/27 or 11,1 %) and absent in asymptomatic HBsAg
carriers (0/63).
Acute δ-infection was very common (13/36 or 36.1 %) in
drug addicts with benign acute viral hepatitis. Acute δ-
superinfection was detected in one HBsAg carrier, while
acute δ- and B coinfection was diagnosed in the remaining
12 drug addict patients. Clinical and biochemical
characteristics did not differ significantly between δ-
infection positive and negative cases. Acute δ-infection
was also diagnosed in two (one drug addict and one transfused patient) of the studied 32 (6.3 %) fulminant hepatitis type B cases. In contrast δ-infection was not found in
anyone of the studied 76 benign acute viral hepatitis B
patients without a history of drug addiction.
It is concluded that δ-infection is very common only in
drug addicts and in patients using imported commercial
blood products. Epidemiologic surveyance should be
considered for preventing its extensive spread in the
future.

DELTA ANTIGEN-ANTIBODY SYSTEM IN CHRONIC PERSISTENT OR
ACTIVE HEPATITIS B

Antonino Picciotto,Guido Celle.
Chair of Gastroenterology of the University of Genoa,Italy.

Serum markers associated with hepatitis B-virus (HBV)infection (HBeAg,anti-HBe,anti-δ)were tested by radioimmunoassay of serum of 106 patients of both sexes with ages ranging from 9 to 70,selected from a larger group of chronic hepatitis patients on the basis of their positivity for serum HBsAg.The corresponding liver biopsies,histologically classified in both chronic persistent hepatitis (CPH,40 patients)and chronic active hepatitis (CAH,66 patients)were examined by means of direct immunofluorescence in order to detect the presence of HBsAg,HBcAg and delta antigen.Delta and/or anti-delta positivity were present in 19 patients (17.9%)for the most part having CAH (15/19,78.9%).In their liver biopsies there was poor morphological expression both of HBsAg (6/19, 31.5%) and of HBcAg (2/19,10.5%).Whereas HBeAg was present only in 2 patients,anti-HBe occurred almost in all cases associated with delta/anti-delta system (17/19,89.4%).These findings seem to confirm that the delta agent requires helper function of HBV,and at the same time inhibits the antigens of the virus.The epidemiological data of the delta and/ or anti-delta positive patients underlined a peculiar geographic distribution.In fact the delta/anti-delta system was very frequent in patients from Southern Italy (14/19,73.7%). Further,the mean age of patients positive for delta and/or anti delta (27.7±13.3)was significantly lower (p < 0.01)than that of the remaining patients (37.3±13.6).This seems to show that superinfection caused by the delta agent often occurs in young HBsAg chronic carriers and can develop into chronic evolutive hepatitis that often leads to untimely death.

ANTIBODY TO DELTA AGENT IN COMMERCIAL IMMUNOGLOBULINS.

Antonio Ponzetto[1], John L. Gerin[2], Barbara Forzani[1],
Robert H. Purcell[3], Giorgio Verme[1] [1]Dept. of
Gastroenterology, Osp. Molinette, [2]Georgetown Univ.,
Washington, DC, and [3]NIH, Bethesda, Maryland.

Passive immunoprophylaxis with human
immunoglobulins (Ig) is widely used for the prevention
of diseases such as Hepatitis A, rabies, tetanus, etc.

Immunoglobulin (IgG) and other plasma derivatives
are prepared from pooled human plasma from multiple
donors. Although properly prepared Ig has an
established record of safety, other plasma derivatives
(e.g. anti-haemophilic factor) may transmit hepatitis
viruses.

Since viral antibodies in Ig are a measure of the
collective virus exposure of the donors, and the
possible presence of viruses in blood products, we have
tested commercial Ig for the presence of antibody to the
delta antigen (anti-delta), the only available serum
marker of infection with the delta agent.

Forty-nine lots of Ig from 10 American (USA) and 7
Italian manufacturers were tested for anti-delta by RIA:
21/42 (50%) American lots, and 3/7 (43%) Italian lots
contained anti-delta at low titer (1:5 to 1:64).

Anti-delta in Ig indicates that one or more plasma
units used to prepare the positive Ig lots were obtained
from individuals exposed to the delta agent. Though it
is presently impossible to ascertain whether the
antibody represented past or current infection, these
results raise the possibility that the IgG source
material contained the transmissible delta agent.
Further studies are required to determine whether the
use of anti-delta positive IgG represents a risk in
patients infected with HBV.

DETERMINATION OF ANTIBODIES TO DELTA ANTIGEN IN VARIOUS
HBsAg POSITIVE POPULATION GROUPS IN WESTERN GERMANY

Michael Roggendorf, Ulla Schlipköter, Friedrich Deinhardt,
Gerd Zoulek, Karl Gmelin* Petra Wolf*, Max von Pettenkofer-
Institute, University of Munich, *Medical Clinic Heidelberg

Sera from various HBsAg carrier populations in Western
Germany have been tested for antibodies to the Delta agent
(anti-δ) (Table 1). To determine anti-δ , a solid phase
enzyme immunoassay was used. The 211 sera from blood
donors who were HBsAg positive were collected from
different blood banks (Bonn, Düsseldorf, Frankfurt,
Munich, Ulm). Only one serum was positive for anti-δ. One
of 278 sera from hemodialysis patients was found positive
for anti-Delta. 658 Sera from 303 patients with acute
hepatitis B and 17 sera of 17 patients with chronic active
hepatitis were all negative for anti-Delta, but it could
be detected in the sera of 4 out of 8 HBsAg positive drug
addicts. However, the percentage of HBsAg carriers in our
study population of drug addicts was only about 1%. Two of
these anti-Delta positive carriers of HBsAg had at the
same time antibodies of the IgM class against hepatitis A
virus, indicating acute hepatitis A. From these data it
can be concluded that in Western Germany Delta infection
is a rare event but drug addicts are the main risk group
for acquiring it.

Table 1. Determination of anti-δ in HBsAg carriers

population	No.tested	No.positive
blood donors	211	1 (0.5%)
hemodialysis patients	278	1 (0.4%)
patients with acute hepatitis B	303	0
patients with CAH	17	0
drug addicts	8	4 (50%)

DELTA INFECTION IN SAUDI ARABIA. A GENERAL POPULATION STUDY.

M. Shuja Shafi, Antonio Ponzetto, Barbara Forzani. Dept Microbiology, King Khalid Hospital, Jeddah, Saudi Arabia and Dpt. Gastroenterology, Osp. Molinette, Torino, Italy.

We tested for antibody to the delta antigen (anti-delta) 169 Saudi patients. They were a part of the 210 Hepatitis B Surface Antigen (HBsAg) positive patients attending the National Guard King Khalid Hospital since its opening in July 1982 (7.4% of the whole Hospital population).
Anti-delta was found in 34 patients (20%). This figure in unselected HBsAg carriers ranks among the highest reported worldwide and points to Saudi Arabia as a likely focus of Delta Agent endemicity.
In this series the majority os patients with anti-delta had anti-HBe (30 of **34**).
Admission to Hospital was motivated by liver disease-related symptoms in 47% of the HBsAg positive patients with anti delta. Liver disease, instead, was the admission cause for only 19.3% of the HBsAg positive patients without anti-delta.
These data suggest a higher pathogenicity of HBV infection accompanied by delta infection than HBV infection alone.

DELTA INFECTION IN IRELAND

A.G. Shattock
Dept. of Medical Microbiology, University College, Dublin.

An outbreak of hepatitis B in parenteral drug-abusers in
Dublin, coinciding with a very large increase in the use of
heroin, commenced in October 1980 and has continued. A
sample of 50 of the initial cases had delta antigenaemia at
a rate of 31% and a low (4%) incidence of anti-delta.

A sensitive enzyme-immunoassay (ELISA) was developed for
the detection of delta antigen, and serum from the outbreak
cases was used as the source of delta antigen for the anti-
delta assays. Using these tests it was found that the over-
all delta marker rate was 35%, 71% of which had detectable
delta antigenaemia in the acute phase. The majority of over
320 cases detected since the start of the outbreak were
diagnosed as acute hepatitis B and delta was acquired simultaneously, in most cases, in those with delta markers. No
significant difference was seen, clinically, biochemically
of serologically, between those with or without delta markers. Of two deaths which have occurred in the group to
date, one was anti-delta positive and died one year after
his apparently acute episode of hepatitis B and becoming an
HBsAg carrier. The other was a case of fulminant hepatitis
B, negative for delta markers.

On the basis of our results so far, it does not appear
that simultaneously acquired delta and hepatitis B infection increases the risk of severe infection, compared
with hepatitis B alone.

SENSITIVE ENZYME-IMMUNOASSAY FOR THE DETECTION OF
DELTA ANTIGEN AND ANTI-DELTA USING SERUM AS THE
DELTA ANTIGEN SOURCE.

Alan G. Shattock and Bridget M. Morgan, Dept. of
Medical Microbiology, University College Dublin 4.

A sensitive enzyme-immunoassay (ELISA) was developed for the detection of delta antigen in serum
treated with 3% Tween 20.   The serum delta antigen so derived was used in ELISA techniques for
the detection of anti-delta of IgG (and later,
IgM) class, with a yield of between 800 to 2400
tests per 10 mls of delta antigen positive serum.
Both tests had comparable or better sensitivity
than radio-immunoassay (RIA, using liver derived
delta antigen) when applied to testing parenteral
drug-abusers with simultaneously acquired hepatitis B and delta infection (IgM anti-HBc positive).
Specificity was confirmed by blocking assays with
anti-delta and by lack of reactions with anti-HBe
and anti-HBc.   In the case of sera positive by
ELISA but negative by RIA, specificity was also
confirmed by sero-conversion or the previous detection of delta antigenaemia.   It is concluded
that the different sources and/or treatment of
the delta antigen used may account for the different sensitivities noted, and that delta antigenaemia in acute infection may be more frequently
detectable than was first thought, amounting to
71% of those with delta infection in this study,
and that these sera are a practical and convienie-
nt alternative source of antigen.

Viral Hepatitis and Delta Infection, page 285
© **1983 Alan R. Liss, Inc., 150 Fifth Avenue, New York, NY 10011**

FULMINANT TYPE B HEPATITIS AND DELTA INFECTION IN A
HOMOSEXUAL MAN

James Shorey MD, Dallas VA Medical Center, Dallas, TX.,
and Charles L. Spurr MD, Augusta, GA.

A 28 year old homosexual man developed acute type B
hepatitis in February 1980 while living in San Francisco.
The illness was mild, and he became assymptomatic several
weeks after its onset. In September 1980 he was hospitalized
with fulminant hepatitis complicated by the development of
stage IV hepatic encephalopathy. Plasmapheresis was
performed with the exchange of 20 units of plasma.
After recovering sufficiently to leave the hospital,
he moved to the Dallas area. Because of continued symptoms
and blood test abnormalities, he underwent laparoscopy with
liver biopsy in the Fall of 1981; he was shown to have
severe chronic active hepatitis with early cirrhosis.
The patient remains HBsAg-positive to the present time
but is negative for HBeAg, anti-HBe, and anti-HAV (all by
RIA). His roommate and presumed   sexual partner, whom
he met after moving to Dallas, also has chronic type B
hepatitis. Both he and the patient were shown to have high
titers of anti-δ in their serum as determined independently
by Dr. M. Rizzetto and Drs. R. Purcell and A. Ponzetto.
Delta antigen was identified by immunofluorescence in the
patient's liver biopsy (M. Rizzetto).
Although it is possible that this patient's severe
chronic hepatitis is due to a non-A, non-B viral infection
acquired from the plasmapheresis treatment, delta infection
superimposed on a chronic HBV carrier state could account
both for the fulminant hepatitis episode and for the
subsequent progression to chronic active hepatitis, an
unusual sequence of events.
These cases call attention to the possibility that
delta superinfection may be a serious health threat to the
many HBV carriers in the male homosexual community as it
has been shown to be among intravenous drug abusers. This
additional risk adds further emphasis to the importance of
hepatitis B vaccination of susceptible persons in the
gay community.

PREVALENCE OF DELTA Ag AND ANTI DELTA BY RADIOIMMUNOASSAY
AMONG VARIOUS GROUPS OF HBs Ag CARRIERS IN FRANCE

D. TREPO, S. DEROSE, T. FONTANGES, P. CHOSSEGROS, C. TREPO,
Hepatitis Laboratory INSERM U 45 and GIS E.I.V.T.
Faculty of Medicine 69372 LYON France

Delta Ag and anti Delta testing by RIA were carried out as
described by RIZZETTO et al. However, as reported in the
previous abstract, the source of Ag used was a purified
preparation derived from plasma. The source of anti delta
for delta Ag determination was the serum of a patient with
CAH and HBs Ag which serum had a titer of 10^5 for anti delta.
1) Among 70 asymptomatic HBs Ag carriers blood donors (80 %
with anti HBe) none reacted for delta Ag or anti-delta.
2) 28/140 (20 %) patients with HBs Ag who underwent liver
biopsy at our center were found positive
   a. 8 (5,7 %) had delta Ag in the serum, all of whom circulated HBe Ag and had <u>active</u> liver disease (5/55 CAH, 3/24
active cirrhosis, all 79 HBe Ag positives,
   b. 20 (11,2 %) reacted for anti delta (8/29 with CAH and/
or active cirrhosis with HBe Ag ; 9/34 CAH or inactive cirrhosis and 3/14 CPH without HBe Ag).
Most of the reactive patients belonged to high risk group
for delta infection.
3) 12/20 (60 %) HBs Ag carriers drug addicts were positive :
two for delta Ag and ten for anti delta.
The above results suggest that in France Delta infection :
1. plays an important role in the most severe forms of liver
diseases,
2. is highly endemic among drug addicts as everywhere but
has remained sofar absent from the asymptomatic HBs Ag carrier blood donor population.
Testing for delta Ag and anti delta will be necessary in the
future in reference liver centers for a better understanding
and management of patients with severe or acute chronic
hepatitis B.

Viral Hepatitis and Delta Infection, page 289
© 1983 Alan R. Liss, Inc., 150 Fifth Avenue, New York, NY 10011

FEASIBILITY OF USING DELTA Ag DERIVED FROM PLASMA FOR THE
DETECTION OF ANTI DELTA BY RADIOIMMUNOASSAY

D. TREPO, S. DEROSE, C. TREPO,
Hepatitis Laboratory INSERM U 45 and GIS E.I.V.T. Faculty
Carrel 69372 LYON France

One of the crucial limiting factor for the development, by
many laboratories, of the specific serology for anti Delta
described by RIZZETTO et al. has been the difficulty to obtain sufficient amount of Delta Ag. Indeed delta Ag had so
far to be purified from the liver of patients suffering
from HBV associated infections.
We report here the possibility of using delta Ag obtained
from plasma. Our source was derived from a fulminant hepatitis case due to HB and delta virus coinfections. The patient's serum was positive for HBs Ag, HBe Ag and anti HBc
IgM and was found reactive for delta Ag during a collaborative study (SMEDILE et al. Lancet, 1982, 2 : 945).
Purification of delta Ag from this source was achieved by
density gradient ultracentrifugation followed by 6 M guanidine treatment. Delta Ag reactive fractions were diluted,
aliquoted and frozen before use for testing. The RIA for
anti delta was then carried out exactly as described by
RIZZETTO.
To assess the specificity and sensitivity of this serum
derived anti delta assay we tested under code a serum panel
of 200 liver patients : 50 with anti HBs ; 100 devoid of
any HBV marker and 50 HBs Ag positives, 10 of which previously found positive in Torino (ibid). Only those 10 samples were again found anti delta. Titration of 5 of these
specimen in the RIA using either serum or liver derived
delta Ag (kindly provided by M. RIZZETTO and O. CRIVELLI)
yielded identical results regardless of the source of
delta Ag used.
The clinical and epidemiological relevance of anti delta
testing using serum derived delta Ag as a source of reagent
is further illustrated in the following abstract showing
the prevalence of anti delta among various HBs Ag positive
groups in France.

DELTA INFECTION IN THE U.K.

Diego Vergani, Giorgina Mieli-Vergani, Munther
Jafar Hussain, Bernard Portmann, Roger Williams.
Depts Immunology,Child Health,Liver Unit,King's
College Hospital, London.

It has been inferred from serological studies
that delta infection has arrived in the U.K. only
recently (1) Using fluorescein labelled anti-
antibody in a direct immunofluorescence technique,
we have found δ-antigen in the liver tissue of
seven out of fifteen HBsAg positive drug addicts
referred to the liver unit, King's College
Hospital, between 1976 and 1981. In none of the
seven positive cases could hepatocyte nuclei be
stained with a fluorescein conjugated high titre
anti-HBc/anti-HBe serum,excluding cross-reaction
with this system. One of these patients, White
and British, who died with decompensated cirrhosis
in 1977,had liver biopsies in 1971,1972,and 1973.
δ-antigen was present in the liver cell nuclei on
all occasions. Our findings show that δ-antigen
was present in North European drug addicts as
early as 1971-73, confirming the obervation of
Hansonn er al (2) who found serological evidence
of δ-infection in 1973 in Sweden.

1) Tedder R.S, Briggs M, Howell D.R.
U.K. prevalence of delta infection. Lancet 1982;
2: 764-765.

2) Hansonn B.G, Moestrup T, Widell A, Mordenfelt
E. Infection with delta agent in Sweden: Introduction of a new hepatitis agent. J.Infect Dis
1982; 146: 472-78.

Viral Hepatitis and Delta Infection, pages 293–294
© **1983 Alan R. Liss, Inc., 150 Fifth Avenue, New York, NY 10011**

DELTA ANTIGEN IN AUSTRALIA

G.V. Williams, Y.E. Cossart
Dept. of Bacteriology, University of Sidney.

At the end of the war in 1945 the Australian population stood at 7.5 million and was almost entirely British by birth or descent. The hepatitis B carrier rate was very low and the adw subtype predominated. Subsequent immigration policy has produced a multi-cultural society and almost one in 8 of the 14.5 million Australians has emigrated from a country where the HBV carrier rate is high (with correspondingly high prevalence of chronic liver disease) and the HBsAg subtype is different. About 276,000 of these "New Australians" come from Italy and 143,500 from South East Asia, but most other Mediterranean and Middle European countries are also well represented.

It has therefore been of some interest to assess the role of delta antigen in patients with chronic liver disease and to determine the prevalence of this infection in various ethnic and social groups.

Delta antibody in patients' sera was detected by radio-immunoassay and delta antigen in liver sections by immunofluorescence. Both methods were standardised with reagents very kindly given by M. Rizzetto.

The results on liver biopsy samples from patients with chronic liver disease were:

	Patient's Hepatitis B status	
	HBsAg positive	Anti-HBs or Anti-HBc
Delta positive	3	0
Delta negative	27	5

When delta antibody was sought in sera from groups of HBV carriers the following results were obtained:

	Delta positive	Delta negative
Italian	1	10
Other Mediterranean	1	17
Vietnamese	3	40
Melanesian	0	10
Chinese	0	6

Anglo Irish (non narcotic)	0	43
Anglo Irish (narcotic users)	3	5
Aborigines	0	13

All the delta positive patients had chronic liver disease (except one with acute hepatitis) compared with only 39 of the 144 delta negative HBV carriers.

We conclude that Delta antigen is a marker for a world wide infection, that it is not restricted by the sub-type of the primary HBV infection, and that it does produce clinically significant increase in liver damage in HBV carriers.

Viral Hepatitis and Delta Infection, pages 295–296
© 1983 Alan R. Liss, Inc., 150 Fifth Avenue, New York, NY 10011

DELTA INFECTION IN CHINESE CARRIERS OF THE HBsAG

Xu Jian-yin and Yan-bo Xie
National Vaccine and Serum Institute,Beijing,
People's Republic of China.

Delta infection occurs only in HBsAg carriers and
predominates therefore in areas where HBV is endemic (Rizzetto,1981).We report in this study a survey on the prevalence of markers of Delta infection in Chinese,a population
with one of the highest rate of HBsAg carriers in the world
(12-18%).Sera were obtained from 407 carriers recruited in
the Beijing area between 1981 and 1982.There were 163 symptomless individuals with normal levels of serum transaminases and 244 patients with clinical evidence of chronic
liver disease.The mean age was 30 years (range 20-40 years)
in asymptomatic carriers and 35 years (range 20-50 years)in
patients with liver disease.The male/female ratio was 8/2
for asymptomatic carriers and 8.5/1.5 for patients with
chronic hepatitis.Liver biopsy specimens were obtained from
27 carriers with liver disease from the He-Bei province and
Dong-Bei area.HBsAg,anti-HBs,HBeAg and anti-HBe were assayed
by commercial Kits (Ausria II,Ausab,HBe and anti-HBe Kit,
Abbott,North Chicago,Ill.USA).Delta antigen and antibody
were detected by radioimmunoassay (Rizzetto,1980),IgM anti-
HBc by RIA (Core-IgMK,Sorin,Saluggia(Vc),Italy).Liver biopsy
specimens were tested for δAg by immunofluorescence (Rizzetto,1980).
No evidence of Delta infection was observed in the 163
asymptomatic carriers while 5 (2%) of the 244 carriers with
liver disease had serum anti-δ at titers higher than 1/5000.
Delta antigen was not detected in the 27 liver biospies ex-
amined.Serum HBcAg was present in 86%(210/244)of patients
and 54%(88/163) of asymptomatic carriers.IgM anti-HBc was
detected in 3%(5/163) of symptomless individuals and in 22%
(53/244) of patients suggesting that in the great majority
HBV infection was acquired in the remote past.The characteristics of the 5 δ-positive patients were as follow:two were
females and three males,all of them were negative for anti-

HBc ,one had serum HBeAg while the other 4 were negative for
both HBeAg and anti-HBe.Each of them,however,had clinical
evidence of cirrhosis.These results show that δ Agent is present,yet rare,among Chinese despite the high rate of HBV in
this population.The δ Agent might not yet have diffuse in
China;alternatively its infrequent presence might be secondary to genetic resistence or to an inhibitory effect of
active HBV infection on its persistence;in contrast to the
prevalence of anti-HBe in carriers from areas where Delta is
endemic,HBeAg was prevalent in Chinese carriers of HBsAg.

References.

Rizzetto M.,Shih J.W-K.,Gerin J.L.(1980).The hepatitis B virus
  associated delta antigen:isolation from liver,development
  of solid phse radioimmunoassay for delta and anti-delta and
  partial characterization of delta.J.Immunol.125:318-324.
Rizzetto M.,Gerin J.L.,Purcell R.H.(1981).Delta antigen:
  Evidence for a variant of hepatitis B virus or a defective
  Non-A Non-B agent.In Perspectives in Virology XI,M.Pollard
  Editor,Alan R.Liss,New York,N.Y.,195-217.

PATHOGENESIS, PROPHYLAXIS, AND THERAPY

Viral Hepatitis and Delta Infection, pages 299–307
© 1983 Alan R. Liss, Inc., 150 Fifth Avenue, New York, NY 10011

SUPPRESSOR CELLS AND CHRONIC HBV INFECTION

ADRIAN L.W.F. EDDLESTON, D.M., F.R.C.P.

PROFESSOR OF LIVER IMMUNOLOGY
LIVER UNIT, KING'S COLLEGE HOSPITAL,
LONDON, S.E.5, ENGLAND

A concept central to most of the hypotheses which seek
to explain the pathogenesis of the various liver lesions
associated with chronic HBV infection, is that the virus
is not cytopathic to the liver cells it infects and that
the liver damage is due to the patient's immune response.
(Eddleston, Williams 1974 ; Dudley et al 1972 ; Edgington,
Chisari 1975). Control of both immune reactivity and the
intensity of immune responses to host and viral antigens
is likely, therefore, to be of fundamental importance in
determining the type of liver disease in patients who
become chronic carriers of HBV.

Suppressor T-lymphocytes are one element in the complex
network of cellular and humoral interactions which determine
the intensity of an immune response to foreign antigens
and the duration and vigour of autoimmunity. (Pernis, Vogel
1980) Two different approaches have been used to the
investigation of suppressor T-cells in chronic liver
diseases. Direct assessment of the function of these cells
is difficult because of the complexity of the various assays
available, and an easier alternative has been to use
commercially available monoclonal antibody reagents to
determine the proportion of T-cells in the peripheral blood
which have differentiation antigens on their surface specific
for the suppressor/cytotoxic sub-set.

In this communication, I will present some of the
results obtained in our laboratory using these two
approaches and discuss their significance.

SUPPRESSOR CELL FUNCTION

While the investigation of antigen-specific suppressor
cells in man is still in its infancy, several groups have
reported on the activity of non-antigen-specific suppressor
T-cells in chronic liver disease (Eddleston et al. 1982)
The observation that these lymphocytes can be stimulated in
vitro by the mitogen Concanavalin A (Con A) has lead to the
development of several assays of suppressor cell function
based on the ability of Con A-stimulated suppressor cells to
inhibit proliferation of allogenic and autologous T- or B-
cells. Kayhan Nouri-Aria in our laboratory has concentrated
on assessing suppressor T-cell control of proliferating
B-cells (Nouri et al. 1982).

In the assay she has used, peripheral blood lymphocytes
are divided into two portions, one of which is incubated with
Con A for 24 hours and then both exposed to Pokeweed mitogen
(PWM) for 6 days to stimulate B-cell proliferation. The
number of B-cells producing IgG is counted using a haemolytic
plaque assay and the activity of the suppressor cells
assessed by calculating the percentage drop in IgG-producing
B-cells induced by the presence of the Con A activated
lymphocytes.

In normal subjects Con A activated suppressor cells
induce a very substantial reduction in the number of IgG-
producing B-cells after PWM stimulation (Figure I), while
a wide range of values was observed in 43 patients with
HBV infection. Eight of these were healthy carriers with
minimal histopathological changes in the liver on light
microscopy and almost all in this group had normal
%suppression values (Figure I). In contrast, suppressor
cell function was defective in the majority of those with
chronic liver disease, with the degree of abnormality being
unrelated to the presence of viral replication as assessed
by HBeAg status or the intensity of liver inflammation or
necrosis. (cf results in patients with CPH and CAH in
Figure I).

ENUMERATION OF T-CELL SUBSETS

This was carried out using commercially available mouse
monoclonal antibodies (Ortho Pharmaceutical Corporation)
OKT4 (to identify helper/inducer T lymphocytes) and OKT8

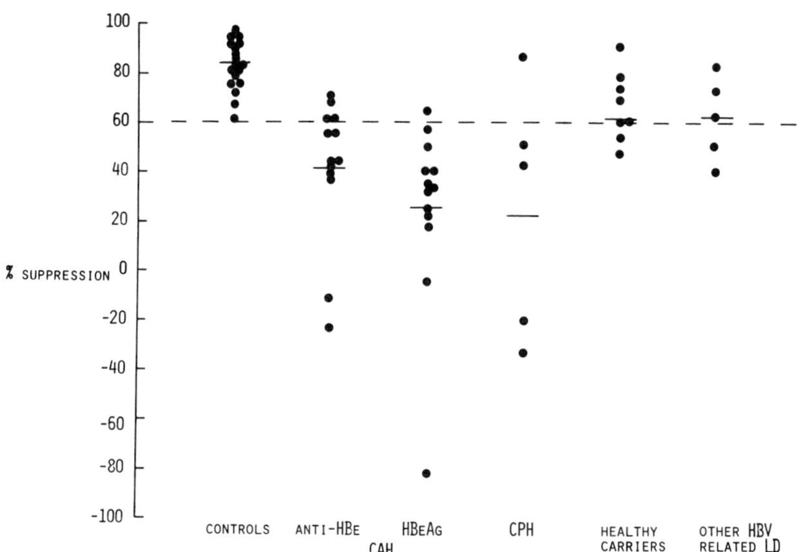

FIGURE 1

Con-A induced lymphocyte suppression of PWM stimulated
B-cell proliferation in 43 patients with HBV infection and
16 normal subjects.

(to identify suppressor/cytotoxic lymphocytes). Cell
surface binding of the monoclonal antibodies was detected
by incubation with fluorescein-labelled goat anti-mouse-
immunoglobulin and examination under UV light microscopy.
(Alexander et al. 1983). The number of positive cells was
expressed as a percentage of total lymphocytes isolated.

To compare number and function of the suppressor cell
population, patients with autoimmune CAH and HBsAg positive
chronic liver disease were studied for the proportion of
OKT4 and OKT8 positive cells and for the activity of
Con A-induced suppressor cells using the assay already
referred to above.

The most severe impairment in suppressor cell function
was observed in active autoimmune chronic active hepatitis
(Table I) while whose whose disease had become inactive
following prednisolone treatment had a mean %suppression
value very similar to that found in the control group. In
spite of these major changes in function, there was no
significant difference between the proportion of suppressor
lymphocytes in these groups (Table I), nor was there any
significant correlation between the proportion of any T
lymphocyte sub-set or the helper/suppressor cell ratio
and suppressor cell function.

In the patients with chronic liver damage associated with
persistent hepatitis B infection, %suppression values were
significantly reduced in all subgroups, while the proportion
of suppressor/cytotoxic T-cells was significantly <u>increased</u>
in those untreated patients with HBeAg in serum (p$<$0.05;
table I) and similar to the control subjects in HBeAg positive
patients receiving prednisolone therapy and in those with
anti-HBe. Furthermore, there was a significant <u>negative</u>
correlation between %suppression and proportions of
suppressor/cytotoxic cells in untreated HBeAg positive
patients (α= -0.62; p$<$0.05), which was not apparent in the
other two subgroups.

RELATION BETWEEN SUPPRESSOR-CELL FUNCTION AND NUMBER

An obvious question at this stage is; how can there be
such discrepancies between the proportion of suppressor/

TABLE I

Results of an assay of suppressor cell function and helper (T4+)
and cytotoxic/suppressor (T8+) lymphocyte proportions together
with the helper/suppressor ratio (T4/T8) in chronic liver disease

	% suppression	%T4+	%T8+	T4/T8
Normal subjects (20)	82.1+10.9*	46.5+4.7	22.7+4.7	2.10+0.50
Autoimmune CAH:				
Active (9)	1.4 +51.5	51.2+10.0	21.0+8.8	2.82+1.48
Inactive (8)	71.6+17.3	44.4+8.7	24.3+7.9	2.03+0.89
HBsAg-positive liver disease:				
HBeAg+ untreated (13)	50.9+39.7	42.7+9.7	32.4+8.3	1.45+0.60
HBeAg+ treated (7)	31.7+50.8	43.7+9.0	24.6+6.6	1.92+0.73
Anti-HBe+ (13)	41.9+39.1	43.2+7.1	25.6+8.8	1.90+0.70

* mean + ISD

cytotoxic cells in the peripheral blood of these patients and
the activity of Con A induced suppressor cells?   You will
notice that I have referred throughout this section to the
OKT8 defined T-cell subset as those having suppressor/
cytotoxic functions and this in itself provides the most
obvious answer to the discrepancy between number and function.
Indeed in the patients with untreated HEeAg positive chronic
liver disease, Mario Mondelli and Graham Alexander have
demonstrated a significant positive correlation between
the proportion of OKT8+ cells and T cell mediated
cytotoxicity for autologous hepatocytes (Figure 2). Mondelli
et al (1982) have shown that hepatitis B core antigen seems
to be the most important viral target antigen for this T
cell attack and this may well explain why the correlation
is restricted to the HBeAg+ cases where viral replication
and expression of core in the liver is more prominent.

     The second possible explanation for the discrepancy
between suppressor cell number and function follows from recent
observations suggesting that the various assays used to
examine suppressor-cell function are looking at independent
subsets of the total suppressor population. (Dwyer, Johnson
1981).   Thus profound disturbances in only one of these
subsets might not be reflected in the total OKT8+ population.
Thus, at least two groups have reported normal function of
suppressor cells in patients with HBsAg+ve chronic active
hepatitis using an assay based on the loss of suppressor
cell function during an initial 24 hour incubation before
mitogen stimulation. (Barnaba, 1983 and Tremolada, 1980).

     Yet a third possibility is that T-cells may carry the
appropriate differentiation antigens but be functionally
defective. Some evidence for this comes from our studies
of the effect of low dose prednisolone in vitro on Con A
induced suppressor cell function (Nouri et al, 1982).
Incubation of peripheral blood lymphocytes from patients
with active autoimmune chronic active hepatitis with
prednisolone for 30 minutes (at a concentration of 5×10^{-8}m)
almost completely corrected the suppressor cell defect while
there was no significant effect on the proportion of OKT8+
cells.   A finding which emphasised the specificity of this
response was that similar treatment of lymphocytes from
HBsAg+ CAH did not lead to any significant change in
suppressor cell function (Nouri et al, 1982). Thus,

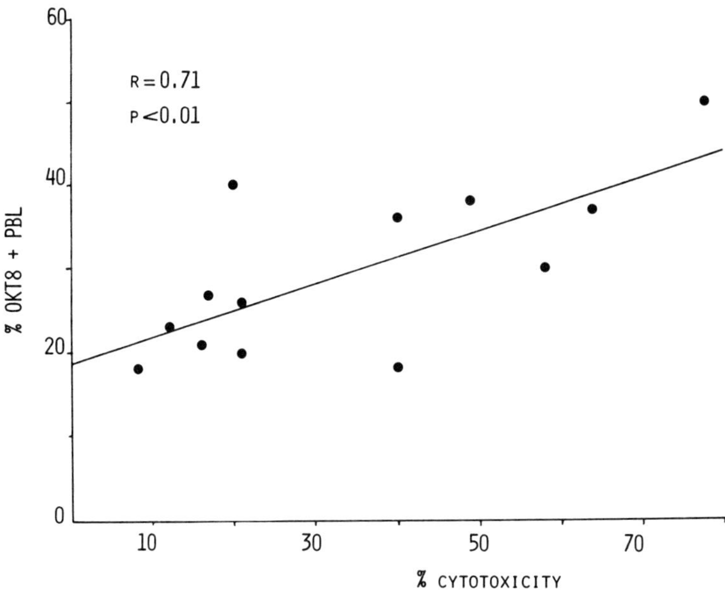

FIGURE 2

The correlation between %OKT8 + peripheral blood lymphocytes
and %cytotoxicity in a T-cell mediated autologous
cytotoxicity system using patients hepatocytes as target
cells.

although both autoimmune and HBsAg positive cases have similar defects in the function of Con A induced suppressor cells, the mechanisms responsible for the defects would seem to be quite different.

CONCLUSION

Despite the brevity of this communication and the selective presentation of just a few of the published studies in this area, it must already be clear that assays of suppressor cell function in chronic liver disease are technically demanding, frequently give apparently contradictory results and are examining only a small part of the immunoregulatory network. On the other hand, enumeration of T-cell subsets gives a more reliable but broader view which may well miss much of the interesting detail. Clarity will only be achieved by application of as many techniques as possible to homogeneous groups of patients and the recognition that the fine tuning of responses to individual antigens will depend on the activity of both antigen-specific suppressor cells and idiotype/anti-idiotype interactions as envisaged by Jerne (1974).

REFERENCES

Alexander GJM, Nouri-Aria KT, Eddleston ALWF, Williams R. (1983) Contrasting relations between suppressor-cell function and suppressor-cell number in chronic liver disease. Lancet i : 1291
Barnaba V, Levrero M, Musca A, Balsano F (1983). Suppressor cell function in chronic liver disease. Lancet ii :342.
Dudley FJ, Fox RA, Sherlock S (1972). Cellular immunity and hepatitis-associated Australia antigen liver disease. Lancet i :723
Dwyer J, Johnson C (1981). The use of Con A to study the immunoregulation of human T cells. Clin. Exp. Immunol. 46 : 237
Eddleston ALWF, Williams R. (1974). Inadequate antibody response to HBAg or suppressor T-cell defect in development of active chronic hepatitis. Lancet ii : 1543.
Eddleston ALWF, Nouri K, Hegarty J, Alexander G, Neuberger J, Williams R. (1982) Immunological responses in liver disease. In Arias IM, Frenkel M, Wilson JHP. (eds.): "The Liver Annual 2", Amsterdam-Oxford-Princeton: Excerpta Medica, p.154.

Edgington TS, Chisari FV (1975) Immunological aspects of
    hepatitis B virus infection. Amer. J. Med. Sci. 270 : 213
Jerne N. (1974) The genetics of immunoglobulins and the
    immune response. Pasteur Institut Symposium CNRS
Mondelli M, Mieli-Vergani G, Alberti A et al. (1982)
    Specificity of T-lymphocyte cytotoxicity to autologous
    hepatocytes in chronic hepatitis B virus infection:
    evidence that T-cells are directed against HBV core
    antigen expressed on hepatocytes. J. Immunol. 129 : 2273
Nouri-Aria KT, Hegarty JE, Alexander GJM, Eddleston ALWF,
    Williams R. (1982) Effect of corticosteroids on suppressor
    cell activity in autoimmune and viral chronic active
    hepatitis. N. Eng. J. Med. 307 : 1310
Pernis B, Vogel HJ (1980) (eds.) "Regulatory T Lymphocytes",
    New York: Academic Press.

Tremolada F, Fattovich G, Panebianco G, Ongaro G, Realdi G.
    (1980) Suppressor cell activity in viral and non-viral
    chronic active hepatitis. Clin. Exp. Immunol. 40 : 89

AUTOLOGOUS HEPATOCYTES IN HEPATITIS B VIRUS (HBV) RELATED
LIVER DISEASE: A PROBLEM OF LIVER CELL CULTURE

Giovanni C. Actis, M.D., Giovanni A. Touscoz, PhD.,
Giorgio Saracco, M.D.
Division of Gastroenterology, Ospedale Molinette
C. Bramante 88, Turin 10126, ITALY

The knowledge of the mechanisms of hepatocyte necrosis
following HBV infection of the humans is fragmentary. Although most patients with HBsAg positive liver disease show
signs of ongoing virus replication, clinical evidence suggests that HBV may not be directly cytopathic, since millions
of HBsAg carriers do exist with a normal liver in the face
of an unchecked virus replication (Levy and Chisari 1981).

The immunological hypothesis put forward by Eddleston
and Williams (1974) has guided research on the field in
the last ten years; according to this proposal, during the
replicative cycle in the hepatocytes HBV induces neoantigens
on the cell membrane, thus creating the conditions for the
rise of an immune attack to the altered cells with the
scope of eliminating the reservoir of virus multiplication;
destruction is likely to be effected by clones of cytotoxic
T cells bearing a receptor for the viral antigen(s) and
for the HLA gene products of the host cells, according to
the theory of the H2 or HLA restriction of T cell cytolysis
of virus-modified cells proposed by Zinkernagel and
Doherty (1974).

In the absence of means of propagating HBV in culture
and of a suitable animal model, attempts were made to
reproduce in-vitro the cytolytic mechanism by separating
different clones of effector lymphocytes from the peripheral blood of the HBsAg carriers to measure their capacity
to lyse in-vitro artificial targets (Alberti et al. 1977)

or cells derived from a human hepatoma line bearing the
integrated HBV genome (Chin et al. 1983). A major alternative
was introduced when isolated human hepatocytes from liver
biopsy were cultured in plastic trays with the corresponding
peripheral blood lymphocytes (Mieli-Vergani et al. 1979;
Eddleston et al. 1982; Mieli-Vergani et al. 1982); the
advantage is that autologous targets are provided for the
blood effectors so that if T cells are to be detected in the
system, the requirement of an histocompatible target is met.

This system entails the attachment of target hepatocytes
to a plastic surface, followed by the incubation with the
blood effectors over two days; the final result of cytotoxicity is read morphologically as number of hepatocytes that
had lost their adherence to the surface of culture because
of lymphocyte-induced damage.

A program was developed in our laboratory aiming at
establishing a reproducible technique for the isolation and
culture of human adult hepatocytes from liver specimens of
different size; collateral to this program was the study of
the specificity and clinical value of the test with regard
to the viability and membrane characteristics of the target
hepatocytes. The data have suggested that alterations of
hepatocyte viability due to pre-existing liver disease or
treatment used to isolate the cells, may profoundly influence
the attainment of specificity with this test (Actis et al.
1983). We report here the results of a group of representative
experiments obtained with the morphologic cytotoxicity system applied to HBsAg positive liver disease.

Details of the technique are reported elsewhere (Actis
et al. 1983). For this study, the liver fragments were subjected to a 4 h incubation with 0.003% SIGMA collagenase
type IV dissolved in pure fetal calf serum.Recovered hepatocytes were washed and deprived of Kupffer cells by three
spins at low speed and seeded in the wells of the Terasaki
tray in number 100-150/10 microliter well. RPMI 1640 or
MEM medium with 10% serum was used as culture medium. In
all cases, hepatocyte viability and yield were recorded;

in some, electron micrographs were also obtained.

Lymphocytes were obtained from heparinized venous blood after sedimentation in Dextran, purification on plastic petri dishes, and final spin on a cushion of Ficoll-Hypaque. In seven experiments, (five culturing autologous patients' hepatocytes and lymphocytes, and two culturing diseased hepatocytes with lymphocytes from normal donors) normal effectors were used in parallel with lymphocytes pre-treated for 45 minutes with 1.2 micrograms/10^6 cells of Actinomycin D.

In all experiments, the test was carried out at a ratio of 400 effectors to one target hepatocyte. In the Terasaki tray, at least ten wells were filled with medium containing hepatocytes alone (controls). In test rows, hepatocytes and lymphocytes were cultured for 48 hrs.; the test was terminated by inverting the plate and washing the detached cells away.

Remaining hepatocytes were fixed, stained and counted under an inverted microscope according to the formula:

$$\frac{\text{hepatocytes in control wells} - \text{hepatocytes in test wells}}{\text{hepatocytes in control wells}} \times 100$$

Six HBsAg positive patients and six controls were studied. Control hepatocytes and lymphocytes were obtained from a patient undergoing liver biopsy for staging of a systemic disease; alternatively, we performed homologous tests by culturing normal donor lymphocytes with normal hepatocytes from the liver of a cholecystectomy patient.

Invariably, the hepatocytes from all preparations showed different degrees of damage, confirming that human hepatocytes recovered after collagenase treatment of liver fragments are particularly "fragile" (Edgington and Mackay 1981). Damage varied from gross alteration of cell shape with frank inclusion of trypan blue, to a pale staining of the nucleus, visible by focusing through the cytoplasm. At the electron microscope, these cells showed membrane erosions and blurring of the cytoplasm. Interestingly, preparations where treatment with uranyl acetate (dissolving glycogen) was avoided, presented nevertheless a complete disappearance of glycogen stores, indicating that, apart from the gross alterations, these cells may show very fine ultrastructural alterations. In table 1 we report in detail the yields and the viabilities of the hepatocytes obtained in the eight separate experiments included in the study.

Table 1. Hepatocyte yields and viabilities in relation to the histological pictures of eight liver biopsies processed for hepatocyte isolation with collagenase.

BIOPSY	HISTOLOGY	CELL YIELD	VIABILITY
1	CLH	1.32	NUCLEAR INCLUSION
2	CPH	0.25	GROSS INCLUSION
3	CPH	0.55	GROSS INCLUSION
4	AC	0.25	NUCLEAR INCLUSION
5	CAH	0.62	NUCLEAR INCLUSION
6	C	0.65	GROSS INCLUSION
7	CPH	0.65	GROSS INCLUSION
8	NL	1.70	NUCLEAR INCLUSION

AC=active cirrhosis; CAH=chronic active hepatitis; CPH= chronic persistent hepatitis; CLH=chronic lobular hepatitis; C=cirrhosis; NL=normal liver. Cell yields are given as number $x10^5$; cell viability was determined by the trypan blue dye exclusion test. The terms "nuclear inclusion and gross inclusion" mean an arbitrary distinction between preparations with an obvious cytoplasmic inclusion, and those where an apparently preserved cell body allowed to focus a stained nucleus. While this microscopic appearance may reflect different degrees of damage, strictly speaking all preparations must be considered as bearing membrane damage enough to allow inclusion of the dye.

Our data confirm that small liver fragments such as those obtained in clinical practice do not usually yield enough hepatocytes to be labeled in a conventional chromium release assay, whilst viabilities assessed by trypan blue exclusion are extremely poor. The best yield was obtained

with the control biopsy, suggesting that the biological damage due to the original liver disease may worsen the ultimate result of the technique. Evaluation of the behavior
of these hepatocytes cultured with the autologous lymphocytes
in the cytotoxicity system showed that HBsAg carriers with
liver disease display a mean cytotoxic index (61.75+18)
twice that of the controls (31+14); cytotoxicity, however,
did not show an obvious cause-effect relationship with the
severity of the liver damage, as of two HBsAg carriers,
one was highly cytotoxic, the other was not cytotoxic at
all (Fig.1).

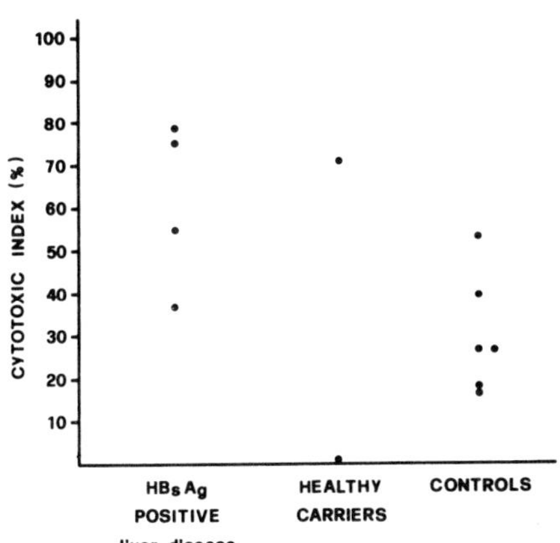

Fig.1 Results of the cytotoxicity assay using peripheral
blood lymphocytes as attackers for the autologous hepatocytes in the three groups of subjects studied.

The demonstration that a leaky hepatocyte membrane
invariably follows collagenase treatment of human liver
biopsies raises the question whether a true lethal hit has
to be released by the effectors for detachment of the hepatocytes to occur, or the system represents simply a trivial
autolytic process where dying hepatocytes are killed by their

own lysosomal bags. To answer this point, experiments were
run in parallel using as effectors normal lymphocytes and
lymphocytes whose protein synthesis was blocked by Actinomycin D. The results (Fig. 2) have shown that a metabolical-
ly active effector is required to release the lethal signal:
whether the specific function inhibited by Actinomycin D is
the formation of effector-target conjugates (Brondz et al.
1973) or the release of a soluble lymphotoxin (Wright and
Bonavida 1983) remains to be elucidated.

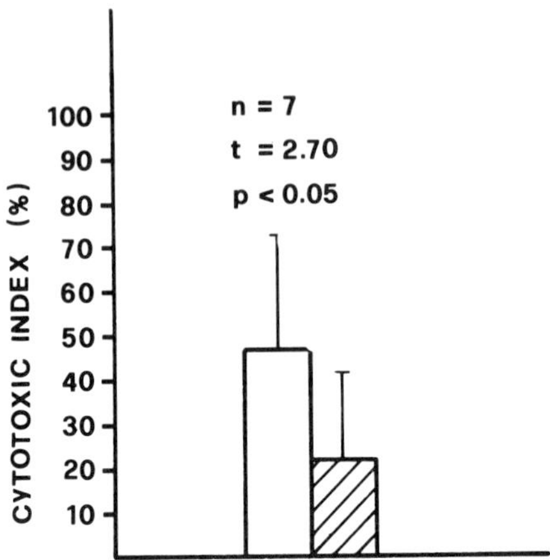

Fig.2 Effect on the cytotoxicity (seven experiments) of
the treatment with Actinomycin D of the effector lymphocytes.
The open histogram indicates control results; the dashed
histogram means the results obtained with the same lymphocyte
samples after treatment with Actinomycin D: effectors with
a blocked protein synthesis are significantly less cytotoxic
in this assay.

The morphologic microcytotoxicity assay represents to
date the best test available to mimick in-vitro the immune
situation of human HBV related liver disease, for it allows
to culture human autologous hepatocytes freshly isolated from

the liver biopsies with the corresponding peripheral blood
effectors. Correctness of design, however, is obscured by
the limits inherent in the procedures of digestion of liver
cores currently available that do not yield autologous hepatocytes with a controlled viability. Since this test measures cytotoxicity as a function of target cell adhesiveness,
membrane integrity seems a logical requirement for specificity: therefore, specificity of this test turns out to be a
problem of liver cell culture. The finding that Actinomycin
D-blocked effectors are no longer active, indicates that,
despite the present inadequacy of the target cells, the
test can still detect the presence of an effector amongst
the cultured lymphocyte population whose release of a lethal
hit causes the detachment of the target hepatocytes. The
culture of intact targets could make it emerge as a distinct
immune recognition event.

Acknowledgments. We wish to thank Dr Santo Landolfo of the
    Microbiology Institute at Turin University for providing
    the Actinomycin D. G.C. Actis is grateful to Dr F. Gilli
    for assistance in the preparation of the manuscript.

REFERENCES

Actis GC, Touscoz GA, Verme G, Poli G (1983). Obtaining
  isolated viable hepatocytes for the study of cell-mediated
  cytotoxicity in chronic liver disease of humans. IRCS
  Medical Science 11:161.
Alberti A, Realdi G, Bortolotti F, Rigoli AM (1977).
  T-lymphocyte cytotoxicity to HBsAg coated target cells
  in hepatitis B virus infection. Gut 18:1004.
Brondz BD, Snegiröva AE, Rassulin YA, Shamborant OG (1973).
  Modification of in-vitro immune lymphocyte-target interactions by some biologically active drugs. Immunochemistry
  10:175.
Chin TW, Hollinger BF, Rich RR, Troisi CL, Dreesman GR,
  Melnick JL (1983). Cytotoxicity by NK-like cells from
  hepatitis B immune patients to a human hepatoma cell line
  secreting HBsAg. J Immunol 130:173.

Eddleston ALWF, Williams R (1974). Inadequate antibody response to HBsAg or suppressor T-cell defect in development of active chronic hepatitis. Lancet 2:1543.

Eddleston ALWF, Mondelli M, Mieli-Vergani G, Williams R (1982). Lymphocyte cytotoxicity to autologous hepatocytes in chronic hepatitis B virus infection. Hepatology 2:122S.

Edgington TS, Mackay IR (1981). Issues in immunologically mediated hepatic injury. Med J Aust 2:606.

Levy GA, Chisari FV (1981). The immunopathogenesis of chronic HBV-induced liver disease. Springer Semin. Immunopathol. 3:439.

Mieli-Vergani G, Vergani D, Jenkins PJ, Portmann B, Mowat AP, Eddleston ALWF, Williams R (1979). Lymphocyte cytotoxicity to autologous hepatocytes in HBsAg-negative chronic active hepatitis. Clin Exp Immunol 38:16.

Mieli-Vergani G, Vergani D, Portmann B, White I, Murray-Lyon I, Marigold JH, Woolf I, Eddleston ALWF, Williams R(1982). Lymphocyte cytotoxicity to autologous hepatocytes in HBsAg positive chronic liver disease. Gut 23:1029.

Wright SC, Bonavida B (1983). YAC-1 variant clones selected for resistance to natural killer cell cytotoxic factors are also resistant to natural killer cell-mediated cytotoxicity. Proc Natl Acad Sci 80:1688.

Zinkernagel RM, Doherty PC (1974). Restriction of in-vitro T-cell mediated cytoxicity in lymphocyte choriomeningitis within a syngeneic or semiallogeneic system. Nature 248:701.

Viral Hepatitis and Delta Infection, pages 317–326
© 1983 Alan R. Liss, Inc., 150 Fifth Avenue, New York, NY 10011

PATHOMORPHOLOGY OF THE FORMATION AND DEPOSITION OF HBV
RELATED IMMUNE COMPLEXES

Krzysztof Krawczynski, M.D.

Department of Immunopathology, National
Institute of Hygiene, Warszawa, Poland

Replication, synthesis and release from hepatocytes
of hepatitis B virus (HBV) and its antigenic components
(HBsAg, HBcAg, HBeAg) induce both cellular and humoral
immune response. These antigens initiate synthesis of
antiviral antibodies of anti-HBs, anti-HBc, and anti-HBe
specificity which are detected in serum in various
stages of the infection. It may be assumed that
anti-HBc occurrence in serum reflects the rate of
humoral response in HBV infection, since free HBcAg is
not released into the circulation. The antiviral
antibodies activity has been found in IgM or IgG class
of immunoglobulins and revealed variable affinity. The
biology of the synthesis of HBV and its antigens leads
to the presence of HBsAg and HBeAg in the circulation.
Their subsequent disappearance may have characteristics
of immunologic clearance. Subsequently, HBsAg/anti-HBs
and HBeAg/anti-HBe immune complexes may be present in
the circulation, removed by the reticuloendothelial
system or deposited in tissue.

Several assays have been devised and applied to
determine the presence of immune complexes in serum.
Anticomplementary activity of hepatitis sera was
observed more than a decade ago (Gitnick et al. 1973).
Subsequently, the Raji cell test, polyethylene glycol
precipitation test, and Clq binding in fluid and solid
phase were applied for identification of immune
complexes in both acute and chronic hepatitis B (Fye et
al. 1977; Abrass et al. 1980). Immune complexes were
also investigated by ultracentrifugation and electron

microscopic examination of the serum pellets including
the use of labeled antibodies for specific
identification of HBV antigens (Almeida, Waterson 1969;
Stannard et al. 1982). Several reports on the
coexistence of HBsAg and anti-HBs in the same serum
samples (Lander et al. 1971; Trepo et al. 1976; Stannard
et al. 1982) suggested that anti-HBs was probably
directed against the subtype different from coexisting
HBsAg. It seems equally conceivable, however, that
anti-HBs of low affinity could dissociate from immune
complexes being detected by highly sensitive assays. A
search for HBV immune complexes was also carried out in
cryoprecipitated from sera of hepatitis B patients both
with acute and chronic liver disease; cryoprecipitins
were found in 77% and 46% of those patients,
respectively (Gocke, McIntosh 1973). HBsAg and anti-HBs
were found in significantly higher concentrations in
cryoprecipitates than in serum and, therefore, were
considered to be components of immune complexes. The
finding of HB antigens in cases of essential mixed
cryoglobulinemia prompted some authors to suggest that
the disease is etiologically linked to HBV infection
(Realdi et al. 1974; Levo et al. 1977).

Pathogenic potential of circulating HBV related
immune complexes plays a role in the extrahepatic
manifestations of the infection. In cases of acute
viral hepatitis a serum sickness-like syndrome is
observed in a proportion of patients. Transient skin
rash and urticaria, arthritis and arthralgia, are
observed in 10 to 20% of patients (Wands et al. 1975;
Schumacher, Gall 1974; Dienstag et al. 1978). The skin
and articular manifestations occur days, sometime weeks,
before the onset of juandice. In serum, HBsAg immune
complexes have been demonstrated, frequently in
cryoprecipitable proteins. HBsAg, immunoglobulins, and
complement deposits were found in synovium and cutaneous
vessel walls. In the skin, morphologic lesions in blood
vessels were compatible with those of necrotizing
venulitis.

It has been generally accepted that circulating
immune complexes do not contribute to parenchymal
lesions in the liver. It has been repeatedly found in
experimental conditions that sinusoidal cells of the
liver remove most of the circulating complexes. In HBV

infection in chimpanzees, nodular lymphoid infiltrations
were observed in portal spaces during the immune
elimination of HBsAg (Krawczynski, unpublished).
Germinal center-like structures in these infiltrations
contained a homogenous mixture of HBsAg,
immunoglobulins, and complement. In the same liver
biopsies, HBsAg was identified in several Kupffer cells.
Similar lymphoid structures have been observed in the
liver tracts of patients with primary biliary cirrhosis
while a number of patients with the disease were shown
to be positive for the presence of immune complexes in
the circulation (Gupta et al. 1978; Wands et al. 1978).

The pathogenic significance of intrahepatic, i.e.
in situ, formation of HBV related immune complexes is
controversial. In hepatocyte nuclei, HBcAg and/or delta
antigen, and immunoglobulins were observed and found to
fix complement in vitro in several cases of chronic
hepatitis B. Formation of these intranuclear immune
complexes remains unclear, especially as the plasma
membranes of viable cells have been considered to be
impermeable to proteins. The hepatocytes containing
immune complexes in the nuclei do not reveal any
evidence of cytolysis or characteristic degeneration.
Although earlier publications suggested pathogenic
significance of intranuclear immune deposits in the
liver (Gerber et al. 1976), a recent study revealed the
intranuclear presence of HBcAg and delta antigen immune
complexes in healthy HBV carriers with a conclusion that
the occurrence of these immune deposits was an
epiphenomenon without pathogenic significance (Rizzetto
et al. 1981). Equally doubtful is the pathogenic role
of HBV antigens located on the surface of hepatocytes.
HBsAg at this location was thought to be a target for
the cell mediated attack (Ray et al. 1976). Further
studies revealed that peripheral localization of the
antigen in the liver cells is not correlated with the
intensity of hepatocellular damage and progression of
liver lesions (Nazarewicz-de Mezer et al. 1980).
Recently, HBcAg demonstrated on the surface of isolated
liver cells was suggested to be a target for the cell
mediated immunity with anti-HBc modulating the course of
illness by masking the target antigen (Realdi et al.
1982). If HBsAg and/or HBcAg are present on the surface
of hepatocytes in vivo, formation of immune complexes on
the liver cells seems inevitable with a subsequent

mediation of the antibody dependent cellular
cytotoxicity (ADCC) (Hopf et al. 1975). This mechanism
could act as a back-up system for T cell killing when
antibody production would otherwise leads to protection
of the target from T cells through blocking of the
surface antigens. However, the number and distribution
of K cells in liver biopsies (Eggink et al. 1982)
responsible for the antibody dependent target cell
killing in vitro does not support the idea of the ADCC
mechanism operating in vivo in cases of chronic liver
disease related to HBV infection. Finally, it has been
suggested that local antigen-antibody reaction in the
liver may lead to massive hepatocytolysis in fulminant
hepatitis related to HBV infection. In a series of
autopsy cases, HBsAg, immunoglobulins, and complement
were found in remnants of necrotic liver cells. HBsAg
immune deposits were also located in germinal centers of
several lymph nodes, kidney glomeruli, and blood vessels
in the majority of these cases (Nowoslawski et al.
1975). Two independent serologic studies demonstrated
anti-HBs in 40% of patients with fulminant hepatitis
(Trepo et al. 1976; Woolf et al. 1976). Electron
microscopic investigations of pellets from serum of a
case of fulminant hepatitis revealed presence of large
HBsAg immune complexes characteristic for antibody
excess (Almeida, Waterson 1969). However, fatal
hepatitis with clinical characteristics of fulminant
hepatitis was observed in a patient with
agammaglobulinemia, although etiologic diagnosis of the
case remains unknown (Good, Page 1960). Taken together,
the immunomorphologic and serologic observations in
fulminant hepatitis should be significantly extended to
establish whether HBsAg related immune complexes formed
in the liver play the central role in the pathogenesis
of massive liver cell necrosis or the presence of HBsAg
immunoglobulin, and complement in necrotic liver cells
is an epiphenomenon without pathogenic significance.

Persistant HBV infection results in a continued
release of viral antigens into the circulation, thus
providing an ideal setting for the development of immune
complex mediated glomerulonephritis. Series of cases of
membranous type of glomerulonephritis were studied in
Poland, Japan, and France and found to be linked with
HBV infection (Brzosko et al. 1974; Takekoshi et al.
1978; Kleinknecht et al. 1979; Slusarczyk et al. 1980).

This association seems to have pathogenic significance since both HBsAg and HBeAg were found in glomeruli in a mixture with immunoglobulins and complement. In cases of membranous glomerulonephritis, nodular deposits of these immune complexes were identified by immunofluorescence and electron microscopy in the subepithelial surface of glomerular basement membrane (Slusarczyk et al. 1980; Ito et al. 1981). The recent studies (Collins et al. 1983) confirmed the presence of HBsAg and HBeAg in kidney glomeruli using monoclonal antibodies and were in agreement with earlier report of anti-HBs located in glomeruli and revealed by differential elution dissociating immune complexes (Ozawa et al. 1976). As in experimental models of glomerulonephritis, the deposition of HBV related immune complexes may depend on their size, net charge, antigen/antibody ratio, and affinity of antibodies. HBeAg/anti-HBe immune complexes of smaller sizes tend to localize in the subepithelial part of glomerular basement membrane. The large size of HBsAg immune complexes makes their localization difficult to explain, unless it is accepted that incomplete particles or nonparticulate antigen can be deposited in kidney glomeruli. Besides deposition from the circulation, immune complexes may be formed in glomeruli, i.e. in situ, with HBV antigens primarily planted in glomeruli (Levy, Kleinknecht 1980). This mechanism has been gaining increasing acceptance as proved to operate in various experimental systems (Hoedmaeker et al. 1982). It is also possible that HBsAg and HBeAg are trapped secondarily in kidneys in immune complexes of different specificities (Levy, Kleinknecht 1980).

The association of persistent HBV infection and polyarteritis nodosa appeared from serologic studies (Treop et al. 1974; Sergent et al. 1976). HBsAg, anti-HBs, or both were detected with incidence varying from 31 to 69%. The first morphologic report which showed HBV immune deposits in the vessel walls of a single case was followed by a study of autopsy material obtained from a substantial group of polyarteritis nodosa cases (Gocke et al. 1970; Krawczynski et al. 1973; Michalak 1978). HBsAg immune deposits were identified in recent fibrinoid lesions in small arteries and arterioles. Healed, fibrotic lesions contained lesser amount or were devoid of these complexes. It

should not be concluded, however, from the demonstration
of circulating immune complexes of HBsAg/anti-HBs and
their presence in the damaged vessel walls that this is
the only or even major antigen-antibody system
contributing to the morphogenesis of vascular lesions.
This might be similar to membranous glomerulonephritis
in which HBs antigenemia is accompanied by
HBeAg/anti-HBe deposition in kidney glomeruli. Several
factors determining pathogenicity of circulating immune
complexes including the integrity and permeability of
blood vessel walls should be considered as only a small
proportion of patients with circulating HBV related
immune complexes develop polyarteritis nodosa.

In conclusion, although there is a coincidence of
HBV infection with clinico-morphologic syndrome related
to immune complex formation and deposition, it is
difficult to conclude which hepatic or extrahepatic
lesions are pathogenically related to HBV antigen(s)
immune complexes and which constitute an epiphenomenon
without pathogenetic significance. Among extrahepatic
features of HBV infection, membranous glomerulonephritis
in children and polyarteritis nodosa provide the
strongest evidence for the existence of the pathogenetic
relationship. It also seems conceivable that HBV
related immune complexes are formed in the liver, on the
surface of the target cells, although their pathogenic
relationship to the liver cell necrosis remains
incertain.

REFERENCES

Abrass CK, Border WA, Hepner G (1980). Non-specificity
  of circulating immune complexes in patients with acute
  and chronic liver disease. Clin exp Immunol 40:292.
Almeida JD, Waterson AP (1969). Immune complexes in
  hepatitis. Lancet 2:983.
Brzosko WJ, Krawczynski K, Nazarewicz T, Morzycka M,
  Nowoslawski A (1974). Glomerulonephritis associated
  with hepatitis B surface antigen immune complexes in
  children. Lancet 2:478.
Collins AB, Bhan AK, Dienstag JL, Colvin RB, Haupert GT,
  Mushahwar IK, McCluskey RT (1983). Hepatitis B immune
  complex glomerulonephritis: Simultaneous glomerular
  deposition of hepatitis B surface and e antigens.

Clin Immunol Immunopathol 26:137.

Dienstag JL, Rhodes AR, Bhan AK, Dvorak AM, Mihm MC, Wands JR (1978). Urticaria associated with acute viral hepatitis type B: Studies of pathogenesis. Ann Intern Med 89:34.

Eggink HF, Houthoff HJ, Huitema S, Gips CH, Poppema S (1982). Cellular and humoral immune reactions in chronic active liver disease. I. Lymphocyte subsets in liver biopsies of patients with untreated idiopathic autoimmune hepatitis, chronic active hepatitis B and primary biliary cirrhosis. Clin exp Immunol 50:17.

Fye KH, Becker MJ, Theofilopoulos AN, Moutsopoulos H, Feldman JL, Talal N (1977). Immune complexes in hepatitis B antigen associated periarteritis nodosa. Detection by antibody dependent cell mediated cytotoxicity and the Raji cell assay. Am J Med 62:783.

Gerber MA, Sarno E, Vernace SJ (1976). Immune complexes in hepatocytic nuclei of HB Ag-positive chronic hepatitis. N Engl J Med 294:922.

Gitnick GL, Summerskill WHJ, Soloway RD, Ritman S, Schoenfield LJ (1973). Anticomplementary hepatitis B antigen. Prognostic importance in chronic active liver disease. Arch Intern Med 132:502.

Gocke DJ, Hsu K, Morgan C, Bombardieri S, Lockshin M, Christian CL (1970). Association between polyarteritis and Australia antigen. Lancet 2:1149.

Gocke DJ, McIntosh RM (1973). Cryoprecipitates containing hepatitis B antigen in patients with liver disease. Gastroenterology 65:542.

Good RA, Page AR (1960). Fatal complications of virus hepatitis in two patients with agammaglobulinemia. Am J Med 29:804.

Gupta RC, Dickson ER, McDuffie FC, Baggenstoss AH (1978). Circulating IgG complexes in primary biliary cirrhosis: A serial study in 40 patients followed for 2 years. Clin exp Immunol 34:19.

Hoedmaeker PJ, Fleuren GJ, Weening JJ (1982). In situ formation of glomerular immune aggregates. Transplant Proc 14:469.

Hopt U, Arnold W, Meyer zum Bushchenfelde KH, Forster E, Bolte JP (1975). Studies on the pathogenesis of chronic inflammatory liver disease. I.Membrane-fixed IgG on isolated hepatocytes from patients. Clin exp Immunol 22:1.

Ito H, Hattori S, Matusda I, Amamiya S, Hajikano H, Yoshizawa H, Miyakawa Y, Mayumi M (1981). Hepatitis B e antigen-mediated membranous glomerulonephritis. Correlation of ultrastructural changes with HBeAg in the serum and glomeruli. Lab Invest 44:214.

Kleinknecht C, Levy M, Peix A, Broyer M, Courtecuisse V (1979). Membranous glomerulonephritis and hepatitis B surface antigen in children. J Pediat 95:946.

Krawczynski K, Slusarczyk J, Brzosko WJ, Nowoslawski A (1974). Viral antigen-antibody complexes and the pathogenesis of degenerative vascular lesions. Adv Biosci 12:435.

Lander JJ, Giles JP, Purcell RH, Krugman S (1971). Viral hepatitis, type B (MS-2 strain): Detection of antibody after primary infection. N Engl J Med 285-303.

Levo Y, Gorevic PD, Kassab HJ, Zucker-Franklin D, Franklin EC (1977). Association between hepatits B virus and essential mixed cryoglobulinemia. N Engl J Med 296:1501.

Levy M, Kleinknecht C (1980). Membranous glomerulonephritis and hepatitis B virus infection. Nephron 26:259.

Michalak T (1978). Immune complexes of hepatitis B surface antigen in the pathogenesis of periarteritis nodosa. Am J Pathol 90:15.

Nazarewicz-de Mezer T, Krawczynski K, Michalak T, Nowoslawski A (1980). Intracellular localization of HB antigens in liver tissue. In Bianchi L, Gerok W, Sickinger K, Stalder G (eds): "Virus and the liver", Falk Symposium 28, Lancaster, MTP Press Limited, p.85.

Nowoslawski A, Krawczynski K, Nazarewicz T, Slusarczyk J (1975). Immunological aspects of hepatitis type B. Am J Med Sci 270:229.

Ozawa T, Levisohn P, Orsini E, McIntosh RM (1976). Acute immune complex disease associated with hepatitis. Arch Pathol Lab Med 100:484.

Ray MB, Desmet VJ, Bradburne AF, Desmyter J, Fevery J, de Groote J (1976). Differential distribution of hepatitis B surface antigen and hepatitis B core antigen in the liver of hepatitis B patients. Gastroenterology 71:462.

Realdi G, Alberti A, Rigoli A, Tremolada F (1974). Immune complexes and Australia antigen in cryoglobulinemic sera. Z Immunitaetsforsch 147:114.

Realdi G, Trevisan A, Alberti A, Noventa F (1982).

Heterogeneity of antigenic expression at the liver
cell surface in hepatitis B virus infection. Liver
2:279.

Rizzetto M, Canese MG, Purcell RH, London WT, Sly LD,
Gerin JL (1981). Experimental HBV and delta
infections of chimpanzees: Occurence and significance
of intrahepatic immune complexes of HBcAg and delta
antigen. Hepatology 1:567.

Schumacher HR, Gall EP (1974). Arthritis in acute
hepatitis and chronic active hepatitis. Am J Med
57:655.

Sergent JS, Lockshin MD, Christian CL, Gocke DJ (1976).
Vasculitis with hepatitis B antigenemia. Medicine
55:1.

Slusarczyk J, Michalak T, Nazarewicz-de Mezer T,
Krawczynski K, Nowoslawski A (1980). Membranous
glomerulopathy associated with hepatitis B core
antigen immune complexes in children. Am J Pathol
98:29.

Stannard ML, Lennon M, Hodgkiss M, Smuts H (1982). An
electron microscopic demonstration of immune complexes
of hepatitis B e-antigen using colloidal gold as a
marker. J Med Virol 9:165.

Takekoshi Y, Tanaka M, Shida N, Satake Y, Saheki Y,
Matsumoto S (1978). Strong association between
membranous nephropathy and hepatitis B surface
antigenaemia in Japanese children. Lancet 2:1065.

Trepo CG, Zuckerman AJ, Bird RC, Prince AM (1974). The
role of circulating hepatitis B antigen/antibody
immune complexes in the pathogenesis of vascular and
hepatic manifestations in polyarteritis nodosa. J
Clin Path 27:863.

Trepo CG, Robert D, Motin J, Sepetjian M, Prince AM
(1976). Hepatitis B antigen (HBsAg) and/or antibodies
(anti-HBs and anti-HBc)in fulminant hepatitis:
Pathogenic and prognostic significance. Gut 17:10.

Wands JR, Mann E, Alpert E, Isselbacher KJ (1975). The
pathogenesis of arthritis associated with acute
hepatitis B surface antigen-positive hepatitis:
Complement activation and characterization of
circulating immune complexes. J Clin Invest 55:930.

Wands JR, Dienstag JL, Bhan AK, Feller ER, Isselbacher
KJ (1978). Circulating immune complexes and
complement activation in primary biliary cirrhosis. N
Engl J Med 298:233.

Woolf IL, el Sheikh N, Cullens H, Lee WM, Eddleston

ALWF, Williams R, Zuckerman AJ (1976). Enhanced HBsAb
production in pathogenesis of fulminant viral
hepatitis type B. Brit Med J 2:669.

Viral Hepatitis and Delta Infection, pages 327–336

VIRUS RECEPTORS FOR POLYMERIZED HUMAN SERUM ALBUMIN AND ANTI-
RECEPTOR ANTIBODY IN HEPATITIS B VIRUS INFECTION

A. Alberti, P. Pontisso, L. Chemello, E. Schiavon
and G. Realdi
Istituto di Medicina Clinica, Patologia Medica I°
Università di Padova,
Padova (Italy)

INTRODUCTION

The existence in hepatitis B surface antigen (HBsAg) positive sera of factors that react with polymerized human serum albumin (pHSA) has been known since 1972 (Matuhasi, Hosoka-
wa 1972) and was initially explained as related to the presence of autoantibodies to denatured HSA (Lenkei et al. 1974).
Indeed there is evidence that antibodies to altered or denatured albumin may develop during the course of acute and chronic liver disease, independently of an ethiologic relation to
hepatitis B virus infection (Lenkei et al. 1977). These antibodies have been found to be directed against species-nonspe-
cific antigenic determinants, related to pyridinium rings that
are formed in albumins of different species as the result of
cross-linking reactions (Onica et al. 1981). Although these
anti-albumin antibodies may develop in the course of hepatitis B, several studies have more recently indicated that they
probably do not represent the major reactants responsible for
serum pHSA binding. These concepts have emerged in 1979 when
Imai et al. have identified on HBV particles a species-specific receptor for polymerized human and chimpanzee albumin. In
these studies evidence was provided indicating that the virus
receptor for pHSA was protein in nature and was distinct from
antibodies. The observation of the species-restriction of the
receptor, toghether with evidence that liver cells bear similar albumin binding sites on their surface membrane (Lenkei
et al. 1977) have led Imai and his coworkers to propose a new
provocative hypothesis. They suggested that the pHSA receptor
could mediate the attachment of the virion to hepatocytes,via
a pHSA bridge, thus explaining the hepatotropism of the virus

and why only humans and chimpanzees are susceptible to HBV infection. Imai et al. also speculated that, on the basis of their hypothesis, an antibody directed against the pHSA receptor on virus particles could be highly effective in virus neutralization.

Several Authors have confirmed the existence of the species-specific receptor for pHSA on HBV particles, as well as its distinction from anti-pHSA antibodies (Tung, Gerber 1981) and its correlation with the presence of HBeAg in serum (Neurath, Strick 1979; Hansson, Purcell 1979).

We have recently investigated serum binding activity for pHSA in acute and chronic HBV infection and will review here the results obtained on three main aspects, including 1) the behaviour of the pHSA receptor in acute and chronic HBV infection in relation to virus replication activity; 2) the expression of the pHSA receptor on different hepatitis B associated viral particles, such as Dane particles and HBsAg particles; 3) the relationship between the pHSA receptor and the antibody precipitating Dane particles, described by us in 1978 in acute hepatitis B sera (Alberti et al. 1978). This antibody, termed at that time anti-Dane particle (anti-DP) antibody, has been recently proved directed against the pHSA receptor on virus particles (Alberti et al. 1983).

VIRUS RECEPTOR FOR pHSA IN ACUTE HEPATITIS TYPE B

The virus receptor for pHSA was measured in HBsAg positive sera by solid phase RIA, according to Hansson and Purcell (1979), with few modifications(Pontisso et al. 1983). Briefly, 30 mg of essentially globulin-free human serum albumin (HSA) (Sigma) were dissolved in phosphate buffer pH 8.6 and reacted with glutaraldehyde for 2 hours. After dialysis, the solution was chromatographed on Sepharose G-200 and the leading protein peak was pooled and adjusted to 5 mg/ml. Polyvynil microplates were coated with pHSA in carbonate buffer pH 8.6, washed with PBS containing 0.05% Tween 20 (PBS/Tween) and incubated again with 10% fetal calf serum. After 5 washings with PBS/Tween, plate wells were filled with 50 μl of serum (diluted 1:50 or more with FCS), and incubated overnight at 37°C. Plates were then washed with PBS/Tween before the addition of 50 μl of ^{125}I-anti-HBs at 37°C for 4 hours. After the final washings, each well was cut apart with scissors and counted in a gamma counter. Control plates, coated with polymerized

bovine albumin, were set up to assess the species-specificity
of the receptor activity. 50 HBsAg sera from healthy subjects
were used to define the upper limit of the negative range of
the assay, taken at 2 standard deviations above the mean.

Serial serum samples, obtained from 31 patients with a-
cute hepatitis type B, were tested in the pHSA receptor assay. Most patients were positive for the receptor at clinical onset, at the time of HBeAg and HBV-DNApolymerase positivity in serum. Receptor levels then rapidly decreased during
the HBeAg positive phase and were significantly reduced at
the time of anti-HBe seroconversion (figure 1).

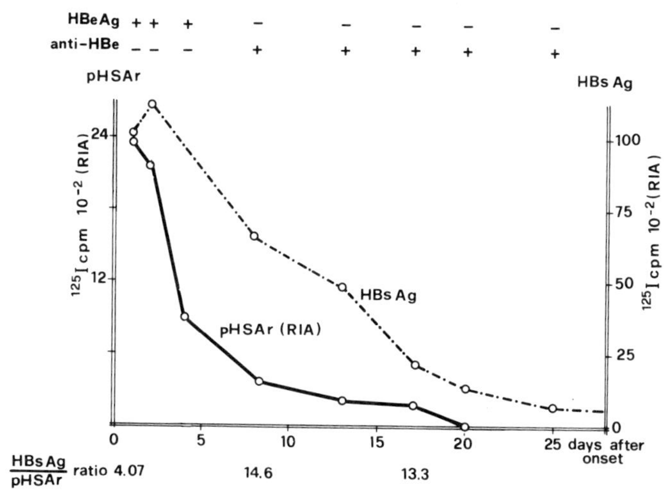

Figure 1 : Levels of pHSA receptor (pHSAr) and HBsAg over
pHSAr ratio in the course of acute hepatitis type B. The
data refer to one of the 31 patients studied.

These changes in receptor activity did not appear to be merely the consequence of variations in HBsAg serum concentration.
In fact, when the ratio of HBsAg over pHSA receptor activity
was calculated to minimize the effect of total HBsAg concentration, its value increased progressively in the course of
the illness, particularly at the time of anti-HBe seroconversion, indicating that a true qualitative change in pHSA receptor expression occurs in this phase on HBsAg particles. These findings were in agreement with the demonstration of loss

of receptor activity by HBsAg particles after anti-HBe seroconversion, described by Imai et al(1979).

pHSA RECEPTOR IN CHRONIC HBV INFECTION:RELATION TO VIRUS RE-
PLICATION ACTIVITY

A large series of HBsAg chronic carriers, including 74
HBeAg positive and 52 anti-HBe positive cases were tested for
pHSA receptor activity by solid phase RIA. As shown in figure 2, 94% of the HBeAg positive patients, but only 39% of
the anti-HBe positive patients showed detectable pHSA receptor activity. Among the HBeAg positive cases, mean receptor

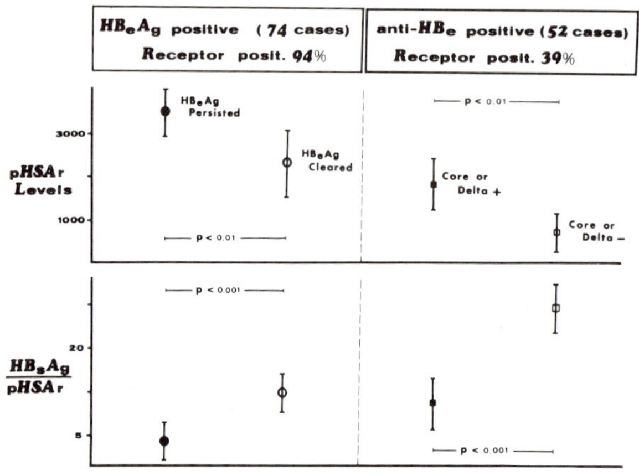

Figure 2: pHSA receptor levels and HBsAg over pHSA receptor
ratio in chronic HBV infection in relation to HBeAg/anti-HBe
status

levels were significantly higher in patients who remained
then persistently HBeAg positive in serum compared to the
cases who eventually seroconverted to anti-HBe during follow-
up. These differences in pHSA receptor levels observed in relation to the outcome of serologic HBeAg status were confirmatory of our earlier results obtained by hemagglutination
(Pontisso et al. 1983) and indicate that testing for the pHSA
receptor may represent a useful prognostic marker in HBeAg
positive chronic hepatitis type B (Alberti et al. 1982).

Among the anti-HBe positive cases pHSA receptor activity
was detected mainly in patients positive for HBcAg or for delta antigen in the liver by immunofluorescence, while patients
negative for these markers usually showed trivial receptor
levels.

These results indicate the existence of a close link between pHSA binding on virus particles and virus replication,
suggesting that expression of the receptor could depend on
presence of complete virions.

pHSA RECEPTOR ON DANE PARTICLES AND HBsAg PARTICLES

HBsAg was purified from HBeAg positive (HBsAg/HBeAg)and
from anti-HBe positive (HBsAg/anti-HBe) serum by affinity
chromatography with monoclonal anti-HBs. Enriched Dane particle pellets were prepared by ultracentrifugation. All preparations were equilibrated for HBsAg titer and tested for
pHSA receptor by RIA. HBsAg/anti-HBe, found to contain only
22 nm HBsAg when examined by electron microscopy, showed trivial pHSA binding (341 cpm), while HBsAg/HBeAg, constituted
mainly by 22 nm HBsAg, had an intermediate value (2179 cpm)
and Dane particle pellets the highest levels(3125-3867 cpm).
Thus, maximum expression of the receptor occurred on Dane particles and this finding was also confirmed by CsCl density
gradient analysis. In these experiments, maximum receptor activity was detected in fractions containing peak HBcAg activity and found to contain almost exclusively Dane particles
when examined by electron microscopy. These fractions had a-
bout 3 times higher receptor levels compared to HBsAg fractions negative for HBcAg and equalized for HBsAg content.

ANTIBODY TO DANE PARTICLE IN ACUTE HEPATITIS B:RELATION TO
pHSA RECEPTOR ON VIRUS PARTICLES

In 1978 (Alberti et al. 1978) we developed a RIP assay
to detect antibody precipitating Dane particles made radioactive by the endogenous DNAP reaction (^{3}H-DP). By this method, an antibody was demonstrated in sera free of anti-HBs
and obtained early in the course of acute hepatitis B, being
absent in patients showing progression to chronic infection.
This observation suggested the possibility that the antibody
could be relevant in virus clearance. The antibody, proved
distinct from anti-HBs, anti-HBc and anti-HBe, was not adsor-

bed by HBsAg particles prepared from anti-HBe positive sera
(Alberti et al. 1980). On the basis of these findings it was
thought specific for Dane particles and termed anti-Dane particle (anti-DP) antibody (Alberti et al. 1979). More recently,
evidence has been provided that HBsAg in HBeAg positive sera
shows structural and antigenic differences compared to HBsAg
in anti-HBe containing sera. Neurath et al. (1980) and Vnek
et al. (1979) reported the detection of new antigenic reactivities on the former but not on the latter particles and Imai
et al. (1979) described pHSA receptor sites on virus particles
in HBeAg positive but not in anti-HBe containing sera. These
reports prompted us to investigate the possible relationship
between the antibody to Dane particles and the pHSA receptor
on virus particles.

INHIBITION OF ANTI-DP ANTIBODY BY HB PARTICLES AND BY pHSA

The precipitation of ^{3}H-DP by the anti-DP antibody was
completely blocked by purified DP while HBsAg from HBeAg positive serum caused 42% inhibition and HBsAg from anti-HBe positive serum had no inhibitory effect, although all three preparations had been equalized for HBsAg content.

Soluble pHSA, but not HSA or pBSA, inhibited the precipitation of ^{3}H-DP by the anti-DP antibody when added in the RIP
assay. This effect was specific since identical concentrations of pHSA had no effect on the precipitation of DP by anti-
HBs sera. Although presence of anti-pHSA antibodies in the
anti-DP positive sera could explain these results, several
data militated against this possibility. Indeed, the inhibition of the anti-DP antibody by polyalbumin was species-res-
tricted, while anti-albumin antibodies are known to cross-
react with albumins of different species (Thung, Gerber 1981).
Furthermore, no anti-pHSA antibody activity could be detected
by conventional methods in the anti-DP positive sera.

To better define the mechanism by which pHSA blocked the
interaction between DP and the anti-DP antibody, affinity
chromatography experiments were performed with IgG prepared
from anti-DP positive sera and insolubilized on Sepharose 4B.

AFFINITY CHROMATOGRAPHY WITH INSOLUBILIZED ANTI-DP ANTIBODY

As shown in figure 3, ^{125}I-HBsAg (Abbott AUSAB reagent)

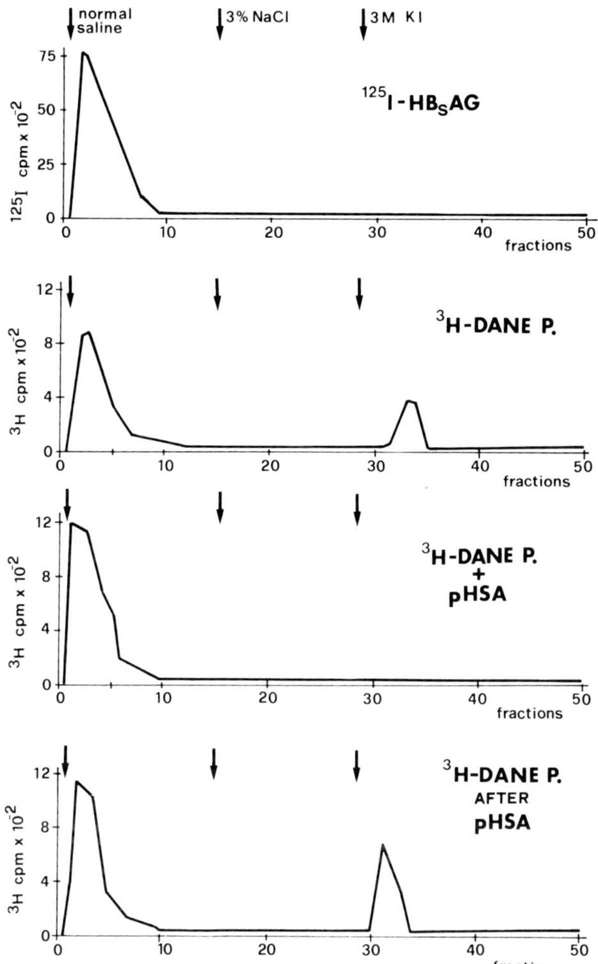

Figure 3 : affinity chromatography experiments with Sepharose 4B coupled with IgG prepared from anti-DP positive serum.

was not adsorbed by anti-DP antibody coupled column, while
about 40% of ^{3}H-DP was retained and could be eluted with 3M
KI. When ^{3}H-DP were mixed with pHSA (1 mg/ml) prior to incubation with the column, binding was prevented while no such
effect was observed if the gel was incubated with pHSA prior
to the addition of ^{3}H-DP. These results provide evidence that
pHSA blocks the interaction of the anti-DP antibody with DP

by reacting with virus particles rather than with the antibody, thus suggesting that pHSA and anti-DP antibody bind to identical sites on Dane particles.

INHIBITION OF VIRUS pHSA RECEPTOR BY ANTI-DP ANTIBODY

To test directly the possibility that anti-DP antibody could interfere with the function of the pHSA receptor, thus behaving as an anti-receptor antibody, purified Dane particles were incubated with anti-DP positive sera or IgG prior to be tested for pHSA receptor by RIA. 200 μl of Dane particles, diluted as to give about 2000 ^{125}I-cpm in the receptor assay, were reacted for 4 hours at room temperature with 200 μl of anti-DP positive serum or IgG, as well as with 200 μl of anti-DP negative serum and IgG. 50 μl of the mixture were then tested for pHSA binding activity. Five sera positive for anti-DP caused from 85 to 100% inhibition of DP-associated pHSA receptor activity while 5 sera negative for anti-DP had no inhibitory effect under the same experimental conditions. IgG (5 mg/ml) obtained from 2 anti-DP positive sera caused 35% and 41% inhibition of the receptor, respectively, while no effect was observed with 5 IgG preparations (5 mg/ml) obtained from anti-DP negative sera. All sera were tested for inhibition after treatment at 56°C for 30', to remove heat-labile unspecific inhibitory factors (Milich et al. 1981)

CONCLUSIONS

Following the original report by Imai et al. (1979) several other Authors have confirmed the existence of a species-specific receptor for pHSA on HBV particles (Hansson, Purcell 1979; Neurath, Strick 1979; Thung, Gerber 1981, Pontisso et al 1983). Although its nature and biologic role remain unknown, there is evidence supporting the viral rather than host specificity of the receptor, that has been detected also on individual HBsAg polypeptides as well as on HBsAg produced "in vitro" by a hepatoma cell line (Ionescu-Matiu et al. 1980).

We have demonstrated that the expression of the receptor on virus particles is higher in sera obtained from patients who are in the phase of active virus replication, as testified by presence of HBeAg in serum or of HBcAg in the liver. These findings suggest that serum levels of the receptor could be dependent on the presence of the complete HB virion. In agree-

ment with this possibility, higher receptor expression was detected on Dane particles compared to HBsAg particles. These
observations, toghether with evidence that normal human hepatocytes bear albumin binding sites on their surface (Trevisan
et al. 1982) support the hypothesis of a pathogenetic role of
the virus receptor in facilitating selective attachment of
complete virus particles to liver cells.

Studies on the characterization of the specificity of the
antibody precipitating Dane particles, described by us in 1978
(Alberti et al. 1978) have now allowed the identification,
early in the course of acute hepatitis type B, of an antibody
activity apparently directed against the pHSA receptor on virus particles. The antibody was found to react not only with
Dane particles, but also with HBsAg in HBeAg positive sera,
according to the expression of pHSA receptors on these particles. The anti-receptor specificity of the antibody was confirmed by the observation that it reduced "in vitro" pHSA receptor expression on purified Dane particles.

The role, if any, that this antibody response could play
in the course of HBV infection remains to be defined. On the
basis of the hypothesis that the virus receptor for pHSA may
mediate virus access to hepatocytes, the anti-receptor antibody could be relevant in the phase of extracellular virus neutralization.

REFERENCES

Alberti A., Diana S., Scullard GH, Eddleston ALWF, Williams
    R (1978). Detection of a new antibody system reacting with
    Dane particles in hepatitis B Virus infection. Brit Med J
    2:1056.
Alberti A, Realdi G, Bortolotti F, Tonel M (1979). Anti-Dane
    particles antibody (anti-DP) and activity of virus replica-
    tion in acute and chronic hepatitis B virus infection.
    Ital J Gastroenterol 11:110.
Alberti A, Realdi G, Bortolotti F, Eddleston ALWF, Williams
    R (1980). Dane particles-precipitating antibodies in hepa-
    titis B virus infection. In Bianchi L, Sickinger K, Gerok
    W (eds):"Virus and the liver" MTP Press Limited, p 59.
Alberti A, Pontisso P, Realdi G (1982). Virus receptors for
    polymerized human serum albumin: a prognostic marker in
    HBeAg positive chronic hepatitis type B? J Med Virol 10:141.
Alberti A, Pontisso P, Schiavon E, Realdi G (1983). Antibody

precipitating Dane particles in acute hepatitis type B:relation to receptor sites that bind polymerized human serum albumin on virus particles. (submitted for publication)

Hansson B, Purcell RH (1979). Sites that bind polymerized albumin on hepatitis B surface antigen particles: detection by radioimmunoassay. Infect Immun 26:125

Imai M, Yanase Y, Nojiri T (1979). A receptor for polymerized human and chimpanzee albumins on hepatitis B virus particles co-occuring with HBeAg. Gastroenterology 76:242

Ionescu I, Sanchez Y, Hollinger B, Melnick J, Dreesman G(1980) Presence of a receptor for albumin on individual HBsAg polypeptides and on HBsAg produced by a hepatoma line. J Med Virol 6:175.

Lenkei R, Mota G, Dan M(1974). The polymerized albumin and anti-albumin antibodies in patients with hepatic diseases. Rev Roum Biochem 11:271

Lenkei R, Onica D, Ghetie V (1977). Receptors for polymerized albumin on liver cells. Experientia 33:1046

Mathuhashi T,Hosokawa Z(1972). Reactants to human serum albumin coated red cells found in Au-positive sera. Jap J Exp Med 42:183

Milich DR, Gottfried T, Vyas G(1981). Characterization of the interaction between polymerized human albumin and hepatitis B surface antigen. Gastroenterology 81:218.

Neurath A,Strick N(1979). Radioimmunoassay for albumin-binding sites associated with e antigen in serum. Intervirol 11:128

Neurath A, Strick N, Huang C(1980). Confirmatory evidence for the association of hepatitis B surface antigen with antigenic determinants reactive with antibodies in some anti-HBe positive sera. J Gen Virol 48:53

Onica D,Margineanu I,Lenkei R(1981). Specificity of anti-albumin antibodies in liver diseases. Molecular Immunol 18:807

Pontisso P, Alberti A, Bortolotti F, Realdi G(1983). Virus receptors for pHSA in acute and chronic HBV infection. Gastroenterology 84:220

Pontisso P, Alberti A,Schiavon E, Realdi G (1983) Receptors for pHSA on HBV particles detected by radioimmunoassay:changes in receptor activity in serum during acute and chronic infection. J Virol Meth 6:151

Trevisan A,Gudat F, Guggenheim R(1982) Demonstration of albumin receptors on isolated human hepatocytes. Hepatology2:832

Thung SN, Gerber MA (1981) Specificities of albumin receptors and albumin antibodies. Infect Immun 32:1292

Vnek J, Prince AM, Trepo C, Chen R (1979). Cryptic association of e antigen (HBeAg) with different morphological forms of HBsAg particles 4:187

OVERT AND LATENT HBV INFECTION

F. Bonino, F. Negro, E. Chiaberge, O. Crivelli

Gastroenterology Dept.,S. Giovanni Hospital,
Turin, Italy

Hepatitis B virus (HBV) behaves like a non cytopathic virus capable of integrating into the host genome; it may prepare the ground for superinfection from other viruses which require helper functions of HBV for their expression. Delta Agent represents the prototype of these viruses and takes advantage of the pre-existing HBV infection, producing liver damage and complicating the initial picture of HBV infection. This evidence entails that in subgroups of HBsAg carriers liver disease disguised as HBV-related is instead induced by other agents.

In order to study the relation between the liver disease and the state of HBV infection in chronic carriers of the HBsAg, HBV and Delta associated markers were analysed in sera and liver biopsies of 125 HBsAg carriers who underwent evaluation of their liver disease at the Gastroenterology Dept. of our Hospital during the last 5 years.

Sera were examined for HBV-DNA, HBV-specific DNA-polymerase (DNA-P), HBeAg, anti-HBe, δ-Ag and anti-δ as reported (Bonino, 1981; Rizzetto, 1980). Liver biopsy specimens were analysed for HBV nucleic acids by spot and Southern blot hybridization of DNAs extracted from liver tissue using a ^{32}P-labeled HBV-DNA probe and for HBcAg, HBsAg and δ-Ag by IFL (Chen, 1982; Bonino, 1981). A liver biopsy was not performed in 63 asymptomatic carriers with persistently normal liver function tests. Patients with liver disease had not received

antiviral or immunosuppressive drugs during the six months
prior to examination. The histological diagnosis are summarized in table n.1 according to presence or absence of HBV-
DNA and HBeAg/anti-HBe in serum.

TABLE 1. HISTOLOGICAL DIAGNOSIS OF 125 CARRIERS OF THE HBsAg
GROUPED ACCORDING TO PRESENCE OR ABSENCE OF HBV-DNA
AND HBeAg/ANTI-HBe IN SERUM.

LIVER		SERUM		
histological diagnosis		HBV-DNA+		HBV-DNA-
		HBeAg+	anti-HBe+	anti-HBe+
Normal liver	2	2	–	–
Chronic Lobular Hepatitis	7	4	3	–
Chronic Persistent Hepatitis	13	3	7	3
Chronic Active Hepatitis	20	6	9	5
Chronic Active Hepatitis with Cirrhosis	20	4	9	7
Asymptomatic Carriers	63	–	–	63
Total	125	19	28	78

All HBeAg positive carriers had HBV-DNA (>1 ng/ml) in
their serum and HBcAg in the liver; only one had also intrahepatic δ-Ag. Most of these patients exhibited chronic hepatitis ; only two had normal liver histology. In 5
of them, after a variable period of time, HBeAg was cleared
from serum with anti-HBe seroconversion. This event occurred
at an approximate rate of 6% per year and was invariably associated with clearance of serum HBV-DNA and reduction of

activity of liver disease (normal levels of serum transferases).

HBV-DNA was not detected in serum of 78 anti-HBe positive carriers; 63 of them were symptomless with persistently normal liver function tests, 15 had histologically proven chronic hepatitis and 7 of these had chronic Delta infection (intrahepatic δ-Ag and serum titers of anti-δ higher than 1/5000).

HBV-DNA was detected in serum of 28 anti-HBe positive carriers, all of them with evidence of liver disease; 18 of these had intrahepatic δ-Ag and serum titers of anti-δ higher than 1/5000. HBcAg was detected in the nuclei of hepatocytes of 9 patients with HBV-DNA and anti-HBe; 5 of these had both nuclear and cytoplasmic fluorescence. Immunofluorescence staining of HBcAg in the cytoplasms was confirmed by detection of 27 nm particles in the Electron Microscope. HBV-DNA and anti-HBe positive sera usually circulated viral nucleic acid at concentrations of about 0.1 ng/ml, even though occasionally HBV-DNA reached levels as high as 0.5 ng/ml, comparable to those detected in sera positive for both HBeAg and DNA-P. The finding of HBV-DNA in DNA-P negative sera with total amounts comparable to those detected in sera positive for DNA-P is intriguing. The DNA-P activity and the concentration of HBV-DNA generally are observed to correlate but do not always maintain a constant quantitative ratio. The higher sensitivity of the hybridization assay for HBV-DNA may explain these results in sera with low levels of HBV-DNA. In other cases, as in sera with relatively high levels of viral nucleic acid, the explanation may reside in either the structure of DNA or in the organization of the viral particle.

The state of HBV-DNA was analysed in 10 liver specimens from 5 carriers with intrahepatic HBcAg (2 of them having serum anti-HBe and 3 HBeAg). Uncut DNAs and Hind III restriction fragments were analysed by Southern blot hybridization (Fig.1). The presence of a hybridization band at the position of the HBV-DNA (3.2 Kb) in both uncut DNA and Hind III restriction patterns revealed free (episomic) forms of viral DNA. A hybridization signal only near the

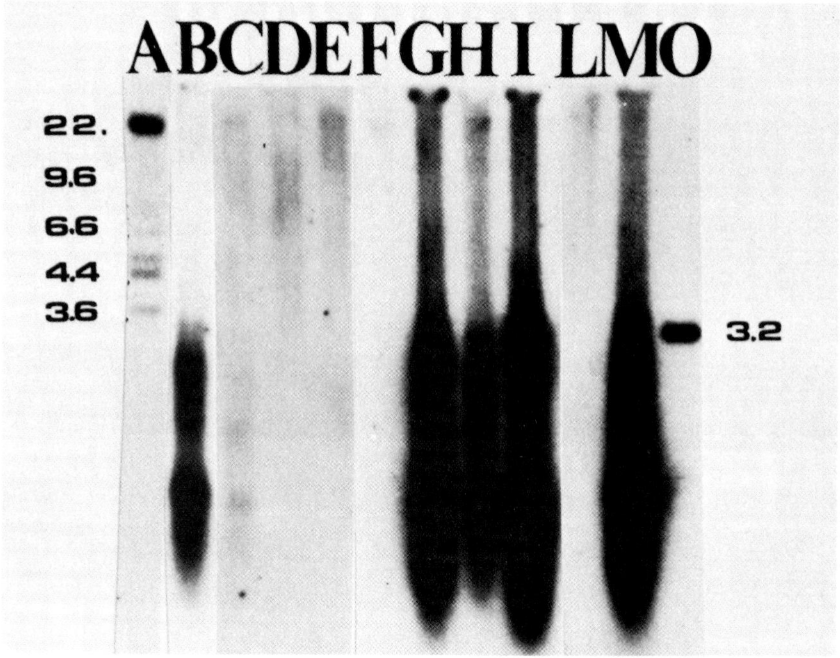

Figure 1. Autoradiography of Southern transferred DNA from liver of chronic HBV carriers after Hind III digestion. Liver tissue obtained from needle biopsies was incubated in 50 mM Tris-HCl pH 8.2, 50 mM Na_3-EDTA, 200 mM NaCl, 2% SDS and 0.5 mg/ml Proteinase K at 37°C overnight. After chloroform-phenol extraction the DNA was digested by Hind III restriction enzyme according to the Manufacturer's specifications (Bethesda Research Laboratories Inc., Gaithersburg, MD, USA) and subjected to electrophoresis in Tris-Acetate buffer for 20 hrs at 30 mA, 37 V in a 20 x 20 x 0.5 agarose gel slab. DNA was transferred to nitrocellulose, hybridized to a ^{32}P-TTP nick-translated HBV-DNA probe (specific activity 2 x 10^8 dpm/ug) and autoradiographed as reported (Bonino, 1981). The band in lane O marks the position of 3.2 Kb linear HBV-DNA.

origin of the lane in the uncut DNA pattern and at positions higher than 3.2 Kb in the Hind III restriction pattern was indicative of HBV-DNA integration.

Replicative forms of HBV-DNA were found in the liver of carriers with intrahepatic HBcAg (lanes B,G,H,I,M; fig.1); all these patients had HBV-DNA in serum in spite of presence or absence of HBeAg. Sequences of viral nucleic acid suggestive of integration could not be excluded because of the intensity of the band in 3.2 Kb region. In Delta positive liver specimens the autoradiograms revealed a hybridization signal of DNA greater than HBV genome size (lanes C,D,E,F,L; fig.1) indicating integration of HBV-DNA sequences. The absence of replicative forms of HBV both in serum and liver of HBsAg carriers with intrahepatic δ-Ag together with the evidence of HBV-DNA integration suggest that liver disease in these individuals is related to Delta superinfection of pre-existing long-lasting carriers of the HBsAg.

Intrahepatic HBV-DNA was also analysed by in situ cito-hybridization. Briefly, frozen sections were fixed in Carnoy's B fixative and a HBV-DNA probe containing the entire HBV genome in a pBR325 plasmid labeled by nick translation with biotinylated dUTP (kindly provided by Dr. M.Berninger, Bethesda Research Laboratories Inc., Gaithersburg, MD, USA) was hybridized to the sections overnight at 37°C. Hybridized nucleic acid was detected by Avidin-Biotin-Peroxidase Complex (ABC) and stained with DAB solution. Sections were counterstained with 0.1% acriflavine or FITC-antiHBc serum. The specificity of the assay was confirmed by negative results obtained using liver biopsy specimens from patients without markers of HBV infection, performing the test with a biotinylated plasmid, using DAB reaction on sections treated only with ABC and suppressing endogenous Avidin-binding activity by pretreatment with free Avidin.

HBV nucleic acid was not detected by this technique in the 5 patients with chronic Delta infection and integrated sequences of HBV-DNA in the liver.

HBV-DNA was found by in situ hybridization in 7 out of 9 (77%) patients with serum HBV-DNA and intrahepatic HBcAg.

The signal detected by in situ hybridization was mainly

intracytoplasmic and perinuclear, in a few cases with diffuse distribution associated with diffuse staining of HBcAg by
IFL and more frequently with focal distribution (Fig.2). In

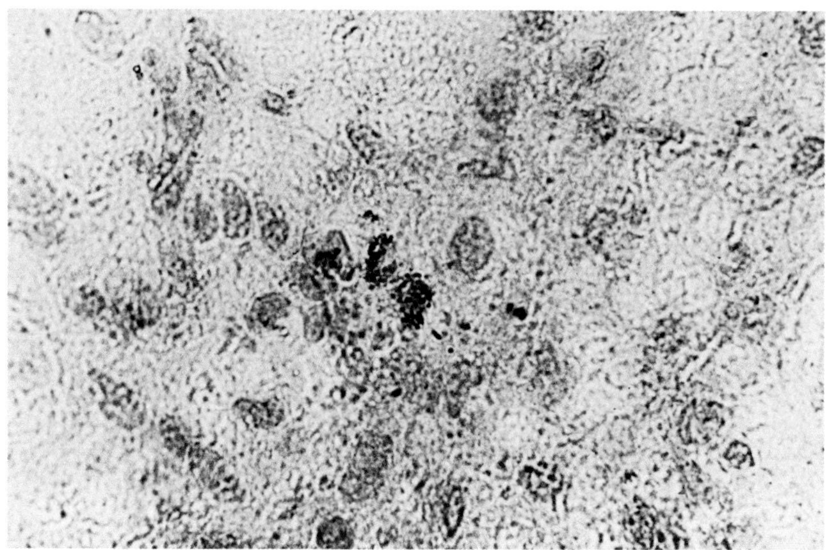

Figure 2. Intracytoplasmic and perinuclear DAB-positive granules with focal distribution in a patient with
chronic active hepatitis, HBcAg positive in the
liver by IFL.

chronic active hepatitis cases positive cells did not show
any particular damage at the light microscope but were sometimes associated with peripolesis. Pretreatment with DNAse
and RNAse and hybridization without denaturing liver tissue
nucleic acids suggest that intracytoplasmic sequences detected by this technique were possibly represented by single
stranded DNA.

The analysis of the state of HBV infection in chronic
HBsAg carriers suggest three main categories of individuals:
1) carriers with overt HBV infection (with only replicative
forms of HBV-DNA into the liver); 2) carriers with latent
HBV infection (with only integrated sequences of HBV-DNA);
3) carriers with characteristics of both previous groups

(with mixed HBV infection).

The natural history of chronic HBV infection is one of slow transition from an early phase of active HBV replication to one of latent HBV infection (Hoofnagle, 1983). It has been hypothesized that hepatocytes with actively replicating HBV express antigens of the viral nucleocapsid on the plasma membrane and become thus target of the host immune response; cells undergoing HBV integration produce only HBsAg and escape instead this immunological aggression (Eddleston, 1982 and Shafritz, 1982). As a consequence carriers with overt HBV infection gradually become carrier with latent infection in parallel with the progressive increase of cells with integrated HBV genome over cells with active HBV replication, eliminated by the host immunity.

The finding of HBV-DNA in regions of agarose gels greater than HBV-DNA genome size is suggestive of integration; however the diffuse autoradiographic signals are difficult to interpret when large quantities of genomic (HBV) DNA are also present. The majority of chronic HBsAg carriers probably have mixed HBV infection, that is with both episomic and integrated sequences of HBV-DNA. The detection of HBeAg and anti-HBe in the sera of these individuals depends on the relative excess of one reactant over the other at the time of sampling and therefore the presence of anti-HBe in serum does not exclude active HBV infection. It is likely, instead, that HBsAg carriers without markers of active HBV infection (both HBeAg and HBV-DNA negative in the serum) have only hepatocytes with integrated forms of HBV genome.

Whereas overt HBV infection is often associated with liver disease (Hoofnagle, 1983), integrated HBV infection usually does not result in liver damage and is indeed the condition typical of the asymptomatic carrier of HBsAg. The occurrence of liver disease in this setting implies a pathogenesis different from HBV. Delta agent may represent a model applying to other infectious agents in the understanding of these cases.

The following partecipated in this study:G.Bussolati,P.
Gugliotta,Institute of Morbid Anatomy,M.G.Canese,Electron
Microscopy Center and E.Lodi,Institute of Zoology,University
of Turin,Turin,Italy.W.Hoyer,J.Nelson,DMVI,Georgetown University,Rockville,MD,USA.

References

Bonino F.,Hoyer B.,Nelson J.,Engle R.,Verme G.,Gerin J.L.
  (1981).Hepatitis B virus DNA in the sera of HBsAg carriers
  a marker of active hepatitis B virus replication in the
  liver.Hepatology 1:386.
Bréchot C.,Pourcel C.,Hadchoucel H.,Dejean A.,Louise A.,
  Scotto J.,Tiollais P.(1982).State of hepatitis B virus DNA
  in liver disease.Hepatology 2:27S.
Chen D.S.,Hoyer B.,Nelson J.,Purcell R.H.,Gerin J.L.(1982).
  Detection and properties of hepatitis B viral DNA in liver
  tissues from patients with hepatocellular carcinoma.
  Hepatology 2:42S.
Eddleston A.L.W.F.,Mondelli M.,Mieli-Vergani G.,Williams R.
  (1982).Lymphocyte cytotoxicity to autologous hepatocytes
  in chronic hepatitis B virus infection.Hepatology 2:128S.
Hoofnagle J.H.(1983).Chronic type B hepatitis.Gastroente-
  rology 84:422.
Rizzetto M.,Shih J.W-K.,Gerin J.L.(1980).The hepatitis B
  virus-associated δ antigen:isolation from liver,develop-
  ment of solid-phase radioimmunoassays for δ antigen and
  anti-δ and partial characterization of δ antigen.J.Immunol.
  125:318.
Shafritz D.A.(1982).Hepatitis B virus DNA molecules in the
  liver of HBsAg carriers:mechanistic considerations in the
  pathogenesis of hepatocellular carcinoma.Hepatology 2:35S

Viral Hepatitis and Delta Infection, pages 345–356
© **1983 Alan R. Liss, Inc., 150 Fifth Avenue, New York, NY 10011**

HEPATITIS B VIRAL DNA SEQUENCES IN THE INFECTED TISSUES

Christian BRECHOT, Anne Dejean, Pierre Tiollais.

Unité de Recombinaison et Expression Génétique
INSERM U.163, CNRS LA 271, Institut Pasteur,
75724 Paris Cedex 15, France.

The cloning in Escherichia coli of the hepatitis B virus
(HBV) DNA has provided a sufficient amount of viral DNA to
label it with 32p and use it as a probe for the detection of
the HBV genome in serum and tissue samples with the transfer-
hybridization technique (Southern 1975). This procedure is
described in figures 1 and 2. It allows to ascertain the presence or absence of HBV DNA sequences in a liver or serum
sample ; in addition, in the liver, it is possible to distinguish between different viral states in the infected cells :
free monomeric viral DNA with viral multiplications, free
monomeric viral DNA without viral multiplication, free viral
oligomers, integration of viral DNA sequences in the genomic
DNA. However two main limitations must be known : the state
of the HBV DNA cannot be determined precisely when only small
needle biopsy samples are available and false positive results
due to bacterial contamination of the liver samples must be
carefully ruled out when autopsy samples are analyzed. For the
serum samples a simplified procedure (the "dot" or "spot" test)
can be applied. Using this approach, we have studied the presence and the state of the HBV genome in the liver and the
serum of patients with HBsAg positive and negative chronic
liver disease with or without hepatocellular carcinoma. In
addition we recently looked for the presence of viral DNA
sequence in extrahepatic tissues.

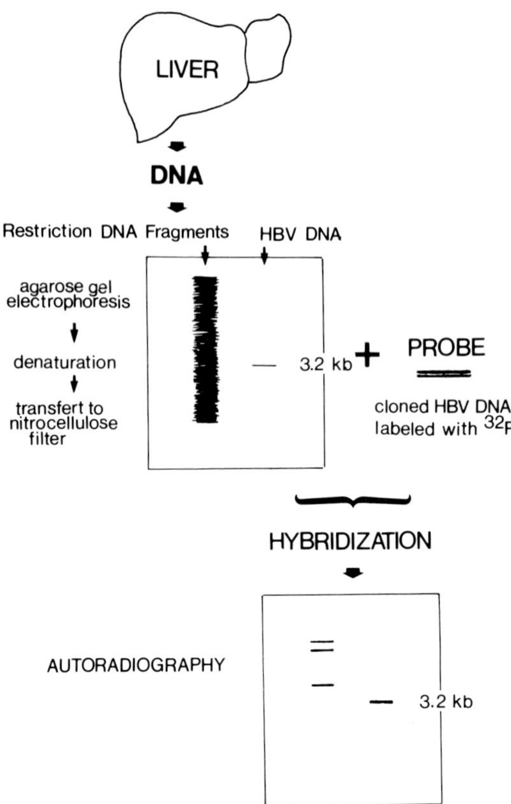

Fig. 1. The technique of transfer-hybridization (Southern blot). Liver DNA was extracted and digested with a restriction endonuclease. DNA fragments were fractionated by agarose-gel electrophoresis, denatured and transferred to a nitrocellulose filter. The denatured DNA fragments immobilized on the filter were hybridized with denatured cloned HBV DNA labeled with 32p. Hybridization was revealed by the presence of bands on an autoradiogram.

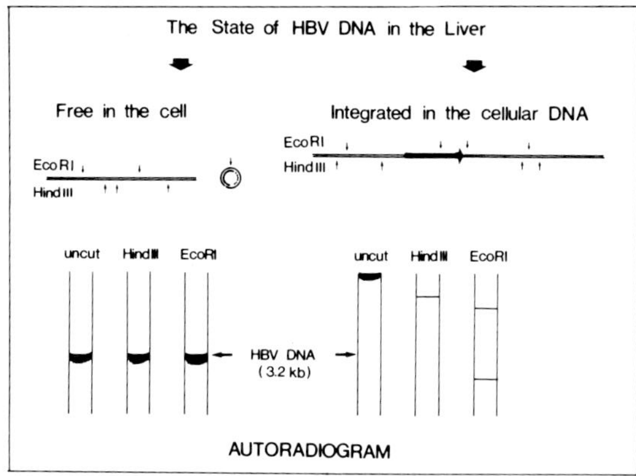

Fig. 2. Determination of the state of HBV DNA in the liver
cells. Because HindIII does not cut HBV DNA and EcoRi cuts
once in the majority of the HBV DNA cloned, uncut DNA, HindIII
and EcoRI restriction fragments were analyzed by Southern
blot. If HBV DNA is free in the cell, analysis of the uncut
DNA, HindIII and EcoRI restriction patterns reveals the presence of a band at the position of the HBV DNA. If HBV DNA
sequences are present in an integrated form, the three patterns are different : a hybridization signal only near the
origin of the lane (without any band) in the uncut DNA pattern, a band at a position higher than 3.2. kb in the HindIII
restriction pattern and two bands in the EcoRI pattern correspond to the existence of one copy of HBV DNA integrated in
one site in liver cell DNA. The presence of three bands, one
of which with a high intensity at 3.2. kb position, suggests
the presence of two or more whole HBV genomes integrated in
a head-to-tail arrangement. Other patterns corresponding to
different genetic organization of the integrated sequences
are possible.

RESULTS

1. Hepatocellular carcinoma.

The patients can be divided into three groups according to
their serological status :
   a) <u>HBsAg and/or anti HBcAg positive, HBeAg negative
patients</u>. Figure 3 shows representative results of this group.
Bands corresponding to DNA fragments of molecular weight higher
than 3.2. kb in the HindIII pattern and a hybridization signal
close to the origin of the lane in the uncut DNA pattern were
observed (Figure 3, Lanes 1 and 2). These results demonstrated

the presence and integration of HBV DNA sequences in the tumorous liver cell DNA. The existence of several bands suggested the existence of several integration sites in the host genome. The EcoRI pattern showed the presence of bands at different positions. The presence of a band of high intensity at the 3.2. kb position suggested the existence of two or more HBV genomes integrated in a head-to-tail arrangement (Figure 3, Lane 3 and see also Figure 2). A similar EcoRI pattern was observed in 6 of the 14 cases studied. The restriction patterns were different for the different patients studied. Moreover, when the tumorous and nontumorous parts of the liver could be clearly distinguished histologically, the restriction patterns corresponding to these two parts were different. In 3 recent cases identical bands were present in the tumorous and non tumorous cell of livers with an early HCC (unpublished data).

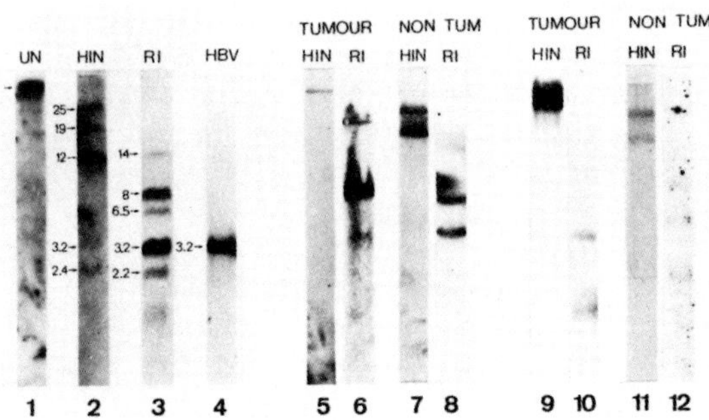

Fig. 3. Autoradiogram of the Southern blot analysis of liver tissue samples of HBeAg negative patients with HCC (representative cases). Lanes 1 to 3 : tumorous part of an autopsy sample of a male patient from the Ivory Coast. HBsAg was present in the serum but undetectable by immunofluorescence in the tumor. Lane 1 : undigested DNA. Lanes 2 and 3 : HindIII and EcoRI restriction DNA patterns. Lane 4 : cloned HBV DNA. Lanes 5 to 8 : tumorous and nontumorous parts of an autopsy sample of a male patient from the Ivory Coast ; HBsAg and anti-HBc positive in the serum. HBsAg and HBcAg were detected in the nontumorous tissue but not in the tumorous part of the liver. Lanes 9 to 12 : another autopsy sample of a male patient from the Ivory Coast, HBsAg and anti-HBc positive in the serum ; HBsAg and HBcAg were detected in the nontumorous tissue. In the tumor, HBsAg was detected in only some scattered cells.

b) <u>HBsAg positive, HBeAg positive patients</u>. In these patients, the autoradiogram patterns are different from those of the two preceding groups. The first case was an early HCC (small tumorous nodule discovered during surgery for portoca- val shunt). The HindIII patterns of the tumor and the nontu- morous part of the liver were identical and showed the pre- sence of an intense band at the 3.2. kb position with a smear downstream. This demonstrated the presence of free viral DNA. Due to the large amount of free viral DNA, integrated sequences were not clearly ascertained. HBV DNA was also detected in the serum. The second case was an autopsy sample of an advanced HCC. Free viral DNA was present only in the nontumorous part, whereas integrated HBV sequences were present both in the tumorous and nontumorous tissues (Figure 5, Lanes 6 and 7).

c) <u>HBsAg negative patients</u>. We focuse on the relationship between HBV and HCC associated with alcoholic cirrhosis be- cause this is the most frequent form of HCC in France. Two groups of alcoholic patients were studied. Group I included 51 prospectively studied alcoholics without appearent tumor, and Group II included 20 retrospectively studied patients with HCC and alcoholic cirrhosis. Integrated HBV DNA sequences were detected in the 20 patients with HCC, but in only 8 of the 51 alcoholics without tumor (Table 1). None of the patients with HCC had HBsAg detectable in the serum. Five had only anti- HBc, 3 had both anti-HBc and anti-HBs, 1 had only anti-HBs and 7 had no HBV serological markers.

GROUP AND PATIENTS NUMBER	SEROLOGIC TESTS			HBV DNA IN THE LIVER	
	HBsAg	ANTI-HBc	ANTI-HBs	FREE	INTEGRATED
GROUP I : ALCOHOLICS WITHOUT HEPATOCELLULAR CARCINOMA (51 CASES).	3/51	16/51	13/51	2/51	6/51
GROUP II : ALCOHOLICS WITH HEPATOCELLULAR CARCINOMA (20 CASES).	0/16	8/16	4/16	0/16	20/20

TABLE 1 : STATE OF HBV DNA IN THE LIVER AND SEROLOGICAL STATUS OF ALCOHOLIC PATIENTS WITH AND WITHOUT HEPATOCELLULAR CARCINOMA (71 CASES).

In addition we recently studied 11 non alcoholic patients
with HBsAg negative HCC (2 Africans,1 Italian, 8 Frenchs).
Only 1 liver sample was obtained at autopsy. HBV DNA was detected in the liver of 10 of these 11 patients. In one case
the restriction DNA pattern suggested the presence of free
oligomeric viral sequences. In 9 cases the restriction DNA
pattern was consistent with the integration of the viral
sequences (Manuscript in preparation).

II. HBV chronic carriers without apparent tumor.

The patients can be divided in three groups according to the
presence or absence of HBsAg and HBeAg.
    a) <u>HBsAg positive, HBeAg negative patients</u>.Eighteen adult
patients were studied. The histology ranged from normal liver
to chronic active hepatitis (CAH) Table 2. Discrete bands
corresponding to DNA fragments of high molecular weight were
observed in the HindIII pattern (Figure 4). When enough DNA
was available, uncut DNA was analyzed and the absence of these
bands were consistent with the presence of integrated HBV DNA
sequences (Figure 4, Lane 2). When the EcoRI digestion was
performed, two different patterns were observed : (i) the
presence of one intense band at the 3.2. kb position, with a
faint band at a higher position in some cases, suggesting the
existence of tandem integration (Figure 4, Lanes 4, 6 and 9)
and (ii) the presence of several bands at variable positions
(Figure 4, Lane 11). In two of the 18 cases analyzed, free
viral DNA was detected in the liver, HBV DNA being detectable
in the serum for one of them.

PATIENTS NUMBER	HISTOLOGY	HBV DNA IN THE LIVER		HBV DNA IN THE SERUM
		FREE	INTEGRATED	
1	NORMAL LIVER	-	+	
2	SLIGHT INFLAMMATORY CHANGES	-	+	-
4	CHRONIC PERSISTENT HEPATITIS (CPH)	-	+	-
11	CHRONIC ACTIVE HEPATITIS (CAH)	-	+	-
1	SLIGHT INFLAMMATORY CHANGES	+	?	-
1	CHRONIC ACTIVE HEPATITIS	+	?	+

TABLE 2 : STATE OF HBV DNA IN THE LIVER AND HISTOLOGY OF HBsAg POSITIVE HBeAg NEGATIVE CHRONIC CARRIERS (20 CASES).

In addition, we recently studied pediatric-aged chronic
HBV carriers for whom the duration of the HBV infection could
be firmly established. Integrated sequences were detected
even for short-term chronic carriers (8 months), demonstrating
that integration of HBV DNA was not related in these cases to
the duration of the chronic carrier state.

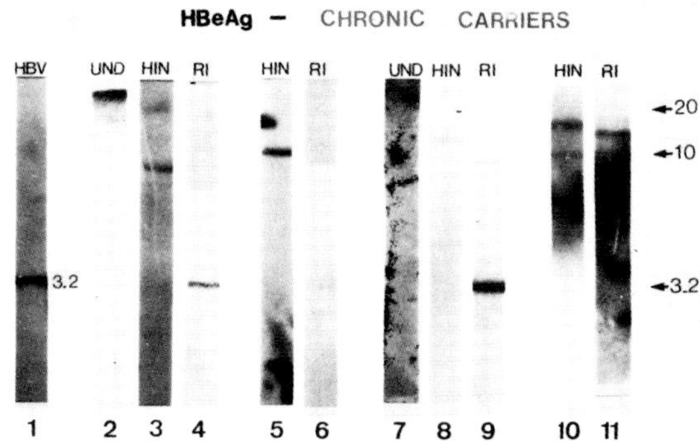

Fig. 4. Autoradiogram of the Southern blot analysis of liver
samples from HBeAg negative HBV chronic carriers (representative cases). Lane 1 : cloned HBV DNA. Lanes 2 to 4 : surgical
biopsy sample of a french patient with CAH without cirrhosis ;
only anti-HBs and anti HBc were detected in the serum although
HBsAg and HBcAg were detected using immunofluorescence in the
liver. Lane 2 : undigested DNA. Lanes 3 and 4 : HindIII and
EcoRI restriction DNA patterns. Lanes 5 to 6 : surgical biopsy
sample of a French patient with HBsAg negative, anti-HBc
positive, and anti-HBs negative inactive cirrhosis. HBsAg and
and HBcAg were detected in the liver. Lanes 7 to 9 : surgical
biopsy sample of a french patient with inactive cirrhosis,
HBsAg in the serum and HBsAg and HBcAg present in the liver.
Lanes 10 and 11 : surgical biopsy sample of a french patient
with CAH ; HBsAg positive, anti-HBc positive in the serum and
HBsAg and HBcAg positive in the liver.

b) <u>HBsAg positive, HBeAg positive</u> patients. Seventeen
adult patients with different liver histology status were
analyzed (Table 3). A long intense smear starting at the
3.2 kb position with few bands superimposed were observed
both in the uncut DNA and the HindIII restriction patterns
HBV DNA was also detected in the serum (Figure 5). These
results demonstrated the presence of free viral DNA in the
liver and production of Dane particles. In three cases,

integrated HBV DNA sequences associated with free HBV DNA were
observed (Figure 5, Lanes 4 and 5). Association of integrated
sequences and free viral DNA was also recently observed for
3 of 8 children who were HBeAg positive, short-term, chronic
carriers (Scotto et al. Gut, 1983. In press).
Comparison of the results obtained with HBeAg negative
and HBeAg positive patients demonstrated the association between free viral DNA in the liver, viral DNA in the serum and
detection of HBeAg in the serum.

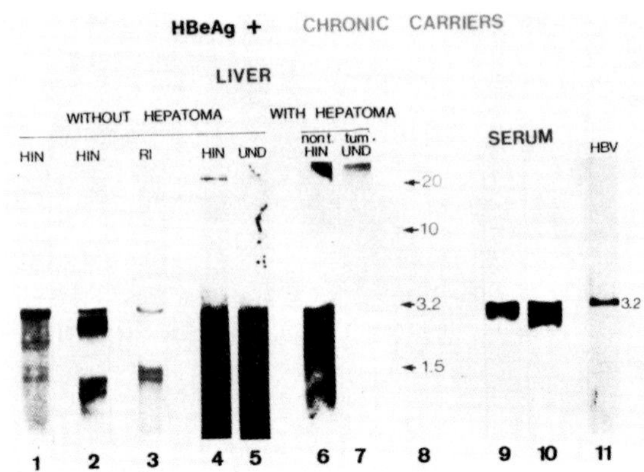

Fig 5. Autoradiogram of the Southern blot analysis of liver
and serum samples from HBeAg positive chronic carriers. Lane
1 : HindIII restriction DNA pattern of a needle biopsy sample
from a french patient with slight inflammatory changes in the
liver. Lane 9 : serum of the same patient. Lanes 2 and 3 :
HindIII and EcoRI patterns of a needle biopsy sample of a
french patient with CAH. Lane 10 : serum of the same patient.
Lanes 4 and 5 : long-term exposure of the HindIII and undigested patterns from a surgical biopsy. The appearance of bands
in the HindIII pattern demonstrated the existence of integrated
sequences in this sample. Lane 6 : HindIII restriction pattern
of the tumor of an autopsy sample of a french patient with
HCC. Lane 7 : undigested DNA pattern of the nontumorous part
of the liver tissue of the same patient. Lane 11 : cloned
HBV DNA.

PATIENTS NUMBER	HISTOLOGY	SEROLOGIC TESTS		HBV DNA IN THE LIVER		HBV DNA IN THE SERUM
		ANTI-HBe	ANTI-HBs	FREE	INTEGRATED	
4	CAH (WITH OR WITHOUT CIRRHOSIS)	+	-	-	+	-
3	CAH (WITH OR WITHOUT CIRRHOSIS)	+	+	-	+	-
1	CAH WITH CIRRHOSIS	-	+	-	+	-
3	CAH WITH CIRRHOSIS	-	-	-	+	-

TABLE 3 : STATE OF HBV DNA IN THE LIVER, PRESENCE OF DNA IN THE SERUM AND SEROLOGICAL STATUS OF HBsAg NEGATIVE CHRONIC HEPATITIS (11 CASES).

In addition we recently identified other restriction DNA patterns in some HBeAg positive patients : free viral DNA without viral multiplication associated with high molecular weight DNA band, and free oligomeric viral DNA sequences (unpublished observation).

c) <u>HBsAg negative patients</u>. The restriction DNA patterns observed for HBsAg positive chronic carriers can also be observed for those patients with HBsAg negative chronic liver disease. Indeed we have now observed the presence of HBV DNA sequences in 23 liver samples from 51 non alcoholic patients with HCA. Moreover HBV DNA was also detectable in 2 of the 29 serum tested from these patients. (Manuscript in preparation). (Table 4).

HBsAg NEGATIVE HCA

NUMBER OF PATIENTS	ANTI HBc	ANTI HBs	HBV DNA LIVER	HBV DNA SERUM
7	+	-	4 + 3 -	0 2
16	+	+	13 + 3 -	1/11
1	-	+	1 -	NT
27	-	-	6 + 21 -	1/16
51	23	17	23	2/29

III. Extrahepatic localisation of HBV DNA.

We have studied extrahepatic samples obtained at autopsy from two patients : a 80 years old woman with an HBsAg positive hepatocellular carcinoma and a 67 years old man with an acute severe protracted hepatitis and a glomerulonephritis (A. Dejean. submitted for publication). HBV DNA sequences unrelated to a blood contamination were demonstrated in the hepatic, pancreatic and renal tissues in the two patients and in the skin in one of them. The restriction DNA patterns were consistent with the integration of the viral DNA at a limited number of sites.

IV. Detection of the HBV DNA in the serum using a "spot"
     test method (Scotto. Hepatology, 1983).

When 86 HBsAg and HBeAg positive sera were analyzed HBV DNA was demonstrated in 72 of them. This confirmed that HBeAg is a marker of active viral multiplication but also showing that its disapearence from the serum is delayed after the viral multiplication as ended. Indeed serological follow up of BHV DNA negative HBeAg positive patients showed a seroconversion to antiHBe in five. When 112 HBsAg negative sera were analyzed HBV DNA was detected in 6 of them. (5 with HBV antibodies, 1 without serological markers).

DISCUSSION

The detection of HBV DNA sequences provides new data on the epidemiology of the HBV infection and the mechanisms of HBV chronic infection. In addition it may have direct clinical implications.

HBV DNA as an epidemiological marker

The finding of HBV DNA sequences in many of our patients with chronic liver disease (including HCC) despite the absence of detectable HBsAg in the serum shows that the viral DNA sequences may persist in a liver when the HBV antibodies are present in the serum or even when no HBV serological markers are detectable. This is in accordance with studies using immunohistochemical technics[*]or very sensitive radioimmunoassays for the detection of the surface antigen (Wands, 1982).
This suggests that such chronic liver disease may be related to an HBV infection (or to a very closely related virus). Epidemiological studies in different countries will allow to compare the frequency of such findings.
[*] Bréchot 1981, Vergagni 1982.

State of HBV DNA in chronic liver disease

The presence of integrated HBV DNA sequences in both the tumorous and nontumorous liver cells of patients with HCC have been reported by several laboratories (Bréchot, 1982. Shafritz, 1982. Chen, 1982. Edman, 1981). The restriction DNA patterns can be identical in the tumorous and nontumorous cells in early HCC but generally differ in advanced HCC. HBV DNA linked to cellular DNA fragments have also been identified in long term HBV chronic carriers without HCC (Bréchot, 1982. Shafritz, 1982. Kim, 1982) but also in short term chronic carriers (Bréchot, Kim). Thus the integration of the viral DNA sequences can be an early event during the HBV infection. At that stage the restriction DNA pattern seems generally consistent with integration of the viral DNA sequences at multiple different sites in the host genome. The finding of discrete bands in the liver DNA pattern from long term chronic carriers may reflect either a clonal proliferation of some infected cells or, more likely, a selection of cells with integration of the viral DNA sequences at particular sites. Promoting factors could be involved in the development of the tumors from these infected cells. The possibility of a non random integration of the viral DNA into the cellular DNA is raised by the finding of discrete bands in the restriction DNA patterns from both hepatic or nonhepatic tissue. The cloning procedures will be necessary to ascertain the presence of integrated viral DNA sequences and to study the specificity of these integration sites. This seems particularly important to distinguish between free oligomers including cellular DNA sequences and a true integration event. The transferhybridization procedure distinguish between several restriction DNA patterns : viral multiplication (generally observed in HBeAg positive patients), free viral DNA without viral multiplication (observed in HBeAg positive or negative patients), free oligomeric viral DNA and incorporation of the viral DNA sequences into cellular DNA sequences (i.e. : integration); Prospective studies are now needed to analyse the prognostic value of the different restriction DNA patterns.

Clinical implication of HBV DNA detection

Antiviral drugs, such as adenine arabinoside or interferon, although possibly effective against the viral multiplication are unlikely to have any effect on integrated sequences. The presence of these integrated sequences in HBeAg positive patients could explain the persistence of HBsAg in the serum after effective treatment with adenine arabinoside. Moreover the comparison between the detection of HBeAg and HBV DNA in

the serum indicates that molecular hybridization not only
provides a more sensitive and more direct method for detecting HBV but also defines serological patterns which can
predict the further appearance of anti-e in serum.

Finally since HBV DNA sequences can be identified in the
pancreas, kidney and skin, it will be important to détermine
if they have a pathogenic role.

Bréchot C, Pourcel C, Dejean A, Louise A, Scotto J, Hadchouel
  M, Tiollais P (1982). State of hepatitis B virus DNA in
  liver diseases. Hepatology 2 : 27S.
Bréchot C, Trépo C, Bradistilova N and al. (1980). Hepatitis
  B core antigen in hepatocytes of patients with chronic ac-
  tive hepatitis. Dig Dis Sci 25 : 593.
Chen DS, Hoyer BH, Nelson J, Purcell RH, Gerin JL (1982).
  Detection and properties of hepatitis B viral DNA in liver
  tissues from patients with hepatocellular carcinoma. Hepa-
  tology 2 : 42S.
Dejean A, Lugassy C, Zafrani S, Tiollais P, Bréchot C. Submitted for publication.
Edman JC, Gray PG, Valenzuela P (1980). Integration of hepatitis B virus sequences and their expression in a human
  hepatoma cell. Nature (Lond) 286 :535.
Kam W, Rall LB, Smuckler EA, Schmid R, Rutter W (1982). Hepatitis B viral DNA in liver and serum of asymptomatic carriers. Proc Natl Acad Sci USA 79 :7522.
Scotto J, Hadchouel M, Hery C, Yvart J, Tiollais P, Bréchot
  C (1983). Detection of hepatitis B virus DNA in serum by a
  simple spot hybridization technique : comparison with
  results for other viral markers. Hepatology 3 : 279.
Shafritz DA (1982). Hepatitis B virus DNA molecules in the
  liver of hepatitis B surface antigen carriers : mechanistic
  considérations in the pathogenesis of hepatocellular car-
  cinoma. Hepatology 2 : 35s.
Shafritz DA, Lieberman HM, Isselbacher KJ, Wands JR (1982).
  Monoclonal radioimmunoassays for hepatitis B surface antigen : Demonstration of hepatitis B virus DNA or related
  sequences in serum and viral epitopes in immune complexes.
  Proc Natl Acad Sci USA 79 : 5675.
Southern EM (1975). Detection of specific sequences among
  DNA fragments separated by gel electrophoresis. J Mol Biol
  98 : 503.
Vergani D, Locasciulli A, Masera G, Alberti A, Moroni G, Tee
  DEH, Portmann B, Mieli Vergani G, Eddleston ALWF (1982).
  Histological evidence of hepatitis-B-virus infection with
  negative serology in children with acute leukaemia who
  develop chronic liver disease. Lancet : 361.

Viral Hepatitis and Delta Infection, pages 357–367
© 1983 Alan R. Liss, Inc., 150 Fifth Avenue, New York, NY 10011

PROPHYLAXIS OF VIRAL HEPATITIS: TRANSFUSION TRANSMITTED DISEASE AND THE HEPATITIS B VACCINE

Paul V. Holland, M.D.

Chief, Blood Bank Department
Clinical Center, N.I.H.
Bethesda, Maryland 20205

Introduction

Prophylaxis is the prevention of disease or the use of preventive treatment to obviate disease. The word prophylaxis comes from the Greek word, prophylassein, which means to keep guard before. For viral hepatitis this would encompass any means to prevent transmission of the viruses as well as specific treatments which would eliminate susceptibility to the hepatitis viruses.

The purpose of this paper is to describe the prophylaxis of viral hepatitis in three areas. The first area is the prevention of transfusion associated viral hepatitis; this involves both specific approaches to the known viruses which cause hepatitis and non-specific means to reduce the risk of transmission of undefined viral hepatitis agents (so called non-A, non-B viruses) which can be transmitted by blood products. The second area is the use of the hepatitis B virus (HBV) vaccine in the immunization of susceptible, high-risk groups to prevent the occurrence of this largely avoidable viral disease before exposure. The third area is the use of the HBV vaccine along with hyper-immune globulin to hepatitis B in susceptible individuals acutely exposed to infectious, HBV-containing material to minimize hepatitis B disease in this situation.

Prevention of Transfusion-transmitted Viral Hepatitis

Specific measures to reduce the risk of transfusion-transmitted viral hepatitis are directed against the known etiologic agents of viral hepatitis. The optimal method is to be able to identify all virus carriers before they donate blood; alternatively, the blood from such individuals should be tested for ability to transmit hepatitis before it is infused. If these two means are not sufficient, then patients at high risk of developing transfusion-transmitted viral hepatitis type B should be immunized to prevent this disease from occuring.

The transmission of viral hepatitis type A by blood transfusion rarely occurs. There does not seem to be a carrier state for the hepatitis A virus (HAV) so this disease can only be transmitted through the blood for a very short period of time. For this to happen a blood donor would have to be in the incubation period for viral hepatitis type A and yet not be symptomatic at the time of blood donation. In addition, most adults who require transfusions have already been exposed to HAV earlier in life and are immune to reinfection; this can be verified by testing for anti-HAV. So, while we cannot easily identify a person who is in the presymptomatic infectious period for HAV infection, transfusion of blood products does not put most recipients at risk of type A hepatitis.

Viral hepatitis type B can easily be transmitted by blood products; however, we have at least three effective approaches to minimize its spread by transfusions. These means have appreciably reduced the risk of HBV transmission through blood despite the fact that there is an asymptomatic carrier state for the HBV. First, in evaluating potential blood donors, they are asked a number of questions about their health and hepatitis history. If they have a history of viral hepatitis or unexplained jaundice, they are permanently rejected as blood donors. If they have had recent exposure to someone with viral hepatitis or if they have been transfused or otherwise exposed to blood products, they are deferred for 6 months (the maximum incubation period) for this disease. Donors who have received hepatitis B immune globulin (HBIG) for exposure to infectious HBV containing material are asked to wait one year before giving blood. Blood donors are also asked about symptoms of viral hepatitis and deferred if it appears they may be

developing this disease. Second, highly sensitive tests
for hepatitis B surface antigen (HBsAg) can identify most
asymptomatic carriers of the hepatitis B virus. It is a
requirement to test all blood products intended for transfusion for HBsAg. Tests for HBsAg are widely available,
specific, easy to perform, and objective; routine screening
of blood donors with the HBsAg test will pick up the vast
majority of HBV carriers as well as individuals in the
presymptomatic phase of acute type B hepatitis. Since a
few HBV carriers appear to be missed by HBsAg testing, it
has been suggested that anti-HBc (antibody to the hepatitis
B core antigen) be used to identify such individuals
(Holland 1982). While this test might further reduce the
risk of HBV transmission through blood transfusion, it is
unclear whether actual anti-HBc testing for this purpose
would be cost effective. The few blood donors with subde-
tectable HBsAg (and thus HBV) who would be identified by
anti-HBc testing would be rejected along with many more
donors with anti-HBc plus antibody to HBsAg (anti-HBs);
these latter donors are not HBV carriers - they are immune
to hepatitis B. Finally, there is a third approach to
prevention of HBV transmission by blood products. Patients
who are going to receive many blood products throughout
their lives, e.g., those with hemophilia or thalassemia
major, should receive the hepatitis B vaccine as early in
life as possible (Krugman 1982). The HBV vaccine will
elicit protective antibody (antibody to the hepatitis B
surface antigen) in most vaccinated individuals and
prevent this type of hepatitis from ever occurring. Thus,
even when these patients receive blood from donors with
HBV missed by routine HBsAg testing, the anti-HBs produced
in response to the vaccine would protect them against viral
hepatitis type B.

At the current time, non-A, non-B viral hepatitis
accounts for most cases of transfusion transmitted viral
hepatitis (Alter et al 1982). Unfortunately as the name
implies, we have not been able to define the virus (or
viruses) which cause this disease. Despite publication of
numerous papers purporting to have a test for non-A, non-B
viral antigens or antibodies, a reproducible test system
is still not here (Alter et al 1982). Only when specific,
verifiable non-A, non-B tests become available will we
be able to effectively reduce the risk of transmission of
this disease by blood products. It is clear that an asymptomatic carrier state exists for the non-A, non-B agent

(or agents) and that this disease is a frequent complication of blood transfusion; however, methods to reduce
the risk of transfusion transmitted non-A, non-B hepatitis
must, at the current time, be nonspecific.

The cytomegalovirus (CMV) is hepatotropic and can
occasionally cause transfusion associated viral hepatitis
(Alter et al 1982). This does not seem to be a major
problem except for some specific patient populations,
e.g., transfused premature neonates born of CMV-antibody-
negative mothers. The use of CMV-antibody negative blood
donors (or better still donors who are not excreting CMV)
can obviate the transmission of CMV to high risk recipients.
The use of white-cell poor blood products (e.g., deglycero-
lized frozen red cells) may be an easier solution to CMV
disease prevention in high risk, transfusion recipients
than obtaining blood from CMV antibody negative donors
(since 50-70% of adult blood donors have CMV antibody).

A number of nonspecific means to reduce transfusion
associated hepatitis have been recommended. These can be
of benefit in reducing the risk of non-A, non-B (NANB)
hepatitis transmission by blood products since no test
exists yet to identify NANB carriers. First of all,
blood products should always be used appropriately and
judiciously. Avoidance of unnecessary transfusions and
use of lower risk (unpooled) blood products will prevent
some transfusion-transmitted viral hepatitis. Auto-
transfusion should be employed wherever possible as this
will provide the safest blood for a patient. Second,
nonspecific tests to identify NANB carriers might be
tried, e.g., alanine amino transferase (ALT) testing and
anti-HBc testing; but these are generally wasteful of
donors, not proven to be effective, and they generate
additional problems for all concerned (Holland 1982).
Third, physicians should be on the lookout for cases
of transfusion transmitted viral hepatitis. By placing
hepatitis implicated blood donors on hepatitis suspect or
hepatitis rejection lists, high risk donors can be identified, and prevented from giving blood. Volunteer blood
donors should be used instead of paid, commercial blood
donors; the commercial blood donor carries a much higher
risk of transmitting viral hepatitis through his blood
than does a volunteer blood donor. Finally, while the use
of immune serum globulin and frozen blood transfusions
have been advocated as means to reduce the risk of trans-

fusion associated hepatitis, neither is well proven
(Holland 1982).

Immunization with the Hepatitis B Virus Vaccine

HBsAg can be purified from the plasma of asymptomatic
hepatitis B virus carriers and prepared into a safe,
immunogenic, and effective vaccine against hepatitis B
virus infections. Thus, HBV vaccine has become the preventive treatment of choice for hepatitis B infections.
Widespread use of this vaccine could interupt transmission
of hepatitis B virus, including HBV infections caused by
blood transfusions (Krugman 1982).

Initial studies with HBV vaccine showed it to be
both safe, immunogenic, and protective against inocula
known to be infectious for hepatitis B. Preliminary trials
were carried out in chimpanzees. Subsequently, safety and
immunogenicity studies were extended to human volunteers.
To date the vaccine has proven to be completely safe and
highly immunogenic. The vast majority of normal individuals
become immunized to the vaccine and develop anti-HBs; this
includes newborns, children, and adults. Three doses of
the vaccine elicit high titered anti-HBs which appears to
last for years.

Numerous efficacy studies on the HBV vaccine illustrate
its marked protective effect in humans too. By all
criteria, the vaccine is highly protective (Szmuness et al
1980). Almost 100% of individuals who develop anti-HBs in
response to the HBV vaccine are protected against overt
and subclinical evidence of hepatitis B infection. This
was true under a variety of high risk situations for HBV
transmission (Szmuness et al 1980, Maupas et al 1981).
There are a number of high risk groups of individuals who
should receive the hepatitis B virus vaccine. All of
these at risk groups have frequent and significant exposure
to blood and excreta from HBsAg-positive patients or are
transfused with many blood products, some of which may
contain sub-detectable quantities of the hepatitis B virus.
Thus, health care workers exposed to blood and specimens
from hospital patients, patients in dialysis and oncology
units, chronically transfused patients such as those with
hemophilia or thalassemia major, and abusers of illicit
intravenous drugs are all at elevated risk of developing
viral hepatitis type B. In addition, sexual contacts of

individuals with acute or chronic type B hepatitis or chronic HBsAg carriers have an increased risk of developing hepatitis B. This includes heterosexual partners, homosexual contacts, and prostitutes. The other major group at high risk is the neonate born of a HBsAg-positive, HBeAg-positive mother. The risk of such newborn babies of becoming HBsAg carriers is close to 100% (Beasley et al 1981); the chance of such a neonate who becomes a chronic carrier of HBsAg to eventually develop hepatocellular cancer is enormously increased over those babies without the HBsAg carrier state.

Anti-HBs testing of members of hepatitis B high risk groups should be performed before HBV vaccination. Individuals who already have anti-HBs are immune and do not need to receive the HBV vaccine. It is cost-effective to perform anti-HBs testing because of the high frequency of prior (often inapparent) HBV infection in the high risk groups and the high cost of the HBV vaccine. While the HBV vaccine is one of the safest, most immunogenic, and most effective vaccines ever made, it is also the most expensive produced to date.

Individuals with high levels of anti-HBs (S/N greater than 10 or more than 50 mIU/ml) will almost always have specific anti-HBs by the generally available tests for this antibody (Tedder 1983). In those individuals with low levels of anti-HBs (S/N from 2.2 to 10 or <50 mIU/ml of antibody to HBsAg), the test may be falsely positive in up to one third of cases (Tedder et al 1980). If the anti-HBs test is falsely positive, then the individual would not be protected against a subsequent HBV infection. To ascertain if a low value for anti-HBs is specific, three techniques may be used, in increasing order of certainty. If the anti-HBs test of low level is repeatable, it is most likely truly positive. If the person with low level anti-HBs also has anti-HBc, it is likely that the anti-HBs is real. Finally, specificity testing can be performed to determine if the anti-HBs test is correctly positive; a serum with HBsAg can be used to neutralize the presumed anti-HBs and compared to the effect of a serum which does not have HBsAg (which should have little effect on the test other than dilution of the anti-HBs).

Since such a high proportion of normal individuals respond with anti-HBs formation to the HBV vaccine,

there is little reason to verify that they have been
immunized. Such testing is not to be recommended unless
there is some reason to believe that anti-HBs has not
formed. This might include the elderly who respond less
well or apply to situations where subsequent overt exposure
to HBsAg occurs, as with a known needle-stick exposure.

When a patient group is known to be less responsive to
the HBV vaccine, testing for anti-HBs is appropriate.
Individuals who do not respond to the standard dose of
the HBV vaccine may still be susceptible to HBV infection.
Patients with renal insufficiency who are undergoing
dialysis may require higher or additional doses of the HBV
vaccine to insure seroconversion to anti-HBs positivity.

The HBV vaccine has now been given to over 200,000
recipients. All studies to date document its remarkable
safety. In the placebo controlled, efficacy trials, except
for an increased frequency of a sore arm, side effects of
the vaccine were no more common than those after the placebo.
Two major concerns have emerged, however: The risk of the
Guillain-Barré syndrome and the risk of the acquired immune
deficiency syndrome (AIDS). Some anecdotal data are available on these two concerns. Two cases of Guillain-Barré
syndrome have occurred in the more than 200,000 HBV vaccine
recipients; one was clearly related to a cytomegalovirus
infection, but the etiology of the other is unexplained.
This frequency of Guillain-Barré Syndrome is, however,
less than that expected to occur by chance alone in any
population of 200,000. Two cases of AIDS have appeared
among the gay men who were part of one of the efficacy
trials for the HBV vaccine; this is a rate of 2.4/1,000.
However, among gay men who did not participate in the
vaccine trial (most already had serologic evidence of
HBV exposure) 16 of 3,646 have developed AIDS; this is a
rate of 4.4/1,000. While the two groups are not strictly
comparable, there does not appear to be an increased
risk of AIDS among recipients of the HBV vaccine. No
health care individuals or non homosexual recipients of
the HBV vaccine have developed AIDS to date.

Recombinant DNA technology offers the promise of HBV
vaccines without the worry of adventitious infectious
agents. Such "synthetic" HBV vaccines should also be
cheaper and thus more available than the current type of
vaccine. The integration of the gene for HBsAg into

vaccinia virus is an example of this novel technology
which holds promise for future applications (Smith et al
1983). It will be some time before such new vaccines have
been similarly proven to be safe, immunogenic and effective,
and then generally available for use.

The HBV vaccine has not been evaluated in the transfusion setting but there is no reason to believe that it
would not be effective. If patients are immunized with HBV
vaccine and develop anti-HBs before transfusion with HBV
containing blood products, they should be protected against
HBV infection. If they are going to receive many transfusions in their lives, HBV immunization should be performed.

Prophylaxis after Acute Exposure to HBV

Individuals without anti-HBs are occasionally acutely
exposed to the HBV. This most commonly means a health care
worker who accidentially sticks himself with a needle used
to draw blood from a patient positive for HBsAg. At this
time prophylaxis with HBIG is the recommended treatment
(Recommendations of the Immunization Practices Advisory
Committee 1981). Two doses of this hyperimmune globulin
with high levels of anti-HBs will provide temporary, passive
protection against overt hepatitis B disease; but HBIG is
not 100% effective in eliminating clinical disease. In
fact, HBIG does not prevent infection but make the disease
more often subclinical (Hoofnagle et al 1979). In addition,
individuals receiving HBIG who do not become infected with
HBV will remain susceptible after the passively administered
anti-HBs is no longer present (four to six months later).

The hepatitis B vaccine is intended to provide pre-
exposure prophylaxis but may be of some benefit as post-
exposure prophylaxis too. In HBV vaccine efficacy trials
among high risk groups, there were fewer overt cases of
hepatitis B in the vaccine groups compared to the placebo
groups during the first two months of the studies (Szmuness
et al 1980). This suggests that the vaccine was of benefit
in minimizing clinical disease but not infection if given
during the incubation phase of hepatitis B. The rates of
infection as measured by serologic tests for hepatitis B
infection were the same in the vaccine and placebo groups
even though there was less clinical disease in the former.

Newborn infants with passively acquired anti-HBs from
their mothers will respond as well to the HBV vaccine as
infants without such antibody (Barin et al 1982). In addition, volunteers given HBIG in one arm and HBV vaccine in
the other had the same frequency of immunization and level
of anti-HBs response as volunteers given just the vaccine
alone (Szmuness et al 1981). So, since the HBV vaccine
will elicit anti-HBs even in the face of exogenous anti-
HBs, the optimal prophylaxis for susceptible individuals
acutely exposed to infectious, HBV containing material may
be the simultaneous use of vaccine and hyperimmune globulin.
The beneficial effects of both may then be realized, without
the worry of interference, and long term protection will
also result. The HBIG will provide immediate, circulating
anti-HBs and the vaccine will elicit long-term production
of this antibody in the recipient. The beneficial effects
of both measures should be additive. HBIG plus HBV vaccine
should afford maximal prophylaxis when susceptible individuals are exposed to HBV containing material. This
combination has not been proven effective yet in humans
exposed to infections HBV containing material but it would
appear to be the treatment of choice in this situation.

Conclusion

Transmission of viral hepatitis can be minimized by
prophylaxis in many situations. In the transfusion setting
the risk of hepatitis can be reduced by several specific
and some nonspecific measures. The hepatitis B virus
vaccine provides effective prophylaxis against this viral
agent in most circumstances of exposure. For individuals
without anti-HBs who are acutely exposed to hepatitis B
virus containing material, the combination of vaccine and
HBIG should provide the most effective treatment for
disease prevention, in this situation where it is too late
for the more usual preventive measure.

References

Alter HJ, Purcell RH, Feinstone SM, Tegtmeier GE (1982).
Non-A, non-B hepatitis: Its relationship to cytomegalo-
virus, to chronic hepatitis, and to direct and indirect test
methods. In Szmuness W, Alter HJ, Maynard JE (eds): "Viral
Hepatitis: 1981 International Symposium," Philadelphia,
Franklin Institute Press, p 279.

Barin F, Goudeau A, Denis F, Yvonnet B, Chiron JP, Coursaget P, Diop Mar I (1982). Immune response in neonates to hepatitis B vaccine. Lancet i:251.

Beasley RP, Hwang L-Y, Lin C-C, Stevens CE, Wang K-Y, Sun T-S, Hsieh F-J, Szmuness W (1981). Hepatitis B immune globulin in the interruption of perinatal transmission of hepatitis B virus carrier state: Initial report of a randomized double-blind placebo-controlled trial. Lancet ii:388.

Holland PV (1982). Available means to further reduce posttransfusion hepatitis. In Szmuness W, Alter HJ, Maynard JE (eds): "Viral Hepatitis: 1981 International Symposium," Philadelphia, Franklin Institute Press, p 563.

Hoofnagle JH, Seeff LB, Bales ZB, Wright EC, Zimmerman HJ, Veterans Administration Cooperative Study Group (1979). Passive-active immunity from hepatitis B immune globulin: Reanalysis of a Veterans Administration cooperative study of needle-stick hepatitis. Ann Int Med 91:813.

Krugman S (1982). The newly licensed hepatitis B vaccine: characteristics and indications for use. JAMA 247:2012.

Maupas P, Chiron J-P, Barin F, Coursaget P, Goudeau A, Perrin J, Denis F, Diop Mar I (1981). Efficacy of hepatitis B vaccine in prevention of early HBsAg carrier state in children: Controlled trial in an endemic area (Senegal). Lancet i:289.

Recommendations of the Immunization Practices Advisory Committee (ACIP) (1981). Immune globulins for protection against viral hepatitis. MMWR 30:423.

Smith GL, Mackett M, Moss B (1983). Infectious vaccinia virus recombinants that express hepatitis B virus surface antigen. Nature 302:490.

Szmuness W, Stevens CE, Harley EJ, Zang EA, Oleszko WR, William DC, Sadovsky R, Morrison JM, Kellner A (1980). Hepatitis B vaccine: Demonstration of efficacy in a controlled trial in a high-risk population in the United States. New Engl J Med 303:833.

Szmuness W, Stevens CE, Oleszko WR, Goodman A (1981).
Passive-active immunization against hepatitis B:
Immunogenicity studies in adult Americans. Lancet
i:575.

Tedder RS (1983). Hepatitis B vaccination policy.
Lancet i:533.

Tedder RS, Cameron CH, Wilson R, Howell DR,
Colgrove A, Barbara JAJ (1980). Contrasting
patterns and frequency of antibodies to the surface,
core and e antigens of hepatitis B virus in blood
donors and in homosexual patients. J Med Virol 6:323.

NEW APPROACHES TO HEPATITIS B VACCINES

John L. Gerin, Ph.D.[1] and Robert H. Purcell, M.D.[2]

[1]Dept. of Microbiology, Georgetown Univ. Med. Ctr., Rockville, MD 20852 [2]National Institute of Allergy & Infectious Diseases, NIH, Bethesda, MD 20205

Hepatitis B virus (HBV) infection places a large burden of liver disease on the world population. The recent availability of vaccines which effectively interdict the transmission of HBV to high risk individuals now provides opportunities for broad control of this serious public health problem.

CURRENT HBV VACCINES

Current HBV vaccines consist of subviral forms (20 nm) of hepatitis B surface antigen (HBsAg) purified from the plasma of chronic HBsAg carriers, inactivated with formalin and absorbed to alum. The purification methods have been described in detail in the literature and are generally based on certain biophysical properties of the 20 nm HBsAg form (e.g., buoyant density and size; Gerin 1975) sometimes coupled with various chemical treatments and enzymatic digestions (Tabor 1983); alternative methods of purification and inactivation have also been used (Reesink 1981). A great deal of analytical data have been accumulated on the purified HBsAg preparations. The NIAID vaccines (McAuliffe 1982), for example, are characterized for uniform biophysical, biochemical and immunological properties (Table 1). A detailed discussion of these properties is beyond the scope of this paper; several points, however, should be emphasized. The extinction coefficient ($A^{1\%}_{280nm}$) is readily determined and represents an important index of purity. Values less than 6.0 usually reflect the contribution of bound albumin to the

---

TABLE 1. HBV VACCINES PREPARED FROM HUMAN PLASMA
   BIOPHYSICAL, BIOCHEMICAL AND IMMUNOLOGICAL
                  CHARACTERISTICS

Buoyant Density	Extinction Coefficient
Sedimentation	Polypeptide Composition
Coefficient	Protein Concentration
Morphology (EM)	

HBsAg Concentration and Subtype
Guinea Pig/Mouse Potency

HBcAg –	HBeAg –
HBV DNA –	Anti-HBc –
HBV DNA Polymearase –	
Delta AG –	

---

final protein content (Shih 1980) and can be confirmed by
conventional polypeptide analysis. The antigenic content
is accurately determined by parallel-line
radioimmunoassays and should agree with the protein data
within assay limits. These analyses show a good
correlation with animal potency data using either guinea
pigs (Hartley Strain) or outbred mice (ICR). In our
experience, final HBV vaccines yield guinea pig and mouse
potency (immunizing dose 50%) endpoints of 100 and 60 ng,
respectively. While such analyses are useful for
lot-to-lot comparisons, there is insufficient data as yet
to establish a predictive correlation between the potency
of vaccines in laboratory animals and humans. Prior to
inactivation, the bulk concentrates are demonstrated to be
free of markers of the hepatitis B virion (HBcAg; Purcell
1974: endogenous DNA polymerase activity; Kaplan 1973:
and, HBV DNA; Berninger 1982) and delta antigen (Rizzetto
1980). Such in vitro analyses would detect gross
contamination of the vaccine with HBV or delta agent prior
to the expensive in vivo safety tests in chimpanzees. We
have used the absence of HBeAg and anti-HBc activities in
the preinactivated concentrate as an indirect measure of
the purification methods.

TABLE 2. HEPATITIS B VACCINE: RISK FACTORS

Pooled Plasma Source of HBsAg

Residual HBV
Delta Agent
Non-A, Non-B Hepatitis Agent(s)
Other Viruses
Putative AIDS Agent

Recipient Response

None or Ineffective
"Auto-immune"
Paradoxical
Idiosyncratic

RISK FACTORS AND ALTERNATIVE VACCINES

While the number of vaccine recipients is still
relatively small by population standards, current HBV
vaccines have to date established an excellent record of
safety, immunogenicity and efficacy in clinical trials.
For purposes of this discussion, risk factors might be
conveniently separated into these associated with (1) the
pooled plasma source of HBsAg and (2) the recipient
response.

No vaccine has been 100% efficacious in the human
population and the HBV vaccines compare very favorably
with other licensed products (e.g., inactivated influenza
vaccine). Importantly, vaccine non-responsiveness does
not appear to identify a predilection of an individual to
chronicity upon natural infection (Szmuness 1980). The
earlier concerns about "autoimmunity" from HBV vaccination
and potential paradoxical effects have clearly been
dispelled by the clinical data and, of course, the
incidence of the rare idiosyncratic response will require
much larger numbers for assessment. The major concerns,
therefore, are associated with the use of pooled plasma as

the source of HBsAg and risk factors associated with the
plasma donor population. Yet, current manufacturing
procedures appear to be entirely successful in the
removal or inactivation of HBV and viruses which are
prevalent in the chronic HBV carrier population (non-A,
non-B, delta agent) and other viruses which are
occasionally transmitted by blood products. What are
the factors, therefore, which account for the current
interest in and pursuit of alternative HBV vaccines?
First, the cost of current vaccines virtually prohibits
their use in those areas of the world where HBV is
endemic and less expensive sources of HBsAg might
greatly alleviate this problem. Second, and possibly
more importantly, is the recent recognition in the
plasma donor population of current HBV vaccines of a
severe illness, known as Acquired Immune Deficiency
Syndrome (AIDS), which may be caused by a transmissible
agent. While studies indicate that vaccine recipients
of the Szmuness trial are at no greater risk to AIDS
than placebo controls (Stevens CE, personal
communication), the possibility that a putative AIDS
agent might be present in more recent lots of vaccine has
greatly inhibited the use of current vaccines.

Fortunately, alternative sources of HBsAg are
available (Table 3). On the basis of cost and safety,
recombinant DNA methods (using the S gene fragment of HBV
in eukaryotic cells) and chemical synthesis of HBsAg
peptides (predicted from the nucleotide sequence of the S
gene) appear to offer the greatest promise for the next
generation of HBV vaccines. Three different approaches
are described below.

NEW APPROACHES

We previously reported the construction and
propagation of a SV 40 virus recombinant carrying a
fragment of HBV DNA; this fragment included the continuous
nucleotide sequence (gene S) encoding HBsAg (Moriarty
1981). Eukaryotic cells infected with this recombinant
expressed and excreted HBsAg indistinguishable from the 20
nm HBsAg form isolated from human plasma. HBsAg purified
from tissue culture, inactivated with formalin and
absorbed to alum stimulated a brisk anti-HBs response in
2 chimpanzees and one animal, available to follow-up, was
protected upon experimental challenge with live virus

TABLE 3. HEPATITIS B VACCINES: SOURCE MATERIAL

HBsAg Source	Product
1. Human Plasma (Pooled)	20 nm
	Polypeptides
2. Hepatoma (Producer) Cell Lines	20 nm
3. Recombinant DNA Methods	
a. Prokaryotic	Polypeptides
b. Eukaryotic	
1. Yeast	20 nm
2. Mammalian	20 nm
4. Chemical Synthesis	Peptides

(Gerin 1983). These data represent the first report of
successful HBV vaccination using recombinant DNA
methodology and establish the validity of this general
approach. Obviously, other vectors must be engineered for
human use but such vaccines are clearly free from residual
HBV or other agents associated with human plasma source
material.

The second approach represents an interesting
variation of the recombinant DNA method for the generation
of HBsAg. Smith, et al (Smith 1983) recently described
the construction of infectious vaccinia virus recombinants
which express HBsAg. A fragment of HBV DNA containing the
S gene, under the control of vaccinia virus early
promoters, was used in the construction. Vaccination of
rabbits with the vaccinia recombinant virus produced
typical local skin lesions and humoral antibodies to
HBsAg. These experiments offer the obvious possibility of

TABLE 4.   EFFICACY OF SYNTHETIC PEPTIDE 49
IMMUNIZATION IN THE CHIMPANZEE MODEL OF HBV INFECTION[a]

Chimpanzee	Incub. Period		Duration		Max Value	
	ALT	HBsAg	ALT	HBsAg	ALT	HBsAg
Controls (X_8)	14	7	15	21	1181	105
Experimental						
#1	12	6	9	14	1390	104
#2	–	9	–	7	–	9
#3	–	–	–	–	–	–

----

[a] Chimpanzees were challenged at time zero with $10^{3.5}$ CID of HBV/ayw, i.v.

[b] Incubation period in weeks to first appearance of abnormal ALT (50 I.U.) or HBsAg (2.1 P/N, Ausria).

[c] Duration of abnormal ALT or HBsAg in weeks.

[d] Alanine aminotransferase values are expressed in international units and HBsAg in P/N ratios by Ausria assay.

[e] Values represent averages of eight animals (X_8).

a live vaccination strategy used so successfully for smallpox eradication. This approach could offer considerable cost as well as safety advantages over current HBV vaccines.

Lastly, Lerner, et al (Lerner 1981) demonstrated that antisera to synthetic peptides predicted from the nucleotide sequence of various regions of the S gene of HBV reacted with native HBsAG. Subsequent studies (Gerin

and Alexander 1983) revealed that one such peptide
(representing amino acid residues 110-137 from the
N-terminal end of the S gene product) stimulated a brisk
but transient anti-HBs response in 3 chimpanzees, the
relevant model of human response. Upon experimental
challenge with live virus (Table 4), one animal was
protected from infection, another was infected without
disease and the third underwent a typical acute HBV
infection when compared with the average response
patterns of 8 experimentally-infected control animals.
Thus, despite the absence of humoral anti-HBs at time of
challenge, immunization with synthetic peptides resulted
in a pattern of partial protection.

SUMMARY

     Current HBV vaccines are composed of subviral forms
of HBsAg purified from pooled human plasma, inactivated
and absorbed to alum. These vaccines have established an
excellent record of safety and efficacy in clinical trials
to date. Economic factors and theoretical safety problems
associated with the plasma donor population, however, have
stimulated an intense interest in the development of
alternative vaccines for HBV. The recombinant DNA and
synthetic peptide approaches appear to offer the greatest
potential for future generations of HBV vaccines.
Such vaccines would be free of the potential safety
problems associated with plasma source material and could
assure the continued supply of uniform HBsAg for vaccine
use.

REFERENCES

Alexander J, McNab G, Saunders R (1978). Studies on in
  vitro production of HBsAg by a human hepatoma cell line.
  In: Pollard M (ed) "Perspectives in Virology 10", New
  York: Raven Press, p. 103.
Berninger M, Hammer M, Hoyer BH, Gerin JL (1982). An
  assay for the detection of the DNA genome of hepatitis B
  virus in serum. J Med Virol 9:57.
Crosnier J, Junger P, Courovce' AM, Laplanche A, Benhamou
  E, Degos F, Lacour B, Prunet P, Cerisier Y, Guesry P.
  (1981). Randomized placebo-controlled trial of
  hepatitis B surface antigen vaccine in French

haemodialysis units: I. Medical Staff. Lancet i:455

Gerin JL, Holland PV, Purcell RH (1971). Australia antigen: large-scale purification from human serum and biochemical studies of its proteins. J Virol 7:569.

Gerin JL, Faust RM, Holland PV (1975). Biophysical characterization of the adr subtype of hepatitis B antigen and preparation of anti-r sera in rabbits. J Immunol 115:100.

Gerin JL, Alexander H, Shih JW-K, Purcell RH, Dapolito G, Engle R, Green N, Sutcliffe JG, Shinnick TM, Lerner RA (1983). Chemically synthesized peptides of hepatitis B surface antigen duplicate the d/y specificities and induce subtype-specific antibodies in chimpanzees. Proc Natl Acad Sci USA 80:2365.

Gerin JL, Lerner RA, Purcell RH. Alternative sources of hepatitis B vaccine. In: Second IABS Symposium on Viral Hepatitis, Athens Greece, In Press, 1983.

Kaplan PM, Greenman RL, Gerin JL, Purcell RH, Robinson WS (1973). DNA polymerase associated with human hepatitis B antigen. J Virol 12:995.

Lerner RA, Green N, Alexander H, Liu F-T, Sutcliffe JG, Shinnick TM (1981). Chemically synthesized peptides predicted from the nucleotide sequence of the hepatitis B virus genome elicit antibodies reactive with the native envelope protein of Dane particles. Proc Natl Acad Sci USA 78:3403.

Maupas P, Chiron J-P, Barin F, Coursaget P, Goudeau A, Perrin J, Denis F, Diop Mar I (1981). Efficacy of hepatitis B vaccine in prevention of early HBsAg carrier state in children: controlled trial in an endemic area (Senegal). Lancet i:289.

McAuliffe V, Purcell RH, Gerin JL (1980). Type B hepatitis: a review of current prospects for a safe and effective vaccine. Rev Infect Dis 2:470.

McAuliffe VJ, Purcell RH, Gerin JL, Tyeryar FJ (1982). In Szmuness W, Alter HJ, Maynard JE (eds): "Viral Hepatitis: 1981 International Symposium," Philadelphia: The Franklin Institute Press, p. 425.

Moriarty AM, Hoyer BH, Shih JW-K, Gerin JL, Hamer DH (1981). Expression of the hepatitis B surface antigen gene in cell culture using a simian virus 40 vector. Proc Natl Acad Sci, USA 78:2606.

Purcell RH, Gerin JL, Almeida JB, Holland PV (1974). Radioimmunoassay for the detection of the core of the Dane particle and antibody to it. Intervirology 2:231.

Purcell RH, Gerin JL (1978). Hepatitis B vaccines: on the

threshold. Am J Clin Pathol 70:159.
Reesink HW, Reerink-Brongers EE, Brummelhuis HGJ,
  Lafeberschut LJTh, Van Elven EH, Duimel WJ, Balner H,
  Stitz LW, Vanden Ende MC, Fletkamp-Vroom TLM, Cohen HH
  (1981). Heat-inactivated HBsAg as a vaccine against
  hepatitis B. Antiviral Research 1:13.
Rizzetto M, Shih JW-K, Gerin JL (1980). The hepatitis B
  virus-associated delta antigen: isolation from liver,
  development of solid-phase radioimmunoassays for antigen
  and anti-delta and parital characterization of delta
  antigen. J Immunol 125:318.
Shih JW-K, Tan PL, Gerin JL (1980). Relationship of the
  large hepatitis B surface antigen polypeptide to human
  serum albumin. Infection and Immunity 28:459.
Smith GL, Mackett M, Moss B (1983). Infectious vaccinia
  virus recombinants that express hepatitis B virus
  surface antigen. Nature 302:490.
Szmuness W, Stevens CE, Harley EJ, Zang EA, Oleszko WR,
  William DC, Sadovsky R, Morrison JM, Kellner A (1980).
  Hepatitis B vaccine: demonstration of efficacy in a
  controlled clinical trial in a high-risk population in
  the United States. N Engl J Med 303:833.
Tabor E, Buynak E, Smallwood LA, Snoy P, Hilleman M and
  Gerety RJ (1983). Inactivation of hepatitis B virus by
  three methods: treatement with pepsin, urea or
  formalin. J Med Virol 11:1.
Zuckerman, AJ (1982). Virological approach to the
  prevention of primary liver cancer. Hepatology 2:67S.

Viral Hepatitis and Delta Infection, pages 379–393
© 1983 Alan R. Liss, Inc., 150 Fifth Avenue, New York, NY 10011

APPROACHES TO THE TREATMENT OF CHRONIC HEPATITIS B VIRAL INFECTION

H C THOMAS BSc PhD FRCP and A S F Lok MBBS MRCP

Reader in Medicine and Honorary Consultant
Physician : Honorary Lecturer in Medicine
Royal Free Hospital and Medical School

INTRODUCTION

Chronic infection with the hepatitis B virus (HBV) may result in a variety of hepatic lesions ranging from a carrier state with virtually normal histology, chronic lobular and persistent hepatitis, to chronic active hepatitis leading to cirrhosis. There are two phases of the chronic infection. In the first, which lasts several years and during which the patient's serum contains HBe antigen, the virus replicates and the patient's serum and other body fluids are infectious. During the second stage, viral replication ceases, the patient develops HBe antibody, and clones of hepatocytes containing integrated hepatitis B viral DNA continue to secrete hepatitis B surface antigen (Figure 1).

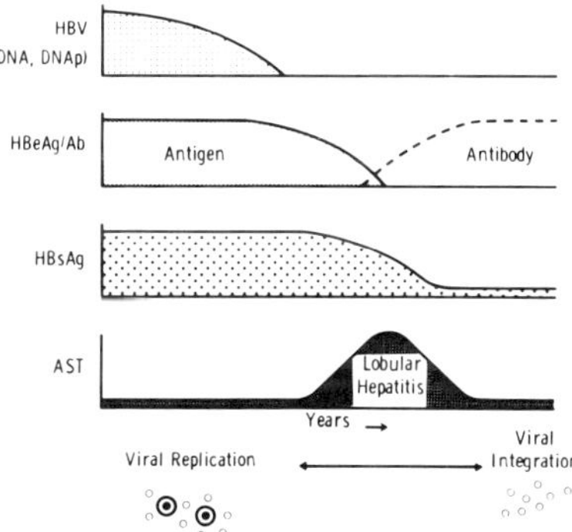

Fig. 1: virological and serological events during chronic HBV infection.

MECHANISMS OF LIVER DAMAGE

Several histological lesions are seen in these patients
at different times during infection (Thomas et al, 1982).
Focal liver cell necrosis, which is seen throughout the
lobule, occurs when there is active viral replication and is
maximal during HBe antigen to antibody seroconversion (Liaw
et al, 1983). At this stage the histological features are
similar to those seen in acute viral hepatitis. It seems
probable that 'focal necrosis' represents immune lysis of
hepatocytes which are actively replicating the virus.
Current evidence suggests that this is mediated by cytotoxic
T-cells (Montano et al, 1983; Eddleston et al, 1982). If
this phase of destruction of hepatocytes containing
replicating virus is protracted then hepatic fibrosis will
ensue. In other individuals elimination of hepatocytes
containing replicating virus is rapidly achieved and these
patients then develop either chronic persistent hepatitis or
become carriers with normal liver histology.

In rare patients viral replication may initiate an autoimmune process similar to that seen in lupoid chronic active
hepatitis (Eddleston and Williams, 1974). These patients,
probably because of a relative deficiency of suppressor cell
function (Thomas et al, 1982) develop liver membrane reactive
antibodies (Thomas et al, 1982) which result in piecemeal
necrosis of periportal hepatocytes. If this process
continues for a prolonged period of time cirrhosis will
develop.

After several years of infection, the patient will
develop clones of cells containing integrated hepatitis B
viral DNA (Shafritz et al, 1981; Brechot et al, 1981;
Fowler et al, 1983). These cells will continue to produce
HBs antigen after elimination of cells which are actively
replicating virus. It is probable that some of these cells
which contain the integrated viral genome will undergo
malignant transformation leading to the development of
primary liver cell cancer.

An additional complication in our understanding of the
pathogenesis of chronic hepatitis B virus infection has been
the presence of co-existant delta agent infection. This
superinfection is an important factor in determining the
severity and rate of progression of the disease. Recent
studies showed a higher proportion of patients with chronic

HBV and delta infection still have active liver disease
despite low level of viral replication and many have
progressed to cirrhosis at a much younger age (Lok et al,
1983; Rizzetto et al, 1983).

<u>THERAPEUTIC APPROACHES</u>

The aim of therapy in patients with chronic HBV
infection is to eradicate the virus in both its replicating
and non-replicating forms, thereby preventing the
development of progressive liver disease and liver cell
cancer. The approach to therapy will be dependent on the
phase of the infection (HBe antigen or antibody positive),
the predominant lesion (Focal lobular or periportal piecemeal
necrosis) and the presence or absence of clones of cells
containing integrated HBV-DNA.

During the HBe antigen positive phase of infection,
when there is active viral replication and focal liver cell
necrosis, attempts at therapy are directed towards
inhibition of viral replication.

Once the patient has ceased to replicate the virus
(HBe antibody positive phase), the level of inflammatory
necrosis of hepatocytes subsides and usually no therapy is
necessary. If the patient has already developed cirrhosis
there is a significant risk of development of primary liver
cell cancer (Beasley et al, 1981) presumably because of the
presence of clones of cells containing integrated HBV-DNA
(Thomas, 1983). Attempts to eliminate these cells usually
involve either stimulation of the host's immune system
(Thomas, 1979) or passive immunisation with antiviral
globulins (Thomas et al, 1982).

In some patients without detectable HBV replication
(HBe antibody positive with negative staining for hBc
antigen in the liver) in whom inflammatory necrosis of liver
cells continues (Hadziyannis et al, 1983), coexistent
delta infection should be suspected (Weller et al, 1983;
Lok et al, 1983). If this is excluded by serological or
immunohistological means, an autoimmune diathesis allowing
the development of liver membrane reactive antibodies should
be suspected (Thomas et al, 1982). This group of patients
may respond to moderate doses of prednisolone (Weller et
al, 1982).

A)   DRUGS USED TO INHIBIT HEPATITIS B VIRAL REPLICATION

1.   <u>Interferon</u>

In uncontrolled studies, human leucocyte interferon
either alone or in combination with adenine arabinoside
(ARA-A) has been used to treat chronic HBV infection
(Scullard et al, 1981). In these studies 37% of patients
lost HBe antigen and DNA polymerase activity and seroconverted to anti-e. Some of these patients cleared HBs
antigen from their serum but this is extremely rare. These
changes in viral markers were accompanied by improvement in
symptoms, biochemistry and histology (Scullard et al, 1981).
These studies were not controlled and we know such changes
may occur spontaneously (Hoofnagle et al, 1981; Realdi et
al, 1980). A controlled study using human leucocyte
interferon alone at a much lower total dose, failed to show
any long term inhibition of viral replication (Schalm et
al, 1982). Controlled studies are still required with more
portracted and higher dose regimens.

Lymphoblastoid interferon is an alpha interferon
produced by stimulation of a human lymphoblastoid cell line
with sendai virus. It consists of a mixture of at least 8
glycoproteins. Inhibition of HBV replication can be
achieved with thrice weekly injections (Weller et al, 1982;
Lok et al, 1983) (Figure 2).

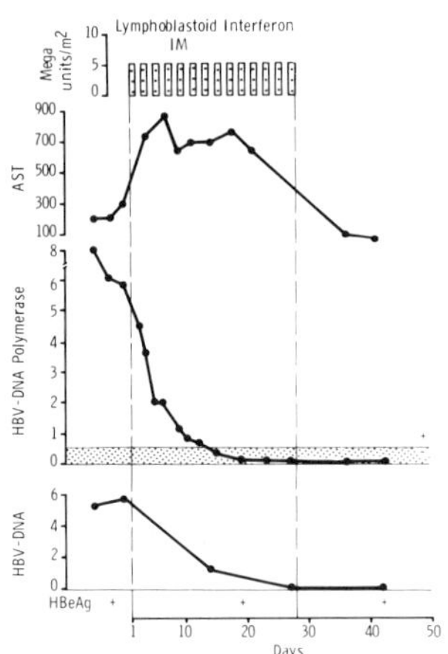

Fig. 2: lymphoblastoid interferon given thrice weekly can
produce permanent inhibition of HBV replication.

5 out of 9 patients who received 7.5 - 10 x 10^6 units of
lymphoblastoid interferon given as thrice weekly intra-
muscular injections, had permanent suppression of HBV
replication. Side-effects, especially the 'flu-like'
syndrome, were uncommon with the thrice weekly regime and
it was well tolerated for periods up to three months
(Lok   et al, 1983). This apparently safe and effective
regimen is now being evaluated in controlled studies.

Fibroblastoid interferon (IFN-β) has been shown to have
no significant antiviral activity in chronic HBV infection
(Weimar et al, 1979). The gamma interferons (IFN-ɣ) have
not yet beem produced in sufficient quantities to be
examined for therapeutic effect.

2.   Synthetic Antiviral Agents

Adenine Arabinoside (ARA-A) is a synthetic purine
nucleoside with a broad spectrum of antiviral activity
against DNA viruses (Shannon, 1975). Early uncontrolled
studies indicated that ARA-A had activity against HBV
(Pollard et al, 1978; Chadwick et al, 1978). In a
randomised controlled study of ARA-A (Bassendine et al, 1981),
4 out of 7 treated HBeAg positive patients lost DNA
polymerase activity with 3 losing HBeAg and showing a
significant decrease in HBsAg concentration and aspartate
transaminase. No such changes occurred in the control
group.

Although ARA-A has a low toxicity relative to other
anti-viral agents (Keeney, 1975), its usefulness is
limited by insolubility and the need for continuous
intravenous administration. Adenine arabinoside
monophosphate (ARA-AMP), the synthetic ester of ARA-A,
is at least four hundred times more water soluble. In 8
HBeAg positive patients with chronic liver disease, ARA-AMP
given intravenously or intramuscularly, six or twelve
hourly, produced inhibition of viral replication
(Weller et al, 1982). In three consecutive cases given a
one month course at a dosage of 5mg/kg/day as twice daily
i.m. injection, inhibition of viral replication was
permanent (Weller et al. 1982: Craxi et al. 1983). ARA-AMP
has now been assessed in a randomised controlled clinical
trial (Weller et al, 1983) in which 4 out of 15 treated
patients showed permanent inhibition of replication and
none of 14 untreated cases.

In attempts to produce higher response rates, more protracted therapeutic regimens are being examined. The limiting factor is the development of a sensory peripheral neuropathy.

Acycloguanosine (acyclovir) inhibits herpes simplex virus replication in vitro and in vivo, its action being dependent on phosphorylation of the drug by a virus coded thymidine kinase (Elion et al, 1977; Fyfe et al, 1978). In vitro studies have also shown activity against cytomegalo and Epstein-Barr viruses but at much higher drug concentrations (Tymes et al, 1981; Colby et al, 1980). However, a relatively high dose is required and extreme care should be taken especially in patients with pre-existing renal impairment or dehydration, as nephrotoxicity may develop (Bridgen et al, 1982). Further studies in chronic HBV infection are needed to establish a suitable regimen.

Intercalating agents such as chloroquine, quinacrine and chlorpromazine, can inhibit the HBV-DNA polymerase reaction in vitro, probably by acting as DNA template blockers (Hirschman and Garfunkel, 1978). They do not seem to be active in vivo (Thomas et al, 1980).

Trisodium Phosphonoformate is a pyrophosphate analogue which inhibits the HBV-DNA polymerase reaction in vitro (Helgstrand et al, 1980), but as yet there has been no report of its use in vivo.

3.   Manipulation of the Immune Response

In chronically infected patients, attempts have been made to manipulate the immune response by active and passive processes, including immunostimulation and immuno-suppression. Our knowledge of the immunopathogenesis of this disease is still incomplete so these approaches to therapy have largely been empirical. BCG seems to be the most promising immunostimulant therapy tried so far (Bassendine et al, 1980) but clearly controlled trials are now required. This form of treatment is of theoretical interest because potentially it would be effective in eliminating hepatocytes containing both replicating and integrated virus (Thomas et al, 1982).

Immunosuppression with prednisolone allows increased HBV replication (Weller et al, 1982; Scullard et al, 1982)

in patients who are already actively replicating the virus.
In patients already on prednisolone, stopping treatment often
resulted in cessation of viral replication. This has led
investigators to consider using a short course of steroid
administration as anti-viral therapy for HBe antigen positive
patients. The danger of precipitating severe liver cell
necrosis on withdrawing prednisolone exists due to sudden
lysis of large numbers of infected hepatocytes.

B)   APPROACHES TO THE ELIMINATION OF HEPATOCYTES CONTAINING
      INTEGRATED HBV-DNA

      The clearance of these cells can only be achieved by
stimulation of the endogenous immune lytic systems or by
administration of specific lytic agents. Their clearance is
necessary in patients who have already developed cirrhosis
but not in carriers with normal histology, since the former,
but not the latter, run the risk of malignant transformation
of these cells.

      Immunostimulation with BCG has produced encouraging
results in uncontrolled studies (Brzosko et al, 1978;
Bassendine et al, 1980) and further efforts are needed.

      More recently, following the observation that native
or toxin conjugated monoclonal anti-HBs will inhibit the
growth of malignantly transformed hepatocytes containing
integrated HBV-DNA (Thomas et al, 1982; Shouval et al,
1982; Oladapo et al, 1983), it has become apparent that
monoclonal anti-HBs may have some role in the elimination of
hepatocytes containing integrated HBV and further studies are
now in progress.

C)   TREATMENT OF AUTO-IMMUNE COMPONENT IN HBe ANTIBODY
      POSITIVE HBs ANTIGEN CARRIERS WITH CHRONIC ACTIVE
      HEPATITIS

      In a minority of patients inflammatory activity
continues after cessation of HBV replication. This may be
caused by superinfection with the delta agent and in others
by an autoimmune reaction initiated by the virus (Montano
et al, 1983; Eddleston and Williams, 1974). Co-existent

delta infection can be excluded by testing for serum anti-
delta or intrahepatic delta-antigen. In the remaining
patients, a trial of prednisolone 10-15 mg daily should
be undertaken.

D)   TREATMENT OF CO-EXISTENT DELTA INFECTION

Delta agent is a defective hepatitis agent dependent
on HBV for its replication, The effect of antiviral therapy
in delta infected carriers is unknown. Interferon is
effective in inhibiting replication of both DNA and RNA
viruses and may be more suitable than the arabinosides
which predominantly influence DNA synthesis. Clearly,
trials evaluating the efficacy of various antiviral
compounds should examine delta infected subjects as a
separate group.

<u>SUMMARY</u>

In HBeAg positive patients with a high level of viral
replication, antiviral therapy is the treatment of choice.
The most promising agents at the moment are ARA-AMP and
Interferon and both are being assessed in controlled clinical
trials. In the anti-HBe positive patients in whom continued
HBs antigenaemia is due to the presence of clones of cells
containing integrated virus, some form of immune
manipulation may be necessary. In rare cases in whom
continuing inflammatory activity is related to an autoimmune
reaction, low dose prednisolone may be beneficial.
Treatment for delta infection has yet to be evaluated but
antiviral agents such as interferon,which inhibit both
DNA and RNA viruses, may prove effective.

Although these forms of therapy are currently experimental, some are now entering phase III clinical trials.
It seems probable that the ultimate regimen will include
antiviral drugs and immune manipulation to adequately
eliminate hepatocytes containing replicating and integrated
virus. The latter is essential if we are to deal with the
problem of neoplasia as well as infectivity and
inflammatory liver disease.

Bassendine MF, Chadwick RG, Salmeron J, Shipton U, Thomas HC, Sherlock S (1981). Adenine arabinoside therapy in HBsAg-positive chronic liver disease : a controlled study. Gastroenterology 80 : 1016-1021.

Bassendine MF, Weller IVD, Murray A, Summers J, Thomas HC Sherlock S (1980). Treatment of HBsAg-positive chronic liver disease with Basicllus Calmetter Guerin (BCG). Gut 21: A915.

Beasley RP, Hwang LY, Lin CC (1981). Hepatocellular carcinoma and hepatitis B virus : a prospective study of 22,707 men in Taiwan. Lancet 2 : 1129-1133.

Brechot C, Scotto J, Charnay P, Hadchouel M, Degos F, Trepo C, Tiollais P (1981) Detection of hepatitis B virus DNA in liver and serum. A direct appraisal of the chronic carrier state. Lancet ii : 765-767.

Bridgen D, Roseling AR, Woods NC. Renal Function following acyclovir intravenous injection.(1982). Am J Med Acyclovir Symposium : 182-185.

Brzosko WJ, Deboski R, Derecka K (1978) Immunostimulation for chronic active hepatitis. Lancet ii : 311.

Chadwick RG, Bassendine MF, Crawford E, Thomas HC, Sherlock S (1978). HBs antigen positive chronic liver disease : inhibition of DNA polymerase activity by vidarabine. Brit Med J ii: 531-537.

Colby BM, Furman PA, Shaw JE, Elion GB, Pagono JS (1980). Abstract of the Fifth Cold Spring Harbour Meeting : Effect of Acyclovir 9-2 (Hydroxyethoxymethyl) guanine of Epstein-Barr virus DNA replication. J of Virology 34 (2) : 560-568.

Cook GC, Mulligan R, Sherlock S (1971). Controlled trial of corticosteroid therapy in chronic active hepatitis. Quarterly Journal of Medicine 40 : 159-185.

Craxi A, Weller IVD, Bassendine MF, Fowler MJF, Monjardino J, Thomas HC, Sherlock S (1983). Relationship between HBV-specific DNA polymerase and HBe antigen/antibody system in chronic HBV infection : factors determining selection of patients and outcome of antiviral therapy. Gut 24 : 143±147.

Eddleston ALWF, Mondelli M, Mieli-Vergani G, Williams R
(1982). Lymphocyte cytotoxicity to autologous hepatocytes
in chronic HBV infection. Hepatology 2 : 122S-127S.

Eddleston ALWF, Williams R (1974). Inadequate antibody
response to HB antigen or suppressor T-cell defect in
development of active chronic hepatitis. Lancet 2: 1543-1545.

Elion GB, Furman PA, Fyfe JA, De Miranda P, Beauchamp L
Schaeffer HJ. (1977). Selectivity of action of an anti-
herpetic agent 9-(2-hydroxye oxymethyl) guanine.
Proceedings of the National Academy of Science USA 74 : 5716-
5720.

Fowler MJF, Monjardino J, Montano L, Weller IVD, Lok ASF,
Oladapo JM, Thomas HC (1983) An analysis of the molecular
state of HBV-DNA in the liver and serum of patients with
chronic hepatitis or primary liver cell carcinoma.and the
effect of therapy with adenine arabinoside. Gut (in press).

Fyfe JA, Keller PM, Furman PA, Miller RL, Elion GB. (1978).
Thymidine kinase from Herpes simplex virus phosphorylates
the new antiviral compound, 9(2-hydroxye oxymethyl) guanine.
Journal of Biology and Chemistry 253 : 8721-8727.

Hadziyannis SJ, Weller IVD, Karvountzis MG, Thomas HC (1983).
Hepatitis B core antigen display in the liver in patients
with chronic hepatitis B virus infection : relationship
to hepatic inflammatory activity and to HBe antigen/antibody
status. Liver (in press).

Helgstrand E, Flodh H, Lernestedt JO, Lundstrom J, Oberg B
(1980). Trisodium phosphonoformate : antiviral activities,
safety evaluation and preliminary clinical results. In :
Collier LH, Oxford J. eds : Developments in antiviral therapy
London :Academic Press, 63-83.

Hirschman SZ, Garfunkel E. (1978). Inhibition of hepatitis
B DNA polymerase by intercalating agents. Nature 271 :
681-683.

Hoofnagel J, Dusheiko GM, Seef LB (1981) Seroconversion from
hepatitis B e antigen to antibody in chronic type B
hepatitis. Annals of Internal Medicine 94 : 744-748.

Keeney RE (1975) Human tolerance of adenine arabinoside
In Pavan-Lagston D, Buchman RA, Alford CA, eds : Adenine
arabinoside : an antiviral agent. New York Raven Press

Kirk AP, Jain S, Pocock S, Thomas HC, Sherlock S (1980).
Late results of the Royal Free Hospital prospective controlled
trial of prednisolone therapy in hepatitis B surface antigen
negative chronic active hepatitis. Gut 21 : 78 - 84.

Lam KC, Lai CL, Ng RP, Trepo C, Wu PC (1981). Deleterious
effect of prednisolone in HBsAg positive chronic active
hepatitis. New England Journal of Medicine 304 : 380-386.

Liaw YF, Chu CM, Su IH, Huang MJ, Lim DY, Chang-Chien CS
(1983). Clinical and histological events preceding
hepatitis B e antigen seroconversion in chronic type B
hepatitis. Gastroenterology 84 : 216-219.

Lok ASF, Lindsay I, Scheuer PJ, Thomas HC (1983). Clinical
and histological features of chronic HBV infection in
HBeAg and anti-HBe positive patients and the imparct of
superimposed delta infection (in preparation).

Lok ASF, Weller IVD, Karayiannis P, Brown D, Fowler MJF,
Monjardino J, Thomas HC, Sherlock S (1983). Thrice weekly
lymphoblastoid interferon is effective in inhibiting
hepatitis B virus replication. Gut (in press).

Montano L, Aranguibel F, BofillM, Goodall A, Janossy G,
Thomas HC (1983). An analysis of the composition of the
inflammatory infiltrate in autoimmune and hepatitis B virus
induced chronic liver disease. Hepatology(in press).

Muller R, Vido I, Schmidt FW. (1981) Rapid withdrawal of
immunosuppressive therapy in chronic active hepatitis B
infection. Lancet 1: 1323-1324.

Oladapo JM, Goodall AH, Parmar J, Brown D, Thomas HC (1983)
In vitro and in vivo cytotoxic activity of native and ricin
conjugated monoclonal antibodies to HBs antigen, for
Alexander primary liver carcinoma cells and tumours.
Gut (in press).

Pollard RB, Smith JL, Neal A, Gregory PB, Merigan TC, Robinson WS (1978). The effect of vidarabine on chronic hepatitis B virus infection. JAMA 239, 1648-1650.

Realdi G, Alberti A, Rugge M, Bortolotti F, Rigoli AM, Tremolada R, Ruol A (1980). Seroconversion from hepatitis B 'e' antigen to anti-HBe in chronic hepatitis B virus infection. Gastroenterology 79 : 195-199.

Rizzetto M, Canese MG, Arico S, Crivelli Q, Trepo C, Bonino F Verme G (1977). Immunofluorescence detection of a new antigen antibody system (delta/anti-delta) associated with he hepatitis B virus in the liver and in the serum of HBsAg carriers. Gut, 18 : 997-1003.

Rizzetto M, Canese MG, Gerin JL, London WT, Sly DL, Purcell RH (1980). Transmission of the hepatitis B virus associated delta antigen to chimpanzees. J. Infect. Dis. 141 : 590-602.

Rizzetto M, Purcell RH, Gerin JL. (1980) Epidemiology of HBV-associated delta antigen. Geographical distribution and prevalence in poly-transfused HBsAg carriers. Lancet i-1215-1218.

Rizzetto M Shih JW, Gocke DJ, Purcell RH, Verme G, Gerin JL (1979) Incidence and significance of antibodies to delta-antigen in hepatitis B virus infection. Lancet ii: 986-990.

Rizzetto M, Verme G, Recchia S, Bonino F, Farci P, Arico S, Calzia R, Picciotto A, Colombo M, Popper H (1983). Chronic hepatitis in carriers of HBsAg with intra-hepatic expression of delta-antigen An anctive and progressive disease unresponsive to immunosuppressive treatment. Ann. Intern. Med. 98 : 437 - 441.

Sagnelli E, Maio G, Felaco FM, Izzo CM, Manzillo G, Pasquale G, Filippini P, Piccinino F (1980). Serum levels of hepatitis B surface and core antigens during immuno-suppressive treatment of HBsAg positive chronic active hepatitis. Lancet 1 : 295 - 297.

Schalm SK, Heigtink RA (1982) Spontaneous disappearance
of viral replication and liver cell inflammation in HBsAg
positive chronic active hepatitis : results of a placebo
versus interferon trial. Hepatology 2: 791-794.

Schalm SW, Summerskill WHJ, Gitnick GL (1976). Contrasting
features and responses to treatment of severe chronic active
liver disease with and without hepatitis B s antigen. Gut
17 : 781-786.

Scullard GH, Andres LL, Greenberg HB (1981). Anti-viral
treatment of chronic hepatitis B virus infection :
improvement in liver disease with interferon and adenine
arabinoside. Hepatology 1 : 228-232.

Scullard GH, Pollard PB, Smith JL, Sacks SL, Gregory PB,
Robinson WS, Merigan TC. (1981) Anti-viral treatment of
chronic hepatitis B virus infection. I changes in viral
markers with interferon combined with adenine arabinoside.
J. Infect. Dis. 143 : 772-783.

Scullard GH, Smith CI, Merigan TC, Robinson WS, Gregory PB
(1981) Effects of immunosuppressive therapy on viral
markers in chronic active hepatitis B. Gastroenterology
81 : 987-991.

Shafritz DA, Shouval D, Sherman HI, Hadziyiannis SJ, Kew MC
(1981). Integration of hepatitis B virus DNA into the genome
of liver cells in chronic liver disease and hepatocellular
carcinoma. New England Journal of Medicine 305, 1067-1073.

Shannon WM (1975). Antiviral activity in vitro. In :
Pavan-Langston D, Buchanan RA, Alford C AJr, eds :
Adenine arabinoside : an antiviral agent. New York
Raven Press.

Shouval D, Wands JR, Zurawski VR, Isselbacher KJ,
Shafritz DA (1982) Protection against experimental hepatoma
formation in nude mice by monoclonal antibodies to hepatitis
B virus surface antigen. Hepatology 2: 128S-133S.

Thomas HC. Pathogenesis of HBV infection. In 'Advanced Medicine 19' Edited by M Lasoursky Published by Pitman (1983).

Thomas HC (1979). Immunostimulants in the treatment of HBs antigen positive chornic active liver disease. Chapter in "Immune reactions in Liver disease" Edited by Eddleston, Weber and Williams. Pitman Press 281-287.

Thomas HC, Bassendine MF, Weller IVD(1980). Treatment of chronic hepatitis b virus infection. In : Collier LH, Oxford J, eds: Developments in anti-viral therapy. London Academic Press 1 : 88-103.

Thomas HC, Brown D, Routhier G, Janossy G, King PC, Goldstein-G, Sherlock S (1982) Inducer and suppressor T-cells in hepatitis B virus induced liver disease. Hepatology 2 : 202-204.

Thomas HC, Montano L, Goodall A, De Koning R, Oladapo J, WiedmannK (1982). Immunoligical mechanisms in chronic HBV infection. Hepatology 2 : 116S-121S.

Tymes AS, Scamons EM, Naim HM (1981) In vitro activity of Acyclovir and related compounds against cytomegalovirus infections. Journal of Antimicrobial Chemotherapy 8: 65-72.

Viola LA, Barrison IG, Coleman JC, Paradinas FJ, Fluker JL Murrey-Lyon IM. (1981) Natural history of liver disease in chronic hepatitis B surface antigen carriers : survey of 100 patients from Great Britain. Lancet 2 : 1156-1159.

Weller IVD, Bassendine MF, Craxi A, Fowler MJF, Monjardino J, Thomas HC, Sherlock S (1982). Successful treatment of HBs and HBeAg positive chronic liver disease : prolonged inhibition of viral replication by highly soluble adenine arabinoside 5'-monophosphate (ARA-AMP). Gut 23 :717-723.

Weller IVD, Bassendine MF, Murray AX, Craxi A, Thomas HC, Sherlock S (1982) The effects of prednisolone/azathioprine in chronic hepatitis B viral infection. Gut 23, 650-655.

Weller IVD, Carreno V, Fowler MJF, Monjardino J, Makinen D,
Vanghese Z, Sweny P, Thomas HC, Sherlock S (1982)
Acycloguanosine in HBeAg-positive chronic liver disease :
inhibition óf viral replication and transient renal
impairment with IV bolus administration. Journal of
Antimicrobial Chemotherapy (in press).

Weller IVD, Carreno V, Fowler MJF, Monjardino J, Makinen D,
Thomas HC, Sherlock S. (1982) Acycloguanosine inhibits
hepatitis B virus replication in man. Lancet 1 : 273.

Weller IVD, Karayiannis P, Lok ASF, Montano L, Bamber M,
Thomas HC, Sherlock S. (1983) The significance of
delta agent infection in chronic hepatitis B viral infection
in Great Britain. Gut (in press).

Weller IVD, Fowler MJF, Monjardino J, Carreno V, Thomas HC
Sherlock S (1982) Inhibition of hepatitis B viral
replication by lymphoblastoid interferon. Philosphical
Transactions of the Royal Society Series B 128-130.

Weller IVD, Lok ASF, Mindel A, Thomas HC, Sherlock S (1983).
Randomsided controlled trial of ARA-AMP in chronic hepatitis
B virus infection (in preparation).

Wu PC, Lai CL, Lam KC, Ho J (1982) Prednisolone in HBsAg-
positive chronic activei,hepatitis : histological evaluation
in a controlled prospective study. Hepatology 2 :777-783.

CONCLUDING REMARKS

Viral Hepatitis and Delta Infection, pages 397–410
© **1983 Alan R. Liss, Inc., 150 Fifth Avenue, New York, NY 10011**

CONCERNING PARTICULARLY DELTA AGENT INFECTION, CHRONIC
HEPATITIS, AND RELATION OF HEPATITIS B INFECTION TO HEPATO-
CELLULAR CARCINOMA

Hans Popper, M.D., Ph.D.

Stratton Laboratory for the Study of Liver Diseases
Mount Sinai School of Medicine of the City
University of New York, New York, N.Y. 10029

The symposium on Viral Hepatitis and Delta Infection was
appropriately held in Turin, where the delta agent (DA) was
discovered by Rizzetto and where its role was explored by his
work with Verme, Bonino and Ponzetto, in cooperation with
Purcell and Gerin in Washington. The symposium surveyed new
knowledge in all forms of viral hepatitis and specifically the
rapidly developing information on the DA .

Progress in Viral Hepatitis. The most remarkable ad-
vances concerned molecular biology, exemplified by the increasing information on the cloning of the genome of the
hepatitis A virus, and the identification of specific sequences coding for hydrophilic immunogenic portions of the
surface antigen of the hepatitis B virus (HBV) which in general are also conserved in the woodchuck virus. These DNA
sequences vary in few nucleotide bases corresponding to the
various subgroups of the HBV surface antigen and to the woodchuck virus surface antigen. Furthermore, in situ hybridization has progressed with detection of perinucleolar and
cytoplasmic DNA sequences and HBV DNA integration was found
to occur in nonalcoholic hepatocellular carcinoma (HCC) even
in the absence of any serum or tisssue markers of HBV infection. Although these investigations were performed on
biopsy specimens, bacterial contamination is not fully excluded since, particularly in cirrhosis, bacteria in portal
blood are not necessarily cleared by Kupffer cells. Finally,
a portion of the delta RNA has been converted into DNA and
cloned. Immunologic studies identified the core antigen of
HBV as the target of the lymphocytotoxicity, although an
attack on liver membrane antigen (LM-Ag) is not excluded.
However, it is still difficult to extrapolate from in vitro

studies incriminating primarily cytotoxic T cells to in vivo processes. The humoral and cellular regulation of the effector cells acting in vivo is still not clear. The role of the various antibodies in protection, including inhibition of viral replication, as well as in antibody dependent lymphocytotoxicity, is not elucidated either except, of course, the protection against infection by surface antibody, which is the basis of the vaccine. The vaccine has now been investigated in the newborn woodchuck model, in which protection against antigenemia was significant.

In hepatitis non-A, non-B (HNANB), the existence of several agents is now confirmed. The epidemic form resembling hepatitis A because of lack of chronicity and fecal/oral spread was originally recognized in India but has now been found in epidemics in various other locations and the designation hepatitis A_2 appears appropriate. However, even in the other forms of HNANB the difference in the evolution between the sporadic cases, with far better long-term prognosis, and those following blood transfusions, characterized by a frequently chronic progressive course and repeated spikes of aminotransferase elevations, suggests different etiologic factors. It is, however, probable that the HNANB transmitting donors had originally been infected under "sporadic" circumstances and not by blood transfusions. Until a reliable antigen/antibody system for all HNANB agents is available, one cannot exclude the possibility that variations in the infective dose or in the route of infection account for different clinical expressions nor disregard the suggested homology between HBV DNA and at least some HNANB agents.

Epidemiology of Delta Agent Infection. The new information about the incidence of DA infection is most exciting. Originally, southern Italy was considered the main and original site of the infection, with spread to other locations, mainly in drug addicts and multitransfused persons and, to a lesser degree, in homosexuals. In families the spread appears to be horizontal and not vertical as in HB. The increasing availability of tests for serum delta antibody and also antigen, as well as the demonstration of delta antigen in liver tissue, has now led to the detection of a localized high incidence in the northern part of South America, for instance in Venezuelan Indians in isolated valleys or in the Amazon basin, as well as in Arabic countries in the Near East. Moreover, the incidence in some regions, such as

southern Italy, Chile and Greece, has apparently decreased.
Finally, in Europe and California, a significant portion of
fatal massive necrotic HB has been found associated with the
DA; the question of co-infection with HBV or superinfection
in previous HBV carriers has not been fully resolved and will
require IgM anti-core studies to indicate an active stage of
HB. Preliminary observations suggest that DA infection associated with HBV is a migrating disease, with possible variations in virulence, already demonstrated by repeated pas-
sages in chimpanzees and from them to virus infected woodchucks. One is reminded of influenza epidemics, although no
evidence exists for genetic variations of the DA itself.

Specific remarks prompted by the reports at the symposium will deal with (1) classification of chronic viral hepatitis and the role of lobular lesions, (2) HBV and HCC, and
(3) future problems of DA infection, attempting to
relate all three.

Classification of Chronic Viral Hepatitis. The term
'chronic hepatitis' has been applied widely only in the last
25 years in the Anglo-American literature, although in
Germany, Kalk (Kalk 1957) had used it earlier; elsewhere the
stress had been on the activity of the underlying cirrhosis.
The widespread use of liver biopsy and of aminotransferase
determinations led to better delineation of chronic hepatitis
and the introduction of immunosupressive therapy called for a
classification to identify the conditions benefited by such
therapy. Chronic persistent or portal hepatitis with inflammation restricted to the portal tracts and little tendency to
progression was distinguished from chronic aggressive or
periportal hepatitis with such tendency and therefore potentially amenable to immunosuppresive therapy (De Groote 1968).
Subsequently, chronic lobular hepatitis was added (Popper
1971), in which diffuse lobular necroinflammation reveals the
features of acute viral hepatitis although the disease lasts
longer than six months, the accepted time limit between acute
and chronic hepatitis. Follow-up observations in part supported this distinction which did not take into account the
type of hepatitis and which was also complicated by additional problems, not the least being the possible detri-
mental effects of immunosuppressive therapy in HB. This
essentially therapeutic classification placed emphasis on the
portal and periportal lesions, although confluent necrosis
was considered part of the severe form of chronic aggressive
hepatitis. The periportal necroinflammation (piecemeal ne-

crosis) may exhibit various histological manifestations, including a lymphocytoid type, possibly reflecting activity of antibody-dependent killer cells, a cytolytic not lymphocyte associated, and furthermore a biliary type. The periportal process alone or accompanied by only minor intralobular lesions only rarely leads to cirrhosis and portal hypertension and the progression is then induced by active septa formation probably caused by fibroplasia inducing interleukines (formed by lymphocytes and monocytes). Such an evolution may be as rare in chronic hepatitis as the development of alcoholic cirrhosis without alcoholic hepatitis. Far more frequent and important in the cirrhotic transformation are episodes of circumscribed lobular degeneration or necrosis of hepatocytes induced either by attack by allogenic restricted T lymphocytes or by cytopathic effects. These acute bouts, described in Germany as chronic necrotizing hepatitis (Selmair 1970) but often also called subacute hepatic necrosis, may be clinically expressed in episodes of more or less severe hepatic failure, sometimes associated with transient ascites, jaundice, and even hepatic coma. Subsequent focal collapse of the parenchyma favors progression to cirrhosis which, however, need not set in. The progression may depend on and be assisted by the periportal necroinflammation. Nevertheless, the evolution of chronic hepatitis depends more on lobular than on periportal processes (Popper 1982).

These lobular processes may represent spontaneous reactivation of chronic HB which may even set in after seroconversion from e to anti-e, accompanied by temporary disappearance of serum HBV DNA and DNA polymerase (Davis 1983). The acute necrotizing episode is characterized by the presence or reappearance of markers of HBV replication. The activation may also result from rapid withdrawal of steroid therapy. In other instances, however, these acute episodes may be induced by superinfection with other viral agents. This is illustrated by the morphologic findings in HBV carrier chimpanzees inoculated with the DA (Dienes 1981). Severe degenerative changes of the hepatocytes are then noted, with temporary destruction of the previously present ground-glass cells rich in surface antigen and with proliferation of macrophages with many PAS-positive granules. In other such inoculated chimpanzees, the lesions are less severe and show features characteristic of HNANB in chimpanzees, which consist of milder toxic alterations of the hepatocytes, including microvesicular steatosis, many acidophilic bodies and

prominence of macrophagic over lymphocytic reaction. The
lesions differ from the ones in chimpanzee HB, in which
lymphocytes predominate and are in close contact with, and
often within, hepatocytes (emperipolesis) (Popper 1980).
During DA reaction in chimpanzees, the previously present HBV
replication is suppressed. The same temporary depression also
develops in chimpanzee HBV carriers inoculated with NANB or
HAV material (Harrison, 1983), in which the respective
typical reactions are far more severe. Thus, in superin-
fections of HBV carrier chimpanzees, the typical morphologic
pattern produced by the superinfecting agent comes through
(Dienes 1981). Moreover, these findings also indicate that
some of the 'acute bouts' in human chronic HB may represent a
superinfection with delta or NANB agent, particularly when
markers of HBV replication are suppressed during the acute
episodes.

These observations also raise the question of a <u>simi-
larity of light-microscopic features induced by the delta and
NANB agents</u>. The characteristic lesions from the DA
(Rizzetto 1983) are being well analyzed by Verme <u>et al.</u> and
the lack of close relation of lymphocytes to the hepatocytes
was emphasized. Autopsy studies on rapidly fatal DA infections showed a predominantly cytopathic effect, but the specificity of the lesion for DA infections remains to be established. At present there is not full agreement as to what
degree the histologic manifestations of HNANB in man are
characteristic and only some tendencies have been described,
which are not necessarily diagnostic in the individual case.
As a rule, the lesions are less severe than DA induced alterations, which moreover, may be complicated by expression
of the underlying HBV infection. The histological alterations in HNANB, suggested by various authors (Bamber 1981, De
Wolf-Peeters 1981, Dienes 1982), in part based on coded read-
ings, include: distinct cell borders of the hepatocytes with
eosinophilic, often granular cytoplasmic changes progressing
to frequently crumbling or granular acidophilic bodies;
sinusoidal cell hyperplasia including excess lymphocytes,
seldom close to hepatocytes but often mixed with macrophages,
results in a picture which has been compared with that in
infectious mononucleosis (Bamber 1981). Although the different alterations are often found in the same liver, it
cannot be excluded that they reflect different NANB agents.
Electron microscopic lesions, both cytoplasmic and nuclear,
have also been described (Shimizu 1979), although their specificity for HNANB is challenged. Similar cytoplasmic lesions

have also been observed in DA infected chimpanzees (Kamimura 1983). The light and electron microscopic features in the lobular parenchyma suggest a cytotoxic rather than a lympho- cytotoxic reaction in both NANB and DA infections. This tentative conclusion cannot be extended to the portal inflam- matory reaction, which in human HNANB includes large ac- cumulations of lymphocytes and bile duct alterations.

At this time one can thus assume a similarity of the main morphological expressions of NANB and DA infections, suggesting similar pathogenetic factors. The assumed cyto- pathic reaction is in keeping with an ineffective or at least low-grade antigen/antibody or lymphocytic reaction. This interferes with the clearance of the agents and explains the repeated spikes of the aminotransferase activities in HNANB, as well as the reappearance of lobular alterations, which makes the histologic separation of human acute from chronic HNANB so difficult. Even in the chimpanzee NANB model lobu- lar alterations may recur for several years (Bradley 1981). Similarly, Redeker's group has reported repeated appearances of delta IgM antibodies, suggesting recurrence of the necro- tizing process. Otherwise, there is no evidence for re-in- fection in DA disease. In DA infection, nuclear antigen is observed in normal-appearing hepatocytes, indicating a latent period before tissue reaction sets in which is then associ- ated with reduction of hepatic delta antigen.

The emphasis on <u>lobular lesions in the evolution of chronic hepatitis</u> also concerns HB, where an antagonism be- tween replication of the virus and its integration into the host genome has been postulated, an antagonism reflected also, but not always, in either e antigen or antibodies. In the e antigen positive stage, lymphocytotoxicity against mem- brane associated HBV antigens, predominantly the core anti- gen, is assumed to cause hepatocellular injury. Such lympho- cytotoxicity, however, may in part also be directed against liver membrane specific antigen (LM-Ag). The latter presum- ably is associated with an antibody dependent killer cell reaction and is not induced by cytotoxic T cells but depends also on cellular and humoral regulation. The killer cell reaction occurs, too, in other, not HB induced, liver in- juries and is characteristic for autoimmune hepatitis. Hepa- tocellular injury of any pathogenesis favors development of cirrhosis over fibroplasia and collapse, but also eliminates hepatocytes with episomal DNA (as well as delta RNA). Thus, it may lead, possibly enhanced by suppression of viral replication by antibodies, to eventual clearance of the antigens, a process which may be inefficient. Antiviral therapy also removes hepatocytes with episomal DNA, reflected in the frequent initial rise of the aminotransferase activity. By contrast, in the e-antibody and HBsAg positive stage, hepatocytes with HBV DNA integrated into the host genome are not removed by lymphocytotoxicity, because they do not express core antigen in the cell membrane. Such hepatocytes are not susceptible to antiviral therapy. The hepatocytes with integrated DNA are supposed to be at risk to develop into HCC. These considerations are in keeping with the clinical observation that HCC usually develops in the absence of active HBV associated liver injury. The simultaneous presence of hepatocytes with active viral replication and others containing integrated DNA, as suggested by the variable quantitative relation between episomal and integrated HBV DNA in the liver of human carriers (Kam 1982), might explain the rare instances of HCC in active viral hepatitis. This, however, is characteristic of the woodchuck model. Available evidence does not support a relation of DA infection to HCC nor is the role of HNANB in HCC established.

Review of the Relation of HBV Infection to HCC. The association between infection and carcinoma is supported by the following observations (Popper 1982):

1. The incidence of HCC runs parallel to the frequency of serum markers of HBV infection in population groups. This includes the areas of high incidence, such as China, Southeast Asia and Sub-Saharan Africa. It also holds true for the areas of medium incidence of both, such as Japan, India and southern Europe, as well as for low incidence areas (central Europe and the United States), although in some groups in the U.S., such as Orientals, the incidence of markers and HCC is high. The parallelism has not been found everywhere. More careful observations, however, have discovered relatively high incidence of HCC in some populations, like the Eskimos and Egyptians, in whom initially high incidence of HBV markers only had been reported.

2. In patients with HCC and also in their mothers, serum markers of HBV infection are frequent, particularly if other etiological factors, such as alcoholism, are excluded. HBV infection precedes HCC as is well illustrated by prospective studies, particulary the extensive ones in Taiwan (Beasley 1981). There carriers with serum HBsAg are at particular risk to develop HCC, usually with cirrhosis, in contrast to persons without surface antigen. Present estimates

from these ongoing studies suggest that such carriers have a 50% lifetime risk to develop cirrhosis and/or HCC. This risk is thus considerably higher than that of 3 pack/day smokers to develop lung cancer.

3. Clusters of hepatitis B infection and HCC have been found in families, suggesting perinatal infection.

4. In the liver around HCC, hepatocytes with much HBsAg in the cytoplasm and only occasionally HBcAg in the nuclei are often abundant and are frequently arranged in nodules in which the hepatocytes are sometimes large (hypertrophic) and sometimes small but in two-cell-thick plates (hyperplastic). Both markers, especially core antigen, are sparse in the carcinoma itself, and it is even claimed (Nakashima 1982) that cells rich in HBsAg are entrapped normal hepatocytes and not real tumor cells, suggesting low, if any viral replication in the HCC.

5. Cell lines developed from human HCC secrete HBsAg but no other antigens, and HBV DNA is integrated into their genome. The same holds true for tumors produced by inoculation of these cell lines into nude mice.

6. The association is also supported by the already mentioned integration of part or the entire viral DNA into host genome, found in the human HCC, in the liver around the HCC and of HBV carriers. Integration of HBV DNA has been demonstrated not only in patients with markers of HBV infection, sometimes only core antibodies, but also occasionally in the absence of any markers, suggesting that HBV DNA integration need not result in expression of markers. This contrasts with the cited experiences in Taiwan which point to a far higher risk of HCC in HBsAg positive carriers. The human HBV carriers frequently have distinct nuclear alterations in ground-glass and other hepatocytes in the absence of other histological lesions, raising the possibility that the nuclear hyperplasia may reflect integration. This is in keeping with the absence of such nuclear alterations in even long-term HBV carrier chimpanzees in which HBV DNA is not integrated (Shouval 1980) and in which HCC has so far not been observed.

7. Various animals persistently infected with Hepadna viruses related to but not identical to HBV develop hepatitis and HCC; the Eastern woodchuck is an outstanding example in which viral integration was first described. In California, ground squirrels infected with a similar virus have hepatits but not HCC, and DNA is not integrated. Pekin ducks infected by another similar virus may have chronic hepatitis and HCC but integration has so far not been established (Omata 1983).

Interestingly, in Qui-dong on the Yang-tze river in China, where the incidence of human HBV infection and HCC is very high, not only ducks but also cats, dogs and pigs (but not rats) have HCC, in part with cirrhosis; virologic studies have so far not been performed.

The major unsolved problem is the <u>pathogenesis</u> of HBV associated HCC. The DNA alteration caused by viral integration could reasonably be a factor in the initiation of the carcinogenesis as assumed for DNA alterations in chemical carcinogenesis. So far, however, a transforming potency of HBV DNA has not been demonstrated in transfection studies. Moreover, an induction period of many years, usually of decades, separates onset of HBV infection from detection of HCC and the carcinogenic processes during this period are unknown. Just as in most forms of chemical carcinogenesis, a selection of single hepatocytes for carcinogenesis seems to take place. This is reflected in Blumberg and London's hypothesis (London 1982) which distinguishes susceptible (S) cells which may express viral disease from resistant (R) cells at risk to become carcinomatous. In analogy to Farber's model (Solt 1977) of chemical carcinogenesis, in which transformed hepatocytes are not susceptible to additional injuries and therefore proliferate upon growth impulses and may become carcinomatous, a similar block preventing destruction of infected but presumably integrated (non-permissive) hepatocytes by immune attack may be a selecting factor (Popper 1982). However, promotion is now considered to be of major significance. The important promoting factor in HBV related carcinogenesis seems to be increased turnover of hepatocytes from prolonged active liver disease, including possibly from exposure to incidental chemicals such as aflatoxin; transformation to cirrhosis is probably the most effective. In HB the balance between necrosis of HBV markers expressing hepatocytes and the cell proliferation stimulated by the necrosis (Popper 1982) may determine the outcome of the disease.

Of major interest in this respect are suggested geographical variations (Okuda 1982). In Africa, large anaplastic HCC is common and cirrhosis formation seems to be less frequent and less extensive. Integration appears to be common and serologic evidence suggests low viral replication. By contrast, in the Orient, minute encapsulated HCC is frequent and often associated with conspicuous cirrhosis which may dominate the clinical picture; viral replication appears to be more intense, but integration may not be as frequent.

In the African form, integration, and in the Oriental form, promotion may be the more important factor in carcinogenesis. To what degree this difference applies to HCC in Western countries is not established. This question also has major clinical significance because in the Far East, surgical removal of the minute, presumably unicentric, HCC detected in the subclinical stage by screening with alpha-fetoprotein determinations and confirmed by imaging methods, has resulted in prolonged survival (Tang 1982). However, existence and frequency of unicentric HCC remains to be established. It joins the other unresolved problems in HBV related carcinogenesis. Foremost among them is the role of integration; this includes the time it occurs during the course of the disease. Mitosis, conspicuous in early hepatitis, may lead to rearrangement of DNA and could favor integration. Moreover, the nature of the integration has to be explored, whether it causes DNA rearrangement and translocation or insertion of promoting sequences which activate cellular oncogenes. As in chemical carcinogenesis, induction of cell proliferation must be distinguished from malignant transformation, reflected in immortality of cells and invasive potential (Weinberg 1983). Today the HBV oncogenicity alone or in combination with other factors appears highly probable, but may only be proved when the incidence of human HCC is significanty lowered by prevention of HBV infection, for instance by successful vaccination. Again, one is reminded of the now established relation of lung carcinoma to smoking.

<u>Unresolved Problems of Delta Agent Infection.</u> In view of the short time the DA has been known, it is no wonder that many questions are still unanswered. The wider availability of testing techniques, including the use of IgM antibodies, should clarify the fascinating problem of geographic spread and the clinical evolution in both co- and superinfection. At this time the latter appears to have a worse prognosis. Further molecular biologic information is required as to the nature of the DA, the mode of replication of delta RNA, and the proteins for which it codes. This includes also a possible homology with NANB agents. The mechanism of the hepatocellular injury induced by DA needs exploration; does the cell damaging process in HBV and DA infections involve the same hepatocyte? HBV replication on one side should favor DA replication, but, on the other side, should support clearance of one or both agents by elimination of infected hepatocytes. Thus anti-HBs may appear in ongoing DA disease (Moestrup 1983). DA induced disease in e antigen positive patients

seems to progress more actively but to have a better long-
term prognosis than in e antigen negative patients. DA carriers appear never to be asymptomatic. The influence of the
expression of the HBV disease on the clinical evolution of
the DA infection requires further study, as does the relation
between delta antigen and antibodies. Since DA infections
seems to inhibit HBV replication and DA infected HBV carriers
usually have e antibodies, it is interesting that they still
may release HBV DNA containing particles (Bonino 1981).
Little is yet known about the humoral and cellular immunological reactions involved in the DA induced injury. Is the
cytotoxicity postulated for the DA the result of viral
toxins, of lymphocyte and monocyte produced interleukines,
or, less probable, of deposition of immune globulins or complexes with delta antigen? For instance, the deposition of
delta antigen and immune globulin in the nuclei seems to be
only an epiphenomenon (Rizzetto 1981). Because of the
similar morphologic expressions caused by NANB and DA
disease, the DA infection may serve as a model to study the
pathogenesis of NANB because DA markers are available. Many
of these questions may be answered at a future symposium
which will be, hopefully, as interesting and well planned as
the one closing now and for which we express deep gratitude
to the organizers.

REFERENCES

See also references to and in the presentations at the
International Symposium: Viral Hepatitis and Delta
Infection.

Bamber M, Murray AK, Waller IVD, Morelli A, Scheuer PJ,
  Thomas HC, Sherlock S (1981). Clinical and histologic
  features of a group of patients with sporadic non-A, non-B
  hepatitis. J Clin Pathol 34:1175.
Beasley RP, Hwana L-Y, Lin CC, Chien C-S (1981). Hepatocellular carcinoma and hepatitis B virus. A prospective
  study of 22707 men in Taiwan. Lancet II:1129
Bonino F, Hoyer B, Nelson H, Engle R, Verme G, Gerin J (1981).
  Hepatitis B virus DNA in the sera of HBsAg carriers: a
  marker of active hepatitis B virus replication in the
  liver. Hepatology 1:386.
Bradley DW, Maynard JE, Popper H, Ebert JW, Cook EH, Fields
  HA, Kemler BJ (1981). Peristent non-A, non-B hepatitis in
  experimentally infected chimpanzees. J Infect Dis 143:210.

Davis GL, Hoofnagle JH, Waggoner JG (1983). Spontaneous re-
activation of chronic type B hepatitis. Gastroenterology
84:1370.
De Groote J, Desmet VJ, Gedick P, Korb G, Popper H, Poulsen H,
Scheuer PJ, Schmid M, Thaler H, Uehlinger E, Wepler W
(1968). A classification of chronic hepatitis. Lancet II:
626.
De Wolf-Peeters C, De Vos R, Desmet V, Ray MB, Desmyter J,
De Groote G, Fevery J, Broeckaert L, De Groote J (1981).
Human non-A, non-B hepatitis: ultrastructural alterations
in hepatocytes. Liver 1:50.
Dienes HP, Purcell RH, Popper H, Bonino F, Ponzetto A (1981).
Simultaneous infection of chimpanzees with more than one
hepatitis virus. Hepatology 1:506.
Dienes HP, Popper H, Arnold W, Lobeck H (1982). Histologic
observations in human hepatitis non-A, non-B. Hepatology
2:562.
Harrison TJ, Tsiguaye KN and Zuckerman AJ (1983). Assay of
HBV DNA in the plasma of HBV-carrier chimpanzees super-
infected with non-A, non-B hepatitis. J Virol Methods 6:
295-302.
Kalk H (1957). Cirrhose und Narbenleber. Entstehung, Klinik
und Therapie. 2. Aufl. Stuttgart: Enke
Kam W, Rall LB, Smuckler EA, Schmid R, Rutter WJ (1982).
Hepatitis B viral DNA in liver and serum of asymptomatic
carriers. Proc Natl Acad Sci USA 79:7522.
Kamimura T, Bonino F, Ponzetto A, Feinstone SM, Gerin JL,
Purcell RH (1983). Cytoplasmic tubular structures in liver
of HBsAg carrier chimpanzees infected with   agent and comparison with cytoplasmic structures in non-A, non-B hepatitis. Hepatology (in press).
London WT, Blumberg BS (1982). A cellular model of the role
of hepatitis B virus in the pathogenesis of primary hepatocellular carcinoma. Hepatology 2:10s.
Moestrup T, Hansson BG, Widell A, Nordenfelt E (1983). Clinical aspects of delta infection. Br Med J 286:87.
Nakashima T, Kojiro M, Kawano Y, Shirai F, Takemoto N,
Tomimatsu H, Kawasaki H, Okuda K (1982). Histologic growth
pattern of hepatocellular carcinoma: relationship to orcein
(hepatitis B surface antigen)-positive cells in cancer tissue. Hum Pathol 13:563.
Okuda K, Nakashima T, Sakamoto K, Ikari T, Hidaka H, Kubo Y,
Sakuma K, Motoike Y, Okuda H, Obata H (1982). Hepatocellular carcinoma arising in noncirrhotic and highly cirrhotic livers: A comparative study of histopathology and frequency of hepatitis B markers. Cancer 49:450.

Omata M, Uchiumi K, Ito Y, Yokosuka O, Mori J, Terao K, Wei-fa Y, O'Connell AP, London WT, Okuda K (1983). Duck hepatitis B virus and liver diseases. Gastroenterology 85: 260-267

Popper H, Schaffner F (1971) The vocabulary of chronic hepatitis. New Engl J Med 284:1154.

Popper H, Dienstag JL, Feinstone SM, Alter HJ, Purcell RH (1980). The pathology of viral hepatitis in chimpanzees. Virchows Arch A Path Anat & Histol 387:91.

Popper H, Thung SN, Gerber MA (1982). Chronic sequelae of viral hepatitis. In Szmuness W, Alter HJ, Maynard JE (eds) "Viral Hepatitis: 1981 Symposium", Philadelphia: The Franklin Institute Press, p 205.

Popper H, Gerber MA, Thung SN (1982). The relation of hepatocellular carcinoma to infections with hepatitis B and related viruses in man and animals. Hepatology 2:1s

Rizzetto M, Canese MG, Purcell RH, London WT, Sly LD. Gerin JL (1981). Experimental HBV and   infection of chimpanzees: Occurrence and significance of intrahepatic immune complexes of HBcAg and   antigen. Hepatology 1:567.

Rizzetto M, Verme G, Recchia S, Bonino F, Farci P, Aricò S, Calzia R, Picciotto A, Colombo M, Popper H (1983). Chronic hepatitis in carriers of hepatitis B surface antigen, with intrahepatic expression of the delta antigen. An active and progressive disease unresponsive to immunosuppressive treatment. An Intern Med 98:437.

Selmair H, Vido I, Wildhirt E, Ortmans H (1970) Die chronisch-nekrotisierende Hepatitis. Dtsch med Wschr 95:1

Shimizu JK, Feinstone SM, Purcell RH, Alter HJ, London WT (1979). Non-A, non-B hepatiis: ultrastructural evidence of two agents in experimenally infected chimpanzees. Science 205:197.

Shouval D, Chakraborty PR, Ruiz-Opazo N, Baum S, Spigland I, Muchmore E, Gerber MA, Thung SN, Popper H, Shafritz DA (1980). Chronic hepatitis in chimpanzee carriers of hepatitis B virus: Morphologic, immunologic and viral DNA studies. Proc Natl Acad Sci USA 77:6147.

Solt DB, Medline A, Farber E (1977). Rapid emergence of carcinogen-induced hyperplastic lesions in a new model for the sequential analysis of liver carcinogenesis. Am J Pathol 88:596.

Tang Z-Y, Ying Y-Y, Gu T-J (1982) Hepatocellular carcinoma:
  Changing concepts in recent years. In Popper H, Schaffner F
  (eds): "Progress in Liver Diseases" Vol 7, New York, Grune &
  Stratton, p 637.
Weinberg RA (1983). Alteration of the genomes of tumor
  cells. Cancer 52:1971.

Index

delta infection with, 203–207
  in children, 226
  hepatitis B virus and, 41
Clq binding, 317
Concanavalin A, 300
Corticosteroids, 216
Counterimmunoelectrophoresis, 29, 32
Creutzfeld-Jacob disease, 32
Cytomegalovirus, 360

Dane particles
  antibodies to, 331–332
    affinity chromatography with
      insolubilized, 332–334
    inhibition of 332
    in pHSA virus receptor inhibition,
      334
  pHSA receptor on, 331
Delta agent
  acquired immune deficiency
    syndrome and, 116
  with acute viral hepatitis, 195, 196,
    197, 200
  antibodies to. *See* Antibodies, delta
    agent
  blood and blood product transmission
    of, 116
  characteristic lesions of, 401
  with chronic active hepatitis, 195,
    196, 198, 200, 210, 273
  with chronic hepatitis infection,
    203–207
  chronic infection of, 209–215
    acute hepatitis preceding, 211–212
    age, sex, and origin in, 210–211
    clinical and laboratory features in,
      213
    liver histology and histochemistry
      in, 214–215
    modes of presentation of, 212
    natural course of, 215–216
  in chronic persistent hepatitis, 210,
    273
  clinical aspects of infection with,
    195–201
  diagnosis of hepatitis from, 169–170

among drug addicts, 155–157,
  245–249
enzyme linked immunoassays of, 263
epidemiology of, 398–399
  among Arabs, 161–164
  in Australia, 293
  in Britain, 219–220
  in China, 29296
  in France, 287
  in Germany, 277
  in Greece, 210, 271
  in Ireland, 281
  in Los Angeles area, 235–236
  in Saudi Arabia, 279
  in Scandinavia, 155–159
  in Southern Italy, 113–117, 195,
    257
  in United Kingdom, 291
familial clustering of infection with,
  133–142
in fulminant hepatitis, 235–236
  clinical features of, 238–239
  epidemiological features of,
    237–238
  serological features of, 239–241
geographic distribution of, 115–116,
  273
in hemodialysis patients, 151–153,
  257
among hemophiliacs, 145–149
in hepatitis B virus infection, 273
hepatocellular carcinoma and, 210,
  231–234
histopathology of hepatitis with,
  169–175
among homosexuals, 155, 156, 285
host range of, 111
infection of, in children, 225–229
  HBe antigen-antibody system and,
    227
  histological diagnosis of, 226
  outcome of, in treated vs untreated
    patients, 228
  prevalence of, 226
in liver disease, 267
  in Greece, 209–216

PROGRESS IN CLINICAL AND BIOLOGICAL RESEARCH